Dual Pathology

The co-occurrence of substance use disorders (addiction) and mental health disorders constitutes a serious challenge in psychiatric practice, not only because of its frequency, but also because of the difficulties it poses for its diagnosis and treatment. Recently, this issue has taken on special importance and debate in the field of mental health because it has gone from being an eventuality to becoming the most common pattern of demand for care in substance use treatment facilities.

Key features:

- An up-to-date, easy-to-read manual with a multidisciplinary approach that provides detailed recommendations on the treatment of dual-diagnosis patients to improve the quality of care provided.
- Covers the basic notions of dual pathology as a clinical entity, as well as its management in professional practice.
- Reviews the scientific literature on essential aspects, facilitating understanding and appropriate guidance of cases, based on evidence, expert consensus, and documented good practices.

Dual Pathology: Recommendations for Improving the Quality of Care is an essential reference for those in psychiatry and other mental health–related disciplines who work to reduce the health and social impact of substance use problems, whether from clinical practice, teaching, or research.

Dual Pathology

Recommendations for Improving the Quality of Care

Edited by

Homero Indalecio Carrera Machado,
Luis Isidoro Alfonzo Bello,
and Adelino Fernando Vale Ferreira

Routledge
Taylor & Francis Group
NEW YORK AND LONDON

Designed cover image: Shutterstock

First edition published 2027
by Routledge
605 Third Avenue, New York, NY 10158

and by Routledge
4 Park Square, Milton Park, Abingdon, Oxon, OX14 4RN

Routledge is an imprint of the Taylor & Francis Group, an Informa business

Translation from the Spanish language edition:

Patología Dual: recomendaciones para mejorar la calidad asistencial by Homero Indalecio Carrera Machado, Luis Isidoro Alfonzo Bello, Adelino Fernando Vale Ferreira

Library of Congress Cataloging-in-Publication Data
Names: Carrera Machado, Homero Indalecio editor | Alfonzo Bello, Luis Isidoro editor | Ferreira, Adelino Fernando Vale editor
Title: Dual pathology : recommendations for improving the quality of care / edited by Homero Indalecio Carrera Machado, Luis Isidoro Alfonzo Bello, and Adelino Fernando Vale Ferreira.
Other titles: Patología dual. English
Description: First edition. | New York, NY : Routledge, 2027. | Original title: Patología dual: recomendaciones para la mejora de calidad del proceso asistencial. | Includes bibliographical references and index.
Identifiers: LCCN 2026008668 (print) | LCCN 2026008669 (ebook) | ISBN 9781041331001 hbk | ISBN 9781041292524 pbk | ISBN 9781003786153 ebk
Subjects: LCSH: Dual diagnosis
Classification: LCC RC564.68 .D8413 2027 (print) | LCC RC564.68 (ebook)
LC record available at https://lccn.loc.gov/2026008668
LC ebook record available at https://lccn.loc.gov/2026008669

ISBN: 978-1-041-33100-1 (hbk)
ISBN: 978-1-041-29252-4 (pbk)
ISBN: 978-1-003-78615-3 (ebk)

DOI: 10.4324/9781003786153

Typeset in Minion
by KnowledgeWorks Global Ltd.

Contents

Health sciences are constantly changing. As new research and clinical experience expand our knowledge, modifications to therapeutic modalities and pharmacological treatments are required. The authors of this work have verified all information with reliable sources to ensure that it is complete and consistent with accepted standards at the time of publication. However, in view of the possibility of human error or changes in the health sciences, neither the authors, the publisher, nor any other person involved in the preparation or publication of this work guarantee that all of the information contained herein is accurate or complete, and they are not responsible for errors or omissions or for the results obtained from the use of this information. Readers are advised to confirm it with other sources. For example, and in particular, readers are advised to review the package insert for each drug they plan to administer to ensure that the information contained in this book is correct and that there have been no changes in the suggested dosages or contraindications for its administration. This recommendation is especially important in relation to new or infrequently used drugs.

AI Usage Statement

DeepL Pro was used to generate a draft translation from the Spanish edition. The text has been subsequently revised.

List of Editors and Coordinators

EDITORS

Homero Indalecio Carrera Machado
Associate Professor, Department of Psychiatry, Faculty of Medicine, University of Santiago de Compostela, Specialist Physician Area, Drug Addiction Care Unit (ACLAD), A Coruña, Spain

Luis Isidoro Alfonzo Bello
Former Regional Advisor on Substance Use for PAHO/WHO and CICAD/OAS, Washington DC, USA

Adelino Fernando Vale Ferreira
Manager, Drug Addiction Prevention Commission of Porto, Portugal

COORDINATORS

America

Gabriel Rossi Gonnet
Specialist Physician, Pediatric Psychiatry Service, British Hospital of Montevideo, Uruguay

Guillermo Alonso Castaño Pérez
Professor, Mental Health Department, Faculty of Medicine, CES University, Medellin; Medical Director, Outpatient Service, Medicann, Medellin, Colombia

Spain

Eduardo Echarri Arrieta
Pharmacist, Pharmacy Service, Conxo Hospital, Santiago de Compostela, Spain

Manuel Conde Amado
Teaching Collaborator, Department of Psychiatry, Faculty of Medicine, University of Santiago de Compostela, Spain; Specialist Physician, Addictive Behaviors Unit Vigo II–Cedro, Psychiatry Service, Vigo University Hospital Complex, Spain

Portugal

Carlos Sena Vasconcelos
Head of Psychiatry Service, Center for Tratamento das Adiçoes (CENTRA), Fernando Pessoa Teaching Hospital, Gondomar, Porto, Portugal

Sara de Jesús Ferreira da Silva Alexandre
Pharmacist, Head of Pharmacy Lisbon Psychiatric Hospital Centre, Portugal

List of Authors

Luis Isidoro Alfonzo Bello Former Regional Advisor on Substance Use for PAHO/WHO and CICAD/OAS, Washington DC, USA

María José Álvarez Alonso Nurse, Cedro Drug Addiction Care Unit, Vigo, Spain

Iván Álvarez Freire Researcher, Institute of Forensic Sciences, Faculty of Medicine, University of Santiago de Compostela, Spain

Angélica Aparicio Zambrano Area Specialist Physician, Torre Intermédica Hospital, Medellín, Colombia

Jacobo Bello Porto Teaching Assistant, Faculty of Medicine, University of Santiago de Compostela; Psychiatrist, ACLAD Service (Drug Addiction Unit), A Coruña, Spain

Ana María Bermejo Barrera Professor, Institute of Forensic Sciences, Faculty of Medicine, University of Santiago de Compostela, Spain

María Luz Bugallo Pardo Nurse, Drug Addiction Care Unit, A Coruña, Spain

Pamela Cabarcos Fernández Contracted Researcher, Institute of Forensic Sciences, Faculty of Medicine, University of Santiago de Compostela, Spain

María Consuelo Carballal Balsa Nurse, Psychiatry Service, Day Unit, Ferrol University Complex–Sergas Naval Hospital, Ferrol, A Coruña, Spain

Homero Indalecio Carrera Machado Associate Professor, Department of Psychiatry, Faculty of Medicine, University of Santiago de Compostela; Specialist Physician, Drug Addiction Care Unit (ACLAD), A Coruña, Spain

Félix Carvalho Professor, Department of Biological Sciences, Faculty of Pharmacy, University of Porto, Portugal

Susana Carvalho Clinical Psychologist, Advisor, Treatment Team Unit at CRI Porto Oriental, DICAD Service - Division of Intervention in Addictive Behaviors and Dependencies, ARS Norte Hospital, Ministry of Health, Porto, Portugal

Guillermo Alonso Castaño Pérez Professor, Mental Health Department, Faculty of Medicine, CES University, Medellin; Medical Director, Outpatient Service, Medicann, Medellin, Colombia

María Auxiliadora Celdrán Hernández Head of Pharmacy Services, Alicante Penitentiary Psychiatric Hospital, Ministry of the Interior, Alicante, Spain

João Augusto Castel-Branco Goulão Head of Service, Directorate, SICAD (Service for Intervention in Addictive Behaviors and Dependencies), Lisbon, Portugal

Manuel Conde Amado Teaching Collaborator, Department of Psychiatry, Faculty of Medicine, University of Santiago de Compostela, Spain; Specialist Physician, Addictive Behaviors Unit Vigo II-Cedro, Psychiatry Service, Vigo University Hospital Complex, Spain

Ana María Coratu Area Specialist Physician, Dual Diagnosis Unit, CAS, Mental Health Institute, Hospital del Mar, Barcelona, Spain

Clara Catalina Cossio Uribe Professor, Department of Psychiatry, Faculty of Medicine, CES University, Medellín, Colombia

António Jorge Da Silva Barbosa Associate Professor, Department of Social Sciences, Faculty of Philosophy and Social Sciences, Braga; Head of Unit, Integrated Response Center (CRI) Porto Oriental, DICAD (Division of Intervention in Addictive Behaviors and Dependencies), ARS Norte Hospital—Northern Regional Health Administration, Porto, Portugal

Ana Isabel Da Silva Tavares Health Technician, Division for Intervention in Addictive Behaviors and Dependencies, Integrated Responses Center Porto Ocidental, Northern Regional Health Administration, IP, Matosinhos, Portugal

Yolanda Diz Chaves Associate Professor, Department of Functional Biology and Health Sciences, CINBIO Faculty, University of Vigo, Spain

António Júlio De Jesús Roque Head of Service, Porto Ocidental Integrated Response Center—ET Porto Ocidental, Health Area—Addictive Behaviors and Dependencies, Northern Regional Health Administration, I.P./DICAD, Porto, Portugal

Eduardo Echarri Arrieta Pharmacist, Pharmacy Service, Conxo Hospital, Santiago de Compostela, Spain

Iria Fernández Baz Associate Professor, Department of Psychiatry, Faculty of Medicine, University of Santiago de Compostela; Specialist Physician, Addiction Unit, Psychiatry Service, University Hospital Complex of A Coruña (CHUAC, Sergas), A Coruña, Spain

José Manuel Fernández Fernández Teaching Collaborator, Addictive Behaviors Seminar, 4th Year Medicine, Department of Psychiatry, Faculty of Medicine, University of Santiago de Compostela; Psychiatrist, Drug Addiction Care Unit, Drug Addiction Service, Ribeira, A Coruña, Spain

Juan Luis Fernández Hierro Area Specialist Physician, Short-Stay Psychiatric Hospitalization Unit, Psychiatry Service, Álvaro Cunqueiro Hospital, Vigo, Spain

Patricia Fernández Palleiro R2 Researcher, Research Unit, Psychiatry Service, Galicia Sur Health Research Institute, Vigo, Spain

Sara de Jesús Ferreira da Silva Alexandre Head of the Psychiatry Service, Lisbon Psychiatric Hospital Center, Portugal

Gerardo Flórez Menéndez Area Specialist Physician, UCA Unit, Mental Health Service, Ourense University Hospital Complex, Spain

Francina Fonseca Casals Associate Professor, Department of Medicine and Life Sciences, Faculty of Medicine, Pompeu Fabra University. Barcelona; Head of Service, Addictions Unit, Mental Health Institute, Hospital del Mar, Barcelona, Spain

Claudia Gama Elías Organic and Flexible Pharmacy Unit, Regional Health Administration of Lisbon and Tagus Valley, Lisbon, Portugal

Daniel García Fuentes Area Specialist Physician, Dual Pathology Unit, Mental Health Service, Parc de Salut Mar Hospital, Santa Coloma de Gramenet, Barcelona, Spain

María del Carmen García Mahía Associate Professor, Department of Psychiatry, Faculty of Medicine, University of Santiago de Compostela; Specialist Physician, Psychiatry Service, Abente y Lago Mental Health Unit, Abente y Lago Hospital, EOXI, A Coruña, Spain

Ana María González López Clinical Psychologist, Head of the Therapeutic Community, ACLAD Unit, Julio Portela Therapeutic Community, Culleredo, A Coruña, Spain

María Teresa Lage López Head of Section, Day Unit, ACLAD Hospital, A Coruña, Spain

Aurelia Mariño Blanco Associate Professor, Department of Psychiatry and Public Health, University of Santiago de Compostela; Social Worker, Psychiatry Service, Drug Addiction Care Unit, ACLAD, A Coruña, Spain

Mónica Martínez Fernández Master's and Doctorate Professor, Department of Biochemistry, Genetics, and Immunology, Faculty of Biology, University of Vigo; Researcher, Research Unit, Medical Oncology Service, Galicia Sur Health Research Institute, Vigo, Spain

Gerard Mateu Codina Director, Mental Health Institute, Hospital del Mar, Barcelona, Spain

José Manuel Olivares Díez Head of Psychiatry, Álvaro Cunqueiro Hospital, Vigo, Spain

Mayra Alejandra Ortega Orozco Head of Addiction Unit, Mental Health Service, Todomed Limited, Palmira, Valle del Cauca, Colombia

Francisco Otero Lamas Medical Director, CEDRO–Drug Addiction Care Unit, Day Unit, Vigo, Spain

César Pereiro Gómez Area Specialist Physician, Drug Addiction Care, A Coruña, Spain

Bartolomé Pérez Gálvez Associate Professor, Clinical Medicine Unit, Faculty of Medicine, Miguel Hernández University, San Juan, Alicante; Specialist Physician, Alcoholism Unit, San Juan University Hospital, San Juan, Alicante, Spain

Manuel Pérez Rivas Prison Health Physician, Ourense Prison, Pereiro de Aguiar, Ourense, Spain

Fátima Cristina das Neves Pessoa Esteves Nurse, CRI Porto Oriental Service, DICAD Norte—ARS Norte, Porto, Portugal

Carla Adriana Carmezim Pinto da Rocha Health Technician, Health Area, Addictive Behaviors and Dependencies, Porto Ocidental Integrated Response Center–ET Matosinhos, Regional Health Administration, North IP—DICAD, Matosinhos, Porto, Portugal

Adolfo Piñón Blanco CEDRO–Vigo Drug Addiction Care Unit, Psychiatry Service of the Vigo Integrated Management Area, Spain

José Manuel Ramos Psychologist, Technical Director, Therapeutic Community, Addictive Behaviors and Mental Illness Area, Vila do Conde, Porto, Portugal

Tania Rivera Baltanás R2 Researcher, Research Unit, Psychiatry Service, Galicia Sur Health Research Institute, Vigo, Spain

Daniela Sofía Rodrigues Amorim Researcher, Picower Institute for Learning and Memory, Massachusetts Institute of Technology, Boston, MA, USA

Tania Rodríguez Barca Teaching Assistant, Department of Psychiatry, Faculty of Medicine, University of Santiago de Compostela; Psychiatrist, Drug Addiction Unit of A Coruña, A Coruña Hospital Complex, Spain

Gabriel Rossi Gonnet Area Specialist Physician, Pediatric Psychiatry Service, British Hospital of Montevideo, Uruguay

Beatriz Salazar Laya Pharmacist, Psychiatric Pharmacy Service, Ferrol University Hospital Complex, A Coruña, Spain

Rosa Blanca Sauras Quetcuti Associate Professor, Department of Psychiatry, Addictions Area, Faculty of Medicine, Pompeu Fabra University, Barcelona; Specialist Physician, Dual Pathology Unit, Forum Center, Mental Health Institute, Hospital del Mar, Barcelona, Spain

Carlos Sena Vasconcelos Head of Psychiatry, Addiction Treatment Center (CENTRA), Fernando Pessoa Teaching Hospital, Gondomar, Porto, Portugal

João Pedro Silva Researcher, Department of Biological Sciences, Faculty of Pharmacy, University of Porto, Portugal

Célia María Sousa Franco Head of Section, Pinhal Interior Norte Community Mental Health Team, Psychiatry Service, University Hospital Center, Coimbra, Portugal

Carlos Spuch Calvar Master's Professor of Neuroscience and Clinical Psychology, Department of Functional Biology and Health Sciences, Faculty of Biology, University of Vigo; R4 Researcher, Research Unit, Psychiatry Service, Neuroscience Area, Galicia Sur Health Research Institute, Vigo, Spain

María Jesús Tabernero Duque Full Professor, Department of Forensic Sciences, Pathological Anatomy, Gynecology, Obstetrics, and Pediatrics, Faculty of Medicine, University of Santiago de Compostela, Spain

Natalia Tailanian Hagopian Pediatric Psychiatrist, Pediatric Psychiatry Clinic, Faculty of Medicine, University of the Republic, Montevideo, Uruguay

Jorge Mario Tamayo Jaramillo Professor, Department of Psychiatry, Faculty of Medicine, CES University, Medellín; Medical Director, Psychiatry Unit, Outpatient Service, Intermédica, Medellín, Colombia

Joana Teixeira Medical Director, Alcoholism and New Addictions Unit, Lisbon Psychiatric Hospital Center, Portugal

Pablo Antonio Tobajas Ruber Specialist Physician, Psychiatry Service, Inca Regional Hospital, Mallorca, Spain

Marta Torrens Melich Professor, Department of Psychiatry, Faculty of Medicine, Autonomous University of Barcelona and University of Vic and Central Catalonia, Barcelona; Head of Service, Mental Health Institute-Hospital del Mar-Barcelona, Spain

Adelino Fernando Vale Ferreira Manager, Drug Addiction Prevention Commission of Porto, Portugal

María del Carmen Vallejo Curto Specialist Nurse in Mental Health, Psychiatric Day Hospital, Nicolás Peña Hospital, Vigo, Spain

María José Veiga Candán Area Specialist Physician, Hospital Psychiatric Rehabilitation Units, Psychiatry Department, Nicolás Peña Hospital, Vigo, Spain

Francisco Javier Vicente Alba Associate Professor, Department of Psychiatry, Radiology, Public Health, Nursing, and Medicine, Faculty of Medicine, University of Santiago de Compostela; Specialist Physician, Psychiatry Service, Salnés Hospital/EOXI Pontevedra-Salnés, Vilagarcía de Arousa, Pontevedra, Spain

María Vidal Millares Associate Professor, Department of Psychiatry, Radiology, Public Health, Nursing, and Medicine, University of Santiago de Compostela; Specialist Physician, Mental Health Unit of Conxo, Psychiatry Service, Santiago de Compostela Hospital Complex, Spain

Ilda María Vieira Murta Head of Service, Dual Pathology Unit, Psychiatry Service, Coimbra University Hospital Center, Portugal

María Lucía Villalba Ambrosoni Associate Professor, Department of Pediatric Psychiatry, Faculty of Medicine, Udelar University, Montevideo; Emergency Psychiatrist and Ward Psychiatrist, Pediatric Psychiatry Service, Italian Hospital of Montevideo, Uruguay

María Villarino González Area Specialist Physician, Drug Addiction Care Unit of A Coruña, Psychiatry Service, ACLAD A Coruña, Spain

João Vitor Marques Psychiatrist, Medical Director, Addictive Behaviors and Mental Illness Unit, Therapeutic Community, Clínica do Outeiro, Vila do Conde, Porto, Portugal

Foreword I

This book concerns **dual pathology**, a topic on which many more works are needed to update and bring up to date the scientific evidence in the field. It has been authored by the Luso-Galaico Research Group, which comprises mental health experts and other healthcare professionals drawn from the north of the Iberian Peninsula, Spain, and Portugal, Under their leadership, other prestigious colleagues from the Iberian Peninsula and Latin America, all experts in dual diagnosis, addiction, mental health, and hospital pharmacy, have joined forces to make this project a reality. It will be useful in addressing this clinical condition, which continues to lack comparable educational initiatives. Although there is now much more talk about dual pathology, it is not certain that knowledge of its meaning has increased in the same proportion.

For the uninitiated, dual pathology is the norm rather than the exception when treating people with various mental disorders, with prevalence increasing as the severity of mental disorders increases. More than 75% of severe mental disorders occur alongside other mental disorders, such as substance use disorders or other addictions. If we look at people who seek treatment for addiction, all of them will have another mental disorder. These are overwhelming data that are unknown to most mental health experts, whether they work in the mental health network or the addiction network.

This is the first obstacle faced by people suffering from dual pathology who are treated by some of these networks and who, on occasions, when they cannot find the right door, are expelled from the system, which increases morbidity and mortality. These two different networks, which should be treated as a single entity, are based on different philosophies and schools of thought, despite the epidemiological and neuroscientific evidence that points to the close relationship and connection between these different symptomatic expressions.

Clinical neuroscience clearly indicates that all mental manifestations, in health and disease, are based in the human brain—a brain that has evolved to survive, for which genetics has structured circuits and connections that support the main functions.

If these basic connections are altered by genetic or environmental causes, dysfunctions occur that, when they impact vital functioning, are called *mental disorders*.

The most widely-known examples of potentially addictive substances (tobacco, alcohol, cannabis, stimulants, and opioids) act as psychotropic drugs and impact different brain systems, such as the opioid, cannabinoid, and cholinergic/nicotinic. But this impact is not always related to the onset of addiction. Only 10% or less of those exposed will develop a severe addiction phenotype.

Identifying these vulnerable individuals is a challenge in prevention.

The effect of these substances differs between individuals and brains. The clearest example is stimulants, which increase impulsivity and hyperactivity in some people with these clinical characteristics and have a different effect on others. When people experience a different effect, this can trigger compulsive or addictive behaviors, which can be very destructive.

Although we await the arrival of biological markers, perhaps genetic polymorphisms that identify these vulnerable individuals, we currently have clinical markers that are other mental disorders or symptoms or abnormal personality traits, a clinical condition known as dual pathology.

Although this term is not precise and is due to historical reasons, it does have the virtue that clinicians who treat people with mental disorders, including addictions, should always consider dual pathology.

Dual diagnosis, whose scientific update is brought to us by this book, is a concept that can significantly improve the quality of care for people with mental disorders.

Néstor Szerman
Psychiatrist, Mental Health Service, Gregorio Marañón University Hospital, Madrid.
Founding President of the Spanish Society of Dual Disorders and
President of the World Association of Dual Disorders

Foreword II

The publication of a textbook on **dual pathology** is an event I welcome with satisfaction as a psychiatrist, because it will allow the scientific and clinical community, which is dedicated to the area of addictive behaviors and addictions, to pay increasing attention to the problem of drug use and mental health, incorporating the updated knowledge this book provides.

The explosion in the use of psychoactive substances that occurred in the second half of the 20th century throughout Portugal and the rest of the world led psychiatrists (and later alerted politicians, when they encountered this scourge among their close relatives) to recognize the association between drug addiction and mental and behavioral disorders. These problems have become priorities on political agendas, particularly their prevention and treatment.

Although the concept of dual pathology had not yet been introduced as clearly as it is today, my colleague Romildo Bueno (at that time a professor of Psychiatry at the Federal University of Rio de Janeiro) and I, in a preface to the book *Dependência de Drogas* by Seibel and Toscano (2000), we drew attention to the problems of diagnosis, considering the integration of the psychopathological dimension and its repercussions on the orientation of treatment. That same book already highlighted the need for specialized training in this area of psychiatric comorbidities associated with drug use for medical and nursing staff at institutions responsible for the treatment and rehabilitation of addicts.

As a university assistant in Psychiatry with Professor António Fernandes da Fonseca, I started a unit dedicated to addressing drug addiction (diagnosis, treatment, and prevention) in the Psychiatry Service of the Hospital de São João in Porto in the 1980s, with the support of the young intern Carlos Vasconcelos, now a renowned specialist in the field of dual pathology.

Other psychiatrists were trained in this pioneering unit, including Drs. Arnaldo Droux, Helena Dias, Carlos Sousa, Douteiro Sá, Manuel Esteves, Luís Castelo Branco, Teixeira de Sousa, Medeiros Paiva, and later João Marques, who, as directors and coordinators of structures dedicated to addiction, made an important contribution to the consolidation of this care network in northern Portugal.

At that time, this pioneering unit already had close ties with the University of Santiago de Compostela, specifically with Professor of Psychiatry Dr. Antonio Rodríguez López, and the psychiatric dimension of the problem of drug addiction was already being discussed.

It is very interesting to note that this proximity has borne fruit over time, facilitating contacts between the two addiction treatment networks in Galicia and northern Portugal, one of the fruits of which has been the creation of the Luso-Galician Research Group (Grupo Luso Galaico de Investigación en Adicciones, GLIA), which gave rise to the initiative for this book on dual pathology.

This first module of the book is a ten-chapter work covering some of the main problems of the disorder, understood as one in which mental illness is intertwined with the use of psychoactive substances.

This module addresses topics such as the concept and diagnosis of dual pathology, the care approach, and pharmacological treatment. It highlights the important work of nursing, as well as social work and the process of "destigmatization." The legal and ethical aspects are covered extensively, including the so-called Portuguese model for addressing the problem of addiction in a comprehensive and integrated manner. There is also a chapter dedicated to prevention. The final chapter is titled "Other Topics of Interest in Dual Pathology"—referring to topics no less important than the first, such as neurobiology, genetics, proteomics, gender, age, and substances and psychopathology.

It is very difficult to find such a variety and depth of topics in a single volume.

This work, edited by Dr. Indalecio Carrera, Dr. Luis Alfonzo, and Dr. Adelino Ferreira, is a clear, well-documented, and engaging contribution that is essential for the training of new and future generations of professionals interested in dual pathology, as well as for those who are already involved in the prevention, treatment, and rehabilitation of dual patients.

We eagerly await the next modules of this work.

Antonio Pacheco Palha
Retired Professor of Psychiatry at the Faculty of Medicine of Porto, Portugal

Foreword III

We understand dual pathology as the co-occurrence of a mental disorder with a substance use disorder. This pathology is associated with poor adherence to treatment, increased risk of contracting sexually transmitted infections, increased suicidal behavior and relapse and rehospitalization rates, increased biopsychosocial deterioration (school dropout, job loss, and legal problems), and, finally, increased use of general and specialized medical services, which leads to higher public healthcare costs.

Although people with dual diagnosis require treatments that integrate care for both conditions, Latin American health systems generally have a structural divide between mental health care and substance use care, which means that patients must navigate a variety of ineffective institutions. Furthermore, barriers to accessing treatment for dual diagnosis include a lack of comprehensive treatment programs and a shortage of qualified personnel to provide adequate diagnosis and treatment. In this regard, this paper gives us the opportunity to delve into dual pathology by addressing, through an international group of experts, various concepts, aspects, and issues that contribute to the analysis of the problem, with the aim of making specific recommendations for the training of human resources and improving the quality of the care process.

The text consists of ten chapters that address different areas of dual pathology. Chapter 1 describes the concept of dual pathology, from basic definitions to its relevance in prognosis. Of particular note here is the interesting etiopathogenic model, in which there are etiological and neurobiological explanations that are not mutually exclusive to justify comorbidity, highlighting the hypotheses of risk factor accumulation, self-medication, the interaction between individual vulnerability and environmental stressors, and, finally, the hypothesis of common vulnerability. Chapter 2 covers the complexity of diagnosing dual pathology, emphasizing the importance of a complete medical history as the basis for diagnosis. Chapter 3 presents the principles for the dual pathology care model, understanding that this is a complex phenomenon that requires social, therapeutic, and pharmacological resources provided by a multidisciplinary team trained in the subject. Chapter 4 provides information on how care is provided to people with dual pathology, with the aim of ideally providing it in their personal and social context, moving away from the asylum model and highlighting the importance of outpatient care provided in the community. However, due to the complexity of dual pathology, sometimes an approach in emergency services, general hospitals, and even mental health hospitals is required. Chapter 5 addresses the art of pharmacologically treating people with dual pathology, which is why this section covers specifiers in different mental disorders, such as schizophrenia, bipolar disorder, depression, anxiety, attention deficit hyperactivity disorder, and personality disorders. Chapter 6 provides an accurate description of the care given to people with dual pathology from the nursing perspective and offers a proposal for standardizing such care. Chapter 7 provides recommendations for reducing the stigma attached to people with dual pathology, actively involving the social work team as a fundamental part of providing support in the therapeutic process and monitoring people in treatment. Fighting the stigma attached to these people means restoring a dignified life to a vulnerable sector of society. Chapter 8 presents the legal and ethical aspects of dual pathology, including an analysis of the criminal capacity of people with mental disorders and their criminal responsibility. It also discusses the process of voluntary or involuntary hospitalization, understanding that respect for human rights is fundamental. Chapter 9 addresses the issue of prevention in dual pathology and proposes interventions for it. Finally, Chapter 10 presents a selection of various important topics.

I would like to highlight and thank Drs. Alfonzo, Carrera, and Ferreira for their leadership efforts, as well as the editors in the three regions of Ibero-America: Latin America, Galicia/Spain, and Portugal. Without a doubt, this book provides knowledge, but more importantly, it offers practical recommendations for improving care for people with dual pathology, who have historically been extremely neglected.

Dr. Eduardo A. Madrigal de León
Director General of the Ramón de la Fuente Muñiz National Institute of Psychiatry, Ramón de la Fuente Muñiz, Mexico City, Mexico

Preface

This monograph reflects the state of available scientific evidence and consensus on various aspects of dual diagnosis, which is the co-occurrence of substance use disorders and other mental disorders, in different contexts of care for these patients. The team of authors, belonging to different scientific societies in the fields of Addiction, Dual Diagnosis, Mental Health, and Hospital Pharmacy, intends to continue developing a series of recommendations in the form of other volumes to improve the quality of care provided to patients.

This is a project initiated by the Luso-Galician Addiction Research Group (GLIA) but which quickly took on an Iberian and later Latin American dimension with the incorporation of the respective directors to formalize the constitution of the working teams that, in each country, are joining the project and adapting this work to the respective national context, as the current team has been doing in the Iberian sphere, given that the reality of the situation regarding the approach to dual pathology is quite different between Spain and Portugal.

Therefore, this publication is aimed at members of teams providing social and health services to this socially marginalized and stigmatized group of patients, as well as at the planners and coordinators of these services and various community actors who may have a special interest in this topic (educational and social institutions, etc.).

The editorial work is structured around a series of modules, starting with a general module (the first in the series) and covering the different comorbid pathologies in specific modules. Dual patients with severe mental disorders have been selected as the priority target group for these recommendations to improve the care process.

The Editors

CHAPTER 1

Conceptual Approach to Dual Pathology

H. I. Carrera Machado, L. I. Alfonzo Bello, A. F. Vale Ferreira, J. M. Fernández Fernández, C. Sena Vasconcelos, E. Echarri Arrieta, S. J. Ferreira da Silva Alexandre, G. A. Castaño Pérez, and M. Conde Amado

BASIC CONCEPTS

Since the dawn of history, humans have resorted to the use of psychoactive substances for different purposes (relief from ailments, magical-religious rituals, mood enhancement, recreation, creativity enhancement, etc.), mainly within the framework of socially accepted use. However, there have always been individuals who deviated from these norms, whether in terms of quantity, timing, type of substance, and/or situation of consumption, decontextualizing these consumption behaviors from their sociocultural rituals and generating problems of drug abuse/dependence.

Furthermore, sometimes, it might be the case that the subjects, due either to their vulnerability or to their previous pathology (self-medication hypothesis), engaged in drug use behaviors that can give rise to complex conditions, according to the severity of the substance use disorder and other, associated psychiatric disorders, and the interaction between the two.

This comorbidity between addictive behaviors and other psychopathological disorders, whose high prevalence was already evident at the end of the last century in various epidemiological studies, is so significant from a neurobiological, diagnostic, and therapeutic point of view that it has given rise to a new clinical concept called **dual diagnosis**, **dual disorder**, or **dual pathology**. In recent years, this concept has also been referred to as "concurrent disorders or comorbidities."[1,2] Throughout this text, we will use the term *dual pathology*.

We note that in recent years the term "dual pathology" has been used to define the coexistence in the same individual of a clinical picture of drug abuse/dependence alongside another psychiatric disorder defined in the psychiatric classifications currently in use.[1,3,4]

DOI: 10.4324/9781003786153-1

We will continue to use the term "dual pathology," despite its controversial nature, as the concept can be considered a tautology in itself (any drug dependence is also a mental disorder), and furthermore, it is not uncommon for not only dual diagnoses to coexist, but triple or quadruple diagnoses, which would constitute a true "**plural disorder**."[2,5]

However, the term *dual diagnosis* has gained in popularity because it fills a latent need in the field of mental health and addiction, describing a prevalent but underdiagnosed condition with specific clinical, diagnostic, and therapeutic characteristics. Furthermore, such disorder is a significant health problem,[2,5] given the widespread lack of specific resources for its treatment, both in the field of mental health care and in the field of addiction treatment.

The concept of *dual pathology*, unlike that of dual disorder or diagnosis, implies an interdependence between addictive disorders and other psychopathological disturbances when they occur simultaneously, which leads to the acceptance that the diagnosis, treatment, evolution, and prognosis of both disorders become inextricably linked from the moment they co-occur in a given patient.

For this reason, we believe that it is not effective to take an individualized approach to each pathology separately, since we are dealing with a single patient who has "two diseases," thus avoiding absurd care pathways such as the so-called wrong door syndrome, in which the patient is sent from one healthcare network to another (like a "ping pong ball") without finding a solution to their problem.

On the other hand, this disease can present symptoms of varying severity, such as association with serious mental disorders (psychotic spectrum disorders, bipolar disorder, personality disorders, etc.), reflecting a degree of poor adaptation to life, with a major impact on functionality, given the complexity of its effects in both the psychiatric and physical fields (HIV, HCV, COPD, etc.) and the social field (lack of family support, employment, housing, legal complications, etc.). For this reason, it is one of the core areas of so-called complex chronic patients, whose care needs require continuous reassessment and close coordination between different levels of health and social services[6–8] and constitutes one of the care paradigms of the "difficult patient."

The clinical relevance of dual pathology is reflected in the differences presented by the "prototype" of the dual schizophrenic patient:[1,9,10]

- The predominance in males is more pronounced, and patients are younger, with a lower socioeconomic status and a first hospitalization at an earlier age.
- Clinically, there is a greater presence of positive and affective symptoms, with a higher risk of consummated suicidal behavior, but with less presence of negative psychotic symptoms.
- It is also important to highlight the higher prevalence of impulsivity, sensation seeking, and risky behaviors (higher rate of comorbidities) on axis III (HCV, HIV), personality disorders (antisocial), and poly-drug use, and also a higher rate of violent and criminal behavior.

- As a result, patients tend to have poorer social functioning and greater social marginalization.
- At the healthcare level, there is a lack of access to the healthcare network, poorer therapeutic compliance with lower rates of "monotherapy" and, logically, more secondary conditions and interactions.

We thus find that dual pathology, understood as comorbidity between addictive disorders and other mental disorders, has become one of the most prevalent pathologies in the field of mental health. It is clear that it is not feasible to develop quality clinical practice without accepting that, progressively and above all in terms of chronic processes, the most frequent clinical form will be the coexistence in the same individual of different psychopathological disorders, always including one or more addictive conditions, in addition to other organic and social comorbidities.[2,5]

EPIDEMIOLOGICAL DIMENSION

Since the end of the last century, epidemiological studies have clarified the significant relationship between other mental disorders and addictive behaviors, showing that the *odds* ratio between psychiatric disorders and drug use is higher for dependence than for drug abuse.[11]

Recent reviews by scientific societies such as Socidrogalcohol,[12,13] the Spanish Society of Dual Disorders,[14,15] the Society of Drug Addiction, the Society of Psychiatry, and the European Monitoring Centre for Drugs and Drug Addiction (EMCDDA)[16] have confirmed the epidemiological reality of this phenomenon, and we will now present the main conclusions:

- The estimated prevalence of these conditions varies greatly, depending, among other factors, on methodological factors, the location of the studies, and the substances consumed: the highest prevalence rates tend to be concentrated in the addiction network rather than the mental health network, in inpatient centers rather than outpatient centers, and in prison and homeless populations. The figures can vary from 7% of dual pathology in the general population to around 75% of the homeless population.
- In the latest study conducted in Spain, in the Mental Health and Addiction networks,[13] a high prevalence of some other diagnosis of comorbid mental disorder was recorded in patients treated in the addiction network (71%), with affective and personality disorders predominating. However, 68.9% of patients treated in the mental health network had a diagnosis of some type of substance use disorder (59% if we exclude smoking).
- In Spain, in the 2013 "Madrid study" (n = 837 patients, MINI and PDQ4+ interview), the overall prevalence of dual diagnosis was 62% in the healthcare network of the Autonomous Community of Madrid: 36% in outpatient mental health facilities (n = 208) compared to 70% in addiction treatment facilities (n = 629).

- However, in another study in the Autonomous Community of Madrid in 2011 (n = 400 patients), which retrospectively assessed the last 20 medical records available in outpatient addiction and mental health centers, the overall prevalence was lower (34%), being higher in addiction centers (37%) than in mental health centers (29%).
- In a 2015 study by the Luso-Galaico Addiction Research Group (GLIA),[17] the rates of dual pathology observed in outpatient addiction centers in Coruña and Porto were 48% and 56%, respectively.
- In Galicia, in the COPSIAD study[18] conducted in addiction centers, the overall prevalence of dual pathology rose to 56.3% of the sample (n = 2,300 patients).

One of the general conclusions of these studies is that the epidemiological dimension of dual pathology tends to be underdiagnosed.

ETIOPATHOGENIC FACTORS: THE SUBSTANCE FACTOR IN THE GENESIS OF DUAL DISORDER

From the point of view of the **etiopathogenic model**, there are a number of mutually non-exclusive etiological and neurobiological explanations that justify this high psychiatric comorbidity among substance users, with the following hypotheses standing out:[1,2,5,12]

- **Hypothesis of the accumulation of risk factors**: The combination of genetic, neurobiological, environmental, sociocultural, and other factors would be decisive in the coexistence of dual disorders.
- **Self-medication hypothesis**: Substance use among dual patients would minimize symptoms or, at least, alleviate their discomfort, altering their perception of dysphoria.
- **Hypothesis of interaction between individual vulnerability and environmental stressors**: Neurobiological and environmental factors combine, reinforcing each other and predisposing each other.
- **Common vulnerability hypothesis**: Presence of neurobiological mechanisms common to both conditions (true dual disorders).

The authors of the EMCDDA report[16] themselves acknowledge that the relationship between addiction and other, comorbid mental disorders presents difficulties when establishing links between the two problems. A better understanding of the cause-and-effect relationship is needed, and there is always the dilemma of which comes first, substance use or mental disorder—or whether they are two phenomena that go together and occur simultaneously.

In short, the importance of the comorbidity of other mental disorders in people who use drugs lines in their high prevalence, clinical and social severity, difficult management, and association with poor therapeutic outcomes.[16]

PROGNOSTIC RELEVANCE

As already mentioned, in addition to being common in clinical practice, dual patients are prototypical "difficult" patients, as they present complex and chronic conditions with a series of clinical and evolutionary repercussions that cloud the prognosis for both pathologies:[1–3,5,12,16,19,20]

- **Relapses**: Their number and duration increase.
- **Usage of emergency services**: Increased use of emergency health (and social) services.
- **Hospitalization**: More frequent and longer duration.
- **Behavioral disorders**: Impulsivity and heteroaggressive behaviors, which lead to greater social and family maladjustment and legal implications that complicate their developmental course (high prevalence in the prison population); self-aggressive behaviors (self-destructive behavior, more pronounced in dual-diagnosis patients with comorbid personality disorders) with increased morbidity/mortality in this group.
- **Residential instability**: Tendency to change residence due to family and legal problems, leading to social emergency situations, with a high prevalence in the homeless population.
- **Loss of employment status and decline in the functional capacity of the patient**: Difficulties in performing activities of daily living and work-related activities.
- **Risk behaviors**: Increased risk of HIV/HCV infection, etc., which contributes to a decline in overall health.
- **Progression**: Non-compliance with treatment in patients who already have low adherence to treatment, increased resistance, secondary effects, and drug interactions.
- **Usage of mental health and addiction services**: The existence of dual pathology increases both the use of mental health services and addiction services as well as their cost, regardless of the primary diagnosis.

In short, the prognosis for this group is bleak, increasing their social vulnerability and often leading them to situations of marginalization and social emergency. This implies a loss of capacity for the healthcare system to adequately retain dual-diagnosis patients and significantly increases social and healthcare costs, as shown in Figure 1.1.[2,18,21–23] However, despite all these difficulties, it can be seen that the costs of untreated addiction (which affects most of the homeless population, with a high prevalence of dual pathology) or the costs of the associated legal and criminal problems presented by this population group far exceed the costs of any other type of treatment that may be considered.

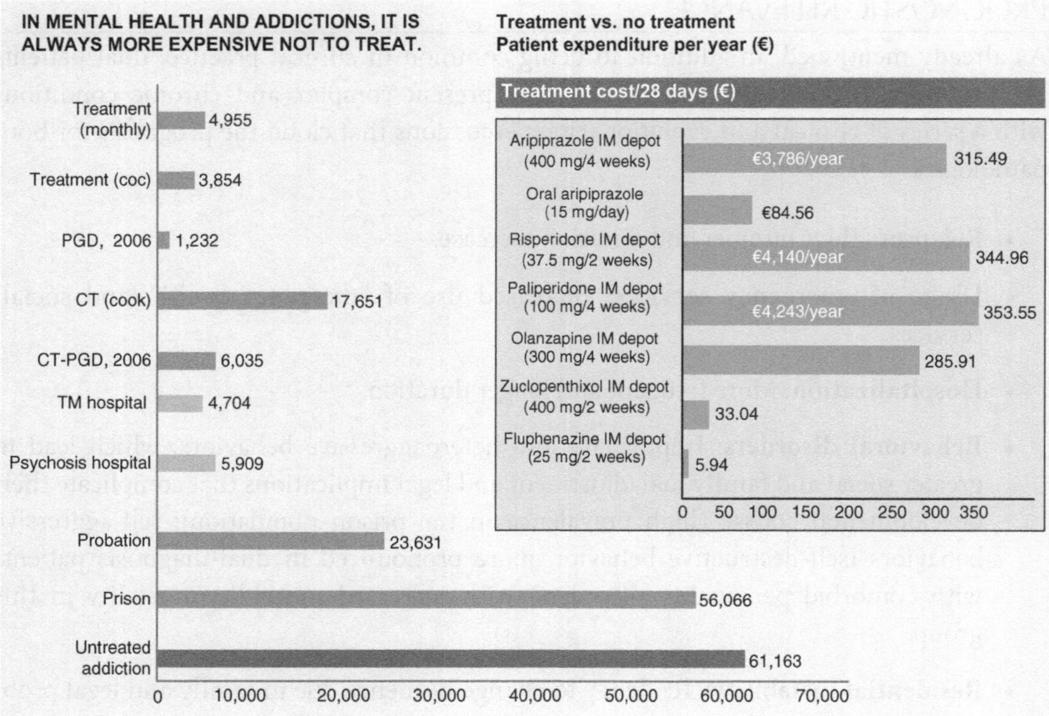

FIGURE 1.1 Analysis of social and healthcare costs.

REFERENCES

1. Haro G, Bobes J, Casas M, Didia J, Rubio G. Tratado sobre Patología Dual. Reintegrando la salud mental. Barcelona: MRA Ediciones, 2010.
2. FGEP-Foro Gallego para el Estudio de la Personalidad. Trastornos de la Personalidad. Un abordaje Integrador. Editorial Pensódromo SL, 2020.
3. Rubio G, López-Muñoz F, Álamo C, Santo-Domingo J. Trastornos psiquiátricos y abuso de sustancias. Madrid: Editorial Médica Panamericana, 2002.
4. NIDA (National Institute on Drug Abuse). Research Report Series. Comorbidity: Addiction and Other Mental Illnesses, 2010.
5. CICAD-Comisión Interamericana para el Control del Abuso de Drogas. Inventario de Recomendaciones sobre Tratamiento GERD 1: Patología Dual. Washington DC: CICAD OAS, 2010.
6. Ministerio de Sanidad, Servicios Sociales e Igualdad. Estrategia para el Abordaje de la Cronicidad en el Sistema Nacional de Salud. Estrategia aprobada por el Consejo Interterritorial del Sistema Nacional de Salud el 27 de junio de 2012.
7. Bengoa R. El reto de la cronicidad en España: mejor transformar que racionar. Gac Sanit. 2015;29(5):323–5.
8. Generalitat de Catalunya-Departament de Salut. Bases para un modelo catalán de atención a las personas con necesidades complejas. Programa de prevención y atención a la cronicidad. Barcelona, 2016.
9. Szerman N, Roncero C, Casas M. Protocolos de intervención en patología dual: Esquizofrenia. Barcelona: Edikamed SL, 2016.
10. Szerman N, Álvarez Vara C, Casas M. Patología dual en esquizofrenia. Opciones terapéuticas. Barcelona: Editorial Glosa, 2007.

11. Compton WM, Thomas YF, Conway KP. Developments in the epidemiology of drug use and drug use disorders. Am J Psychiatry. 2005;162:1494–502.
12. Socidrogalcohol. Comorbilidad psiquiátrica en adicciones. Colección Guías Clínicas Socidrogalcohol. Concepto, epidemiología & diagnóstico. Editorial Socidrogalcohol, 2017 (available on the website socidrogalcohol.org).
13. Socidrogalcohol. Encuesta Nacional sobre Prevención y Tratamiento de la Concurrencia de los Trastornos por uso de sustancias y de otro trastorno mental. Editorial Socidrogalcohol 2020 (available on the website socidrogalcohol.org).
14. Sociedad Española de Patología Dual. Libro Blanco: Recursos y Necesidades Asistenciales en Patología Dual. Editorial Sanidad y Ediciones SL, 2015 (available on the SEpatología dual website).
15. Sociedad Española de Patología Dual. Protocolos de Intervención en Patología Dual. EdikaMed, SL, 2016 (available on the SEpatología dual website).
16. Torrens M, Mestre-Pintó JI, Domingo-Salvany A. Co-morbidity of substance use and mental health disorders in Europe. EMCDDA, 2015.
17. GLIA-Grupo Luso-Galaico de Investigación en Adicciones. Estudio sobre comorbilidad psiquiátrica en las redes asistenciales de adicciones de Porto y A Coruña: propuesta de un modelo asistencial integral. Encuentro Luso Galaico. Las adicciones en siglo XXI. Vigo, 2015.
18. COPSIAD Group. Psychiatric comorbidity in patients from the addiction disorders assistance units of Galicia: The COPSIAD study. PLoS ONE 2013;8(6):e66451. doi:10.1371/journal.pone.0066451
19. Bobes J, Casas M, Gutiérrez M. Manual de Trastornos Adictivos (2nd edition). Enfoque Editorial SC, 2011.
20. Benabarre, A. Trastornos Esquizoafectivos. Madrid: Editorial Médica Panamericana, 2014.
21. ONU-UNODC. Por qué invertir en el tratamiento del abuso de drogas: documento de debate para formulación de políticas. New York: United Nations, 2003.
22. Análise económica de asistencia sanitaria prestada na rede do Plan de Galicia sobre Drogas e impacto económico da súa integración no sistema sanitario galego. Santiago de Compostela, 2009.
23. Campos A, Carrera I, Mateos R. Abordaje del enfermo dual con trastornos de personalidad comórbidos. Trabajo Fin de Grado de Medicina. Faculty of Medicine, USC, 2019.

CHAPTER 2

Diagnostic Approach to Dual Pathology

H. I. Carrera Machado, M. Conde Amado, A. F. Vale Ferreira, C. Sena Vasconcelos, E. Echarri Arrieta, S. J. Ferreira da Silva Alexandre, P. A. Tobajas Ruber, G. A. Castaño Pérez, and L. I. Alfonzo Bello

GUIDELINES FOR PROPER DIAGNOSIS OF DUAL DISORDERS

With regard to diagnostic issues, the NIDA[1] states that due to the high rate of comorbidity between drug abuse disorders and other mental disorders, a comprehensive approach is required with interventions that assess each disorder at the same time. And as far as possible, for a correct diagnosis, it is preferable for the patient to stop substance abuse,[2] as there may be similarities between the symptoms related to consumption/withdrawal and other potentially comorbid mental disorders, so observation of the course of the disorder may be essential to establish a correct diagnosis.[3–5]

The following is a proposal for protocolization for the diagnostic phase of the dual patient care process, seeking to improve the quality of care.[3–11]

Protocolization of Diagnosis

Every intervention plan begins with a diagnosis, and in this sense, it is important to remember that we are dealing with an underdiagnosed disorder in a population with little awareness of the disease and low demand for treatment.[12] Therefore, in addition to promoting access to care facilities and developing individualized treatment plans, we must begin by establishing an accurate diagnosis;[9] to this end, various difficulties that arise during this phase of the intervention must be taken into account:[3–8,10,11,13,14]

- Existence of drug use patterns in psychiatric patients
- Drug use that can produce effects (acute or chronic) similar to certain psychiatric disorders
- Existence of physical complications associated with substance use that can generate or aggravate psychiatric symptoms

DOI: 10.4324/9781003786153-2

- Family history of psychiatric pathology and/or addictive behavior
- Denial of drug use and lack of cooperation on the part of the patient
- Existence of parallel care networks

DIAGNOSTIC TOOLS IN DUAL DISORDERS: BIOLOGICAL MARKERS AND DIAGNOSTIC TESTS

Medical History

The basic element for diagnosing these patients continues to be their medical history, which must be taken into account when considering a series of circumstances:[3–8,10,11,14]

- Given the high frequency of comorbidity, both diagnostic possibilities should always be explored when one of them is present.
- Determine whether there are coexisting physical diseases that may cause certain psychiatric symptoms (thyroid disorders, neurological disorders, etc.) exist.
- It is advisable to allow a period of 3–4 weeks of abstinence before assessing psychiatric symptoms and, if this is not possible, a provisional diagnosis will be established.
- Determine whether there is a family history of psychiatric disorders.
- Determine whether there exist psychomotor development problems (learning difficulties and attention deficit hyperactivity disorder due to the enormous "disease burden" of this pathology, which is underdiagnosed and undertreated).
- Determine whether there exist simulation disorders (possible secondary gains).
- Whenever possible, multiple sources of information should be used and cross-checked with the patient's information.
- Whenever possible, laboratory tests should be requested to monitor drug use.

Psychiatric Interviews

LEAD Method

Although in clinical practice it is sometimes difficult to differentiate between dual pathologies, the longitudinal course of the condition and the response to treatment will provide us with clarifying information about the definitive diagnosis, as postulated by the *LEAD* (*Longitudinal Expert with All Data*) method, the true "gold standard" of psychiatric interviews in this field.[15]

LEAD is an acronym that encompasses three *basic* concepts: **longitudinal assessment, performed by experts, and using all available data**:

- **Longitudinal** implies that the diagnosis is not limited to a single examination, and the longitudinal period may be brief or last several years.

- **Expert** means that such diagnoses are made by trained and experienced clinicians.
- **All data** refers to the fact that clinical experts not only evaluate systematically over time, but also access other key sources of information: family and friends, clinical histories from other services, complementary examinations, etc.

Psychodiagnostic Instruments

Regarding the clinical application of these instruments, there are reviews to this effect,[3,15] and, among the structured interviews, we should highlight the application of the *Psychiatric Research Interview for Substance and Mental Disorders* (PRISM) and the *Structured Clinical Interview for DSM-IV* (SCID).[7,8,15]

In the diagnostic phase, the main dilemma usually centers on the differential diagnosis between an induced and a primary/independent disorder, with decision trees already existing in this regard, such as the one shown in Figure 2.1.[6–9,13]

As we can see, a very useful element in the diagnosis of dual pathology is determining whether the component disorders are primary or secondary, especially considering that medical history remains the main diagnostic tool in the field of dual pathology.

Thus, based on the available evidence, we can make the following considerati ons.[3,4,6,7,11,16,17]

Step One

Establish the relationship between drug use and psychiatric symptoms
- No → Independent disorder
- Yes → Continue exploring the psychopathological characteristics and chronology of disorders

Step Two

Determine whether the psychopathology is more severe than that which usually appears during episodes of intoxication or withdrawal syndrome
- Not more serious → Diagnose drug intoxication or withdrawal syndrome
- More serious → Complete investigations to differentiate between induced and independent disorders

Step Three

Establish the chronology of the onset of the disorders, personal and/or family history of affective disorders, and resolution of the episode after several weeks of abstinence
- Independent disorder
- Induced disorder

FIGURE 2.1 Steps for establishing a differential diagnosis in dual pathology.

Dual Patient with Primary Mental Disorder

- This is more common in males, in young people, and in those of low socioeconomic status.
- There is a family history of drug abuse/dependence and/or exposure to drugs.
- The patient's premorbid adaptation was unsuccessful.
- Comorbidity on axis II (personality disorders) is common.
- The mental disorder precedes drug use.
- The psychiatric symptoms are not accompanied by physical symptoms characteristic of intoxication or withdrawal.
- The mental disorder persists after the withdrawal phase (by consensus, it is recommended to wait a minimum of four weeks of abstinence to assess whether the persistence of symptoms is not due to substance use).
- The psychiatric symptoms are clearly excessive in relation to what would be expected given the type, dose, and duration of drug use.
- There is a family history of psychiatric disorders.
- High doses of psychotropic drugs are needed to obtain relief from symptoms.

Dual Patient with Mental Disorder Secondary to Drug Use

- Polydrug use behaviors and high-consumption indicators
- Late onset of drug use
- Shortened and brief phases of abstinence (< 1 year)
- History of childhood sexual abuse
- Rapid response of psychiatric symptoms to pharmacological treatment
- Excessive sensitivity to psychotropic drugs and/or appearance of side effects with low doses of psychotropic drugs
- Therapeutic failure to reduce addiction when the patient is treated in mental health facilities

We must be aware that the main diagnostic problem in dual pathology is precisely the tendency not to diagnose dual disorders, which may be due to the tendency to conceal, deny, or minimize possible consumption in mental health services, while in the addiction network, there is a tendency to focus attention on the addictive aspect of the problem and not detect other possible psychopathological conditions in addicted patients.

REFERENCES

1. NIDA. Research Report Series. Comorbidity: Addiction and Other Mental Illnesses, 2010.
2. Torrens M, Mestre-Pintó JI, Domingo-Salvany A. Comorbidity of substance use and mental health disorders in Europe. EMCDDA, 2015.
3. Haro G, Bobes J, Casas M, Didia J, Rubio G. Tratado sobre Patología Dual. Reintegrando la salud mental. Barcelona: MRA Ediciones, 2010.
4. CICAD-Comisión Interamericana para el Control del Abuso de Drogas. Inventario de Recomendaciones sobre Tratamiento GERD 1: Patología Dual. Washington DC: CICAD OAS, 2010.
5. Socidrogalcohol. Comorbilidad psiquiátrica en adicciones. Colección Guías Clínicas Socidrogalcohol. Concepto, epidemiología & diagnóstico Editorial Socidrogalcohol, 2017 (available at socidrogalcohol.org).
6. Rubio G, López-Muñoz F, Álamo C, Santo-Domingo J. Trastornos psiquiátricos y abuso de sustancias. Madrid: Editorial Médica Panamericana, 2002.
7. Socidrogalcohol. Manejo clínico del paciente con patología dual. Recomendaciones de expertos. Socidrogalcohol, 2009 (available at socidrogalcohol.org).
8. Socidrogalcohol. Manual de adicciones para medicos especialistas en formación. Socidrogalcohol, 2010 (available at socidrogalcohol.org).
9. Xunta de Galicia-Consellería de Sanidade. Catálogo de Programas Asistenciais do Plan de Galicia sobre Drogas. Santiago de Compostela, 2003 (available at sergas.es).
10. Bobes J, Casas M, Gutiérrez M. Manual de Trastornos Adictivos (2ª edición). Enfoque Editorial SC, 2011.
11. FGEP-Foro Gallego para Estudio de la Personalidad. Trastornos de la Personalidad. Un abordaje Integrador. Editorial Pensódromo SL, 2020.
12. Carrera I, Mateos R, Rodríguez A. Consumo de alcohol, psicopatología y demanda asistencial en Galicia. En: García Rodríguez J, López Sánchez, C. Manual de estudios sobre alcohol. Madrid: Editorial EDAF, 2001: 597–632.
13. Pedrero Pérez E, Ruiz Sánchez de León JM. Los trastornos psicopatológicos y el dilema del diagnóstico. Neuropsicología de la Adicción. Madrid: Editorial Médica Panamericana, 2014.
14. Socidrogalcohol (2019). Comorbilidad psiquiátrica en adicciones. Colección Guías Clínicas Socidrogalcohol, nº 8. Resumen de intervenciones. Summary of interventions. Editorial Socidrogalcohol, 2019 (available at socidrogalcohol.org).
15. Sociedad Española de Toxicomanías (SET). Tratado SET de Trastornos adictivos, tomos I y II. Madrid: Editorial Médica Panamericana, 2006.
16. Solomon J, Zimberg S, Shollar E. Diagnóstico dual. Barcelona: Ediciones en Neurociencias, 1996: 247–66.
17. Sociedad Española de Patología Dual. Protocolos de Intervención en Patología Dual. Editorial EdikaMed SL, 2016 (available on the SEPD website).

CHAPTER 3

Care Approach

Principles, Models, and Proposed Care Pathway for Dual Pathology Patients

H. I. Carrera Machado, L. I. Alfonzo Bello, C. Sena Vasconcelos, A. F. Vale Ferreira, E. Echarri Arrieta, G. Rossi Gonnet, M. A. Ortega Orozco, G. A. Castaño Pérez, and M. Conde Amado

PRINCIPLES FOR EFFECTIVE TREATMENT OF DUAL PATHOLOGY PATIENTS

According to the report by the *European Monitoring Centre for Drugs and Drug Addiction* (EMCDDA),[1] comorbidity between substance use disorders (SUDs) and other mental disorders (MDs), or vice versa, currently represents a significant challenge for diagnosis and treatment, as well as for drug policies. This is mainly due to the high prevalence and complexity of treatment given the limited resources available for this type of patient, and can be considered key to the future of addiction care. Compared to patients suffering from only one disorder, this comorbidity is characterized by the high severity of the psychopathological and/or addictive condition.

Addictive disorders and their comorbidities have a multi-causal etiopathogenesis and, for this reason, the therapeutic approach must always be multidisciplinary, addressing all the repercussions derived from the combination of the different comorbid clinical pictures.

According to the EMCDDA,[1] the following possibilities should be considered:

- SUD and the other psychiatric condition are independent of each other.
- The psychiatric condition is a risk factor for developing SUD.
- Substance abuse may be the cause of the psychiatric condition, influencing its usual course.
- A temporary psychiatric condition may appear as a result of intoxication or withdrawal syndrome caused by a substance, which we would refer to as a substance-induced disorder.
- The symptoms of SUD and MD have a common origin based on individual vulnerability factors, which gives rise to the concept of dual pathology.

DOI: 10.4324/9781003786153-3

The presence of a dual diagnosis complicates treatment and leads to a worse prognosis for both disorders, especially if one of the two disorders is not properly diagnosed and treated.

The problems associated with their treatment relate to mutual interference between specific treatments, non-compliance with prescriptions, lack of social support and specific care resources, and the high frequency of family and legal problems present in these cases.

Treatment must be individualized, taking into account the available care resources and the patient's expectations, and considering the need for more intensive therapeutic interventions, with social and family support being a determining factor for a favorable outcome.

Therefore, these patients with a poorer prognosis and difficult therapeutic management require an integrated care system. The existence of two distinct and parallel care networks poses a serious difficulty for their care, and there is consensus on the greater effectiveness of the integrated treatment, which requires follow-up to be carried out by a multidisciplinary team that addresses the medical, psychological, and social aspects of the patient and their environment.

In short, when planning quality care for dual pathology patients, the following quality criteria should be considered:[2]

- It should be provided in healthcare centers that are accredited and authorized by the competent health authority, avoiding unprofessional models.
- It should be applied by multidisciplinary teams, working in an interdisciplinary manner and with the necessary specialized training, allowing for the application of interventions with scientific evidence: individualized treatment plans, therapeutic flexibility, and gradual exposure to groups.
- Wherever possible, priority should be given to the application of the comprehensive care model, avoiding the "wrong door" syndrome.
- Therapeutic continuity should be enhanced through networking, ensuring coordination between outpatient and inpatient (total/partial) resources to respond to the patient's needs during the course of their therapeutic process.
- The quality of the therapeutic alliance, a key concept in any therapeutic intervention and one of the best predictors of the success of such an intervention, should be enhanced.

CARE MODELS IN DUAL PATHOLOGY

Given the complexity of the phenomenon of dual pathology, it is considered that the most advisable way to offer quality care to this group of patients is to conceptualize them as patients undergoing a complex diagnostic and therapeutic process. This process must combine various psychopharmacological, psychotherapeutic, and sociotherapeutic resources and must be developed by multi- and interdisciplinary teams that undertake a comprehensive and integrated approach to this problem.[3–12] Only in this way will we achieve effective, efficient treatments that can improve the quality of life of these patients, their families, and their community. From the perspective of the therapeutic response to dual pathology patients, different care models have been developed to try to offer a treatment alternative tailored to their biopsychosocial needs. Classically, several alternatives are distinguished, which are outlined below.

Sequential Model

The sequential model is characterized by first treating the patient in the mental health or drug treatment network and then referring them to the other resource to continue their treatment there. The order of treatment is preferably clinical, seeking initial stabilization of the most serious condition.

Although this model has historically been the most widely used, it is now in disuse, because, by not addressing dual pathology comprehensively, it loses effectiveness and reduces therapeutic adherence.

Parallel Model

The parallel model is a therapeutic process in which the patient is included in both networks (addictions and mental health) for a simultaneous approach to the addictive problem and the associated psychiatric disorder.

Its effectiveness and efficiency depend on good coordination of resources, which is not always guaranteed, and therefore it can present the following drawbacks of fostering:

- Mistrust between teams
- The sending of contradictory messages to the patient
- A lack of coordination in interventions
- The patient being "passed around" between different teams

However, despite the drawbacks, this model (with well-designed coordination mechanisms, known as the *coordinated parallel model*) has been the option chosen in certain communities, as it is considered the only viable option due to the prior existence of two parallel care networks (mental health and addiction), with joint action protocols between *mental health* and *drug addiction* having been drawn up for this purpose.[13–14]

OTHER MODELS

In line with this approach of enabling comprehensive therapeutic plans focused on the needs of dual pathology patients, other care models have been implemented.

Matrix Model

It is a therapeutic process in which the patient is treated at the same time and in the same healthcare facility (for either addiction or mental health) by professionals from those services, coordinated in a joint effort in one of the aforementioned facilities and establishing treatment protocols for a single therapeutic plan.

Parallel Care Quadrant Model

It is a therapeutic process in which patients receive tiered care based on the prevalence and severity of comorbid disorders: from less severe cases, which are treated in primary care, to more severe cases, which are treated in more specialized facilities.

Integrated Model

This involves the simultaneous treatment of both disorders by the same care team, in standard units within the mental health or addiction network, or in specific dual pathology units.

Advantages[1,3–8,12–20]

- It promotes the use of outpatient services, reducing the use of hospitalization services, making it the most efficient option.
- It reduces the risk of illegal behavior, promoting the social integration of patients.
- It is the most effective model, but it is currently rarely implemented, a difficulty that is not unrelated to the existence of parallel care networks.

Possibilities for Developing This Model

- Using **standardized mental health or drug addiction resources** (re-integrated, at least functionally) when healthcare teams have training and education in addiction and mental health, respectively. This would correspond to the model of choice, as it allows for therapeutic continuity, even if the patient moves between various resources (depending on the course of their illness: outpatient units, acute care units, day units, therapeutic communities, etc.), while maintaining adherence to treatment.[21,22]
- Through the creation of **specific dual pathology units**. These generally arise in large healthcare areas with a very significant population (large cities). It is a "super-specialization" of mental health resources to respond to the most serious dual cases. It includes the provision of hospital resources for the admission of dual patients in the acute phase and an outpatient clinic for follow-up of cases, which are attended by the same therapeutic team, which is why this clinic is normally located in the same hospital.[10,12,20]

Disadvantages

- Risk to the continuity of referred patients, with the consequent loss of therapeutic adherence
- Hindrance of coordination with primary care and social services
- Incentivization of the creation of professional elites, who act with rigid selection criteria
- Fostering suspicion, mistrust, and discouragement among professionals in standard outpatient units

Characteristics

In developing the integrated model—the one that enjoys the most support according to the available scientific evidence—we must highlight its main characteristics:[3–8,10,11,13–20]

- **Stabilization of acute psychiatric symptoms and/or addictive behavior**, for which hospitalization may be necessary.
- In order to develop a psychiatric diagnosis and individualized long-term treatment plan, it is advisable to observe the patient during a **period of drug abstinence** lasting 3 to 6 weeks, if feasible, since it is always a priority to quickly address the symptoms of withdrawal, intoxication, and/or psychopathological decompensation of the comorbid condition.
- **Concomitant treatment of associated disorders** (and not only psychopathological disorders, as they often present a high rate of associated organic pathologies [HIV, HCV, COPD]) **by a single interdisciplinary care team, with an individualized, long-term, intensive treatment plan** that contemplates the appropriate use of resources based on the dual patient's progress (hospital admissions, therapeutic community, day centers, etc.), thus ensuring the necessary continuity of care.
- From the start of treatment, promote the **establishment of a solid therapeutic alliance** with the dual patient, as this is considered to be a favorable predictor of retention and subsequent therapeutic outcomes.
- It is advisable to perform **periodic urine drug tests** to ensure that abstinence is maintained; however, **treatment plans must be flexible**, setting realistic therapeutic goals to meet the needs of dual-diagnosis patients at different stages of their recovery and taking a **comprehensive, long-term approach** to this condition, including:
    - **Psychopharmacological coverage** tailored to the needs of the addictive disorder and associated mental disorder, as well as the course of the disease (atypical antipsychotics, anticonvulsants, antidepressants, mood stabilizers, etc.). **Psychotropic drugs that may be abused** by this population should be **used with caution**, and **strategies to improve therapeutic adherence** should be implemented:
        - Directly supervised treatments (whenever possible)
        - Use of long-acting drugs with simplified dosing schedules
        - Route of administration that ensures compliance (depot, long-acting injections)
        - Assessment of interactions and side effects
    - **Psychotherapeutic intervention**: Among psychosocial treatments,[23] those recommended most strongly are:
        - **Psychological interventions: multi-component programs** based on the application of motivational and cognitive-behavioral therapy should be highlighted: relapse prevention, contingency management with incentives, and skills training.

- **Personal and family psychoeducation**: Increasing awareness of the illness and the need for long-term treatment, recognizing the symptoms of relapse, promoting adherence to treatment, and actively involving the family in the treatment plan to dispel myths and false beliefs that contribute to the process of "stigmatization" of dual pathology (a double process due to the negative connotations derived from stigmatization, both "for madness and for addiction").
- **Group therapy**: Although it is generally recommended to encourage patient participation in group therapy, except for specific groups not all dual pathology patients are candidates for this type of intervention.
- **Family (and/or couple) therapy**: Especially for families with adolescents, strategies based on family intervention are indicated, encouraging patients' commitment and active participation in treatment, improving family dynamics, and promoting social normalization.
- **There is no scientific evidence that either psychotherapy applied in isolation or self-help groups are effective treatments for dual pathology patients.**

• **Measures for social integration**: In addition to clinical care, dual patients require special attention to their deficits in the social sphere (occupational, labor, legal, housing, etc.), requiring a personalized intervention plan to facilitate their social integration process.[24]

Treatment of the Acute Phase of Dual Pathology

Due to its particular clinical and therapeutic relevance, we will now outline a series of **considerations regarding the treatment of the acute phase of dual pathology**, although most of the treatment of a dual pathology patient can and should be carried out on an outpatient basis in their community.[6–8,10–12]

From this process of rehabilitation and reintegration, and with the specific objective of stabilizingan episode of decompensation or exacerbation of their chronic pathology, it is occasionally necessary to resort to hospital admission.

The particular characteristics of these patients, the complexity of their psychopathology and management, and the occasional existence of parallel care networks can make the coordination of the procedure for their hospital admission extremely complex.

Care Arrangements for Hospitalization During the Acute Phase

Both SUD and any other mental disorder form part of the body of knowledge and care provided by psychiatry, which is why all psychiatrists must have the necessary knowledge and skills to address both disorders, and healthcare facilities must meet the necessary conditions for their management. However, different circumstances have led to the emergence of parallel healthcare circuits, often doomed to disagreement and to "superspecialization," which tends to take precedence over the efficient use of available resources. In this vein, there is a predilection to create specific systems for each pathology, which increases healthcare spending, hinders continuity of care, stigmatizes patients, and fragments care, distancing it from clinical reality (there are few pure pathologies).

Therefore, it seems logical to think that care arrangements for acute dual pathology should include **acute psychiatric hospitalization units**, preferably within general hospitals. This would make better use of facilities and material and human resources, avoiding additional costs and duplication.

In view of the fact that caring for patients with dual pathology requires adequate training of staff and adaptation of care measures to the particular characteristics of these patients, it is desirable to design **specific care programs for dual pathology**,[6,7,9–12,18] following the model of specific programs for other pathologies (e.g., eating disorders, etc.).

In cases such as that of Galicia, Spain, where there are already "hospital detoxification units" that in practice function as a program (they often lack material resources and specific personnel), and given the progressive decline in traditional detoxification demands, these units can take on the dual pathology program, as the staff is trained in the management of both types of disorders (SUD and other MDD).

The creation of specific hospital dual pathology units would only be justified in the case of large cities and/or hospital centers, where the existence of a high volume of care might justify such superspecialization.

Care Process

There are many reasons why patients with dual pathology may need to be admitted to hospital, especially in situations of acute decompensation. As a general rule, it might be said that any clinical situation in which outpatient management is impossible or inadvisable would require admission; the most commonly cited **reasons for admission** are as follows:

- Severe psychiatric disorder: psychosis, major depression, manic episode, decompensated personality disorder, etc.
- Risk of self-harm or harm to others, conditioned by patients' psychopathology
- Diagnostic evaluation in patients with complex clinical presentations, enabling better observation and ensuring substance abstinence
- Initiation of treatment in certain specific situations: lack of awareness of illness and rejection of treatment, possible drug interactions or interactions with drugs of abuse, and use of certain therapeutic techniques (ECT, etc.)
- Stabilization of addictive pathology decompensated by psychiatric comorbidity
- Stabilization of psychiatric pathology decompensated by substance use and/or withdrawal syndromes

On the other hand, it would be useful to highlight **certain situations that do not constitute an indication for admission to an acute psychiatric unit, or that would even make admission inadvisable**: social problems (social admission), organic brain disorders (dementia, confusional states, etc.), serious somatic pathology requiring priority care, etc. However, admission should not be restricted, as unfortunately sometimes happens, due to certain circumstances directly related to the psychopathology of these patients (polydrug use, signs of recent intoxication, lack of social and family support, comorbidity with personality disorder, etc.).

It is also advisable to establish mechanisms with outpatient centers in order to facilitate coordination between outpatient and hospital facilities and vice versa:[18] referral protocols, responsible professionals, discharge reports, and the creation of integrated electronic medical record systems that allow for the unified recording of all clinical information from health-related activities (consultations, surgical procedures, diagnostic tests, drug prescriptions, etc., performed on a citizen at the different levels of care that make up a health system).[22]

The methods for making internal transfers can be made in the following ways:

- **From the outpatient treatment center**: This should be the preferred route, as the patient's psychiatrist is best placed to assess the clinical severity and need for admission, and has the greatest influence on the patient to follow instructions. Furthermore, admission should be part of the overall therapeutic process that each patient is undergoing on an outpatient basis. Once the advisability/necessity of hospital admission has been determined, the patient's psychiatrist should assess whether it should be urgent, preferred, or scheduled and contact the appropriate hospitalization unit to coordinate the referral.
- **From the emergency department**: Unfortunately, it is not always possible to follow the above procedure and, in many cases, the acute situation must be assessed in the emergency department of general hospitals, where patients go or are taken by family members, law enforcement, emergency services, etc., for a wide variety of reasons: suicide attempts, heteroaggressiveness, serious behavioral disorders, etc. In this case, the psychiatrist on duty will be responsible for ordering immediate admission if the severity of the clinical picture so requires.

In both circumstances, admission may be voluntary, if the patient agrees to it and is in psychopathological condition to give consent, or involuntary, if the above conditions are not met and there is a perceived risk to them or to third parties—in which case judicial authorization for admission must be requested, in accordance with the provisions of the legislation currently in force in this area.

With regard to the **specific actions** required for the care of dual pathology patients in an acute psychiatric unit, the following should be noted:

- In general, patients with dual pathology require the same care and benefit from the same therapeutic measures as other patients admitted for any other mental illness:[6,9,10,12,17] They can share rooms, common areas, therapeutic and leisure activities, etc. However, given their particular characteristics, they might require some type of specific measure, generally aimed at preventing substance use: restrictions on leaving the unit, on visits, and on contact with the outside world; greater attention when inspecting their belongings; frequent tests to verify abstinence from use; avoiding the prescription of psychotropic drugs with a high risk of abuse; etc.

- Once the therapeutic objectives that led to admission have been achieved and the clinical picture has stabilized, the patient should be referred back to their outpatient treatment unit.

Given the special characteristics of dual pathology patients (greater severity, poorer compliance, risk of relapse, comorbid personality disorders, etc.), outpatient centers should try not to delay follow-up appointments, in the interests of maintaining the necessary therapeutic continuity.

In short, in the care aspect of the dual pathology treatment process, as opposed to intensive therapeutic approaches focused on abstinence (whose results are difficult to maintain once treatment is completed), treatments based on holistic approaches, focused on the needs of the individual, with low-intensity, low-demand therapies and a low level of structure, tend to facilitate the dual patient's adherence to the care resource, promoting restraint in consumption patterns, and also improvement in the patient's comorbid psychopathology and functionality; reduction of hospitalizations; less use of emergency services; lower crime rates; and improvement in the quality of life of the patient and their social and community environment.

PROPOSED CARE CIRCUIT FOR DUAL PATHOLOGY PATIENTS

As a result of the analysis of these care models, a proposal was made in the A Coruña health area to restructure the different networks[2] to establish a care pathway for dual patients (Figure 3.1), based on the determinants of the integrated care model:

- **TYPE A. Complex chemical dependency**: Dual patients with mild psychopathology and severe dependency. This includes drug-dependent patients who also have mild, non-persistent psychiatric disorders; they are usually treated primarily within the addiction network.
- **TYPE B. Psychiatric patients with drug abuse**: Dual pathology patients with severe psychopathology and mild dependence. These are mentally ill patients who abuse substances. If they use legal drugs, they are usually treated in the mental health network, while those who use illegal drugs and/or have non-chemical addictions (gambling addiction, etc.) are generally referred to the addiction network, especially when their progress is unfavorable (they suffer repeated relapses).
- **TYPE C. Drug-dependent psychiatric patients**: Dual patients with severe psychopathology and severe dependence. These are mentally ill drug addicts who, as in the previous case, can be treated within the mental health network if they are using legal

- Severe dependency and mild psychopathology ➡ UCA <<>> DU/CT
- Mild dependency and severe psychopathology ➡ USM/DH/UHP << >> UCA/DU/CT
- Severe dependence and psychopathology ➡ UHP/CT (UEPD?) <<>> UCA/DU
- Mild depression and psychopathy ➡ CAP <<>> UCA

√ UCA: addictive behaviors unit (outpatient-community: UAA+UAD)
√ DU: day unit (UCA dependency)
√ TC: therapeutic community (UCA dependency)
√ USM: mental health unit (outpatient-community)
√ DH: day hospital (UPA unit)
√ UHP: psychiatric hospital unit (in general hospital), acute cases

FIGURE 3.1 Care circuit for dual-pahtology patients in the A Coruña health area (Galicia).

drugs. In severe cases of addiction, with repeated relapses, use of illegal substances, and non-chemical addictions, these patients are usually referred to addiction treatment facilities.

- **TYPE D. Drug abuse and mild psychopathology**: Patients whose addictive behavior and psychopathology are *minor* and who, in the case of legal drugs (alcohol and tobacco), are treated in primary care, but who use illegal drugs and have behavioral (non-chemical) addictions, are usually referred to the addiction network.

The placement of dual patients at the appropriate level of care depends on an accurate assessment of their treatment needs, which are determined by the complexity of their condition, an adequate analysis of the various factors involved, and knowledge of the care resources available and the ease of access to them.

As a result of this organizational proposal, in the A Coruña health area, the healthcare situation of the dual population (Figure 3.2) is as follows.[2]

If we delve deeper into the analysis and investigate the healthcare distribution of dual patients based on comorbidities, the situation is as follows (Figures 3.3 and 3.4).

We can therefore conclude that, based on these care principles and from an organizational perspective of treatment services for dual pathology patients, it is possible to identify and recommend the type of intervention expected for each level of care in the service network, depending on the type of problems presented by dual pathology patients.

For all the reasons outlined above, and even though the integrated model is currently the most recommended, it should be remembered that *the best is not always possible.* Therefore, in each healthcare area and depending on the resources available, efforts should be made to develop the therapeutic response that provides the best quality of care in addressing the biopsychosocial needs of dual pathology patients.

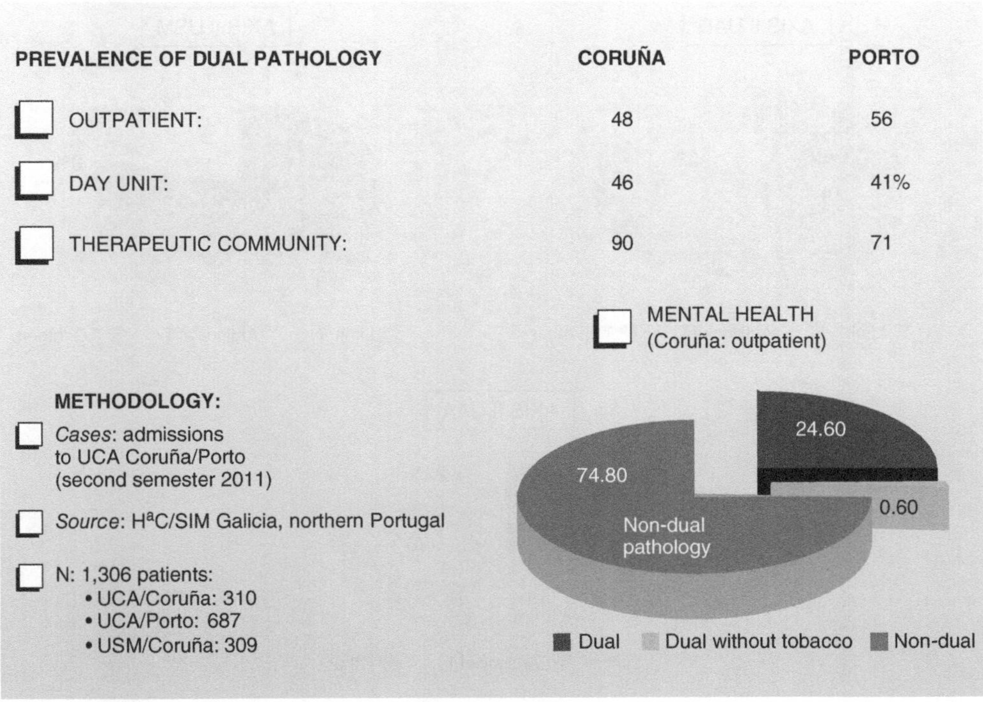

FIGURE 3.2 Distribution of care for the dual population in A Coruña and Porto.

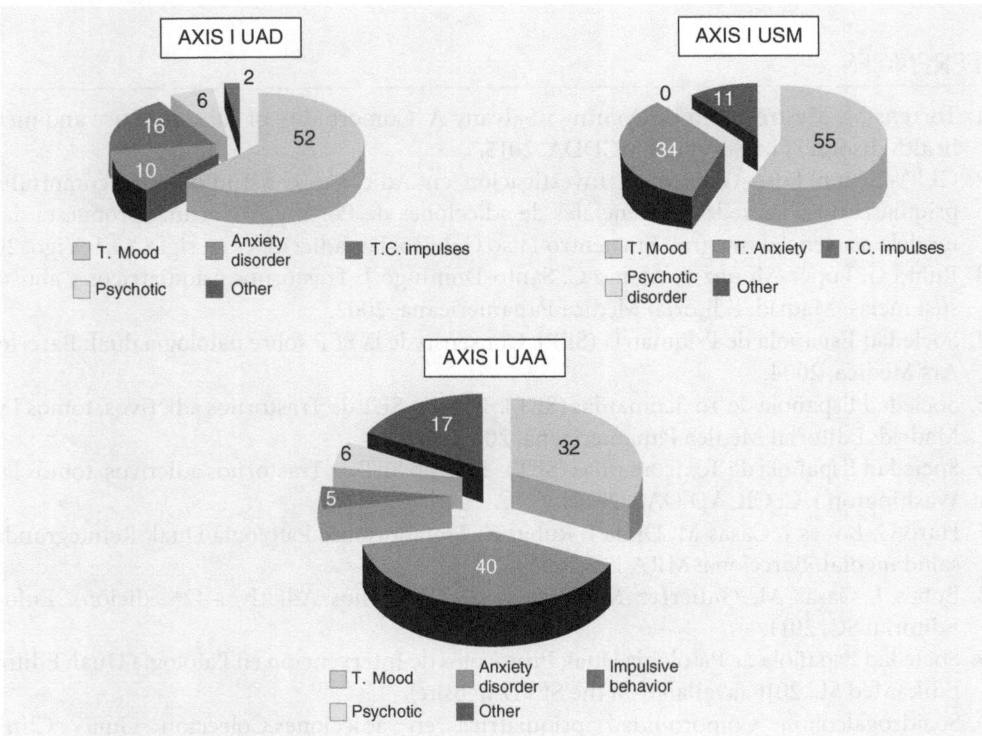

FIGURE 3.3 Distribution of care for the dual population in A Coruña (axis I).

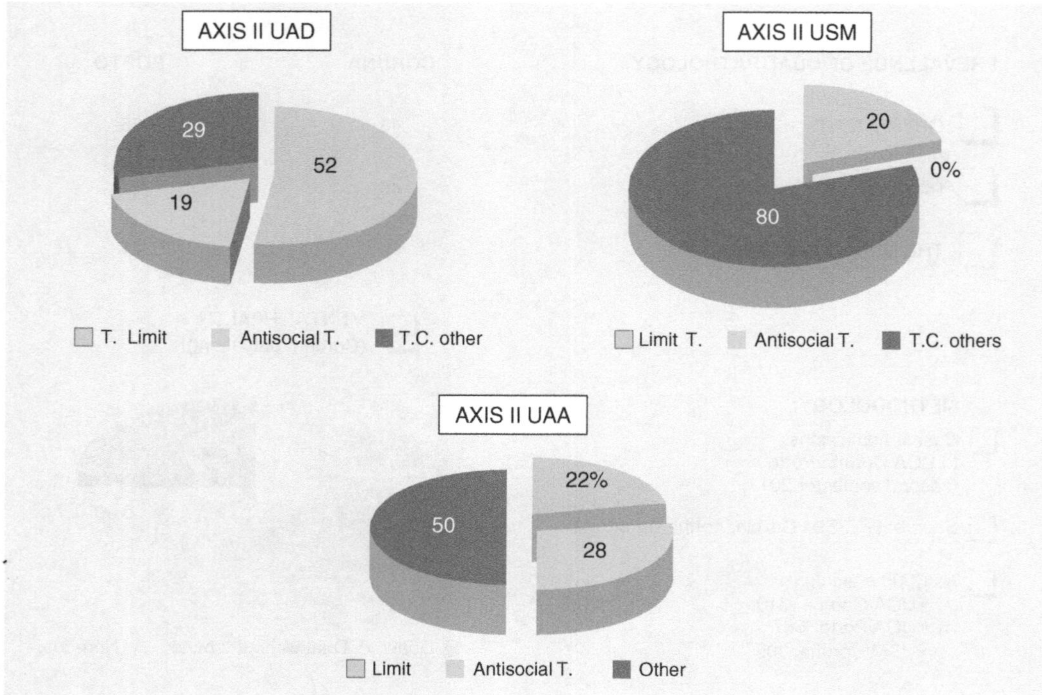

FIGURE 3.4 Distribution of care for the dual population in A Coruña (axis II).

REFERENCES

1. Torrens M, Mestre-Pintó JI, Domingo-Salvany A. Comorbidity of substance use and mental health disorders in Europe. EMCDDA, 2015.
2. GLIA-Grupo Luso-Galaico de Investigación en Adicciones. Estudio sobre comorbilidad psiquiátrica en las redes asistenciales de adicciones de Porto y A Coruña: propuesta de un modelo asistencial integral. Encuentro Luso Galaico. Las adicciones en siglo XXI. Vigo, 2015.
3. Rubio G, López-Muñoz F, Álamo C, Santo-Domingo J. Trastornos psiquiátricos y abuso de sustancias. Madrid: Editorial Médica Panamericana, 2002.
4. Sociedad Española de Psiquiatría (SEP). Consenso de la SEP sobre patología dual. Barcelona: Ars Medica, 2004.
5. Sociedad Española de Toxicomanías (SET). Tratado SET de Trastornos adictivos, tomos I y II. Madrid: Editorial Médica Panamericana, 2006.
6. Sociedad Española de Toxicomanías (SET). Tratado SET de Trastornos adictivos, tomos I y II. Washington DC: CICAD OAS, 2010.
7. Haro G, Bobes J, Casas M, Didia J, Rubio G. Tratado sobre Patología Dual. Reintegrando la salud mental. Barcelona: MRA Ediciones, 2010.
8. Bobes J, Casas M, Gutiérrez M. Manual de Trastornos Adictivos (2ª edición). Enfoque Editorial SC, 2011.
9. Sociedad Española de Patología Dual. Protocolos de Intervención en Patología Dual. Editorial EdikaMed SL, 2016 (available on the SEPD website).
10. Socidrogalcohol. Comorbilidad psiquiátrica en adicciones.Colección Guías Clínicas Socidrogalcohol. Concepto, epidemiología & diagnóstico. Socidrogalcohol Publishing House, 2017 (available at socidrogalcohol.org).

11. Comorbilidad psiquiátrica en adicciones. Colección Guías Clínicas "Socidrogalcohol". Nº 8: Resumen de intervenciones & árboles de decisiones. Socidrogalcohol, 2019 (available on the website socidrogalcohol.org).
12. FGEP-Foro Gallego para Estudio de la Personalidad. Trastornos de la Personalidad. Un abordaje Integrador. Editorial Pensódromo SL, 2020.
13. Junta de Andalucía-Consejería de Igualdad y Bienestar Social. Protocolo de actuación conjunta entre equipos de Salud Mental de Distrito y Centros de Tratamiento Ambulatorio de Drogodependencias, 2002.
14. Junta de Extremadura-Consejería de Sanidad y Dependencia. Protocolo de Coordinación y Atención a la Patología Dual, 2007.
15. Solomon J, Zimberg S, Shollar E. Diagnóstico dual. Barcelona: Ediciones en Neurociencias, 1996.
16. NIDA (National Institute on Drug Abuse). Principios de tratamientos efectivos para Trastornos por Uso de Sustancias, 1999 (available at nida.nih.gov).
17. San L, Casas M. ecomendaciones Terapéuticas en Patología Dual. Barcelona: Ars Medica, 2002.
18. Xunta de Galicia-Consellería de Sanidade. Catálogo de Programas Asistenciais do Plan de Galicia sobre Drogas. Santiago de Compostela, 2003 (available on the website sergas.es).
19. SAMHSA (Substance Abuse and Mental Health Services Administration). Substance Abuse Treatment for Persons with Co-Occurring Disorders Treatment Improvement Protocol (TIP) Series No 42. HHS Publication No. (SMA) 13-3992. Rockville, MD: Substance Abuse and Mental Health Services Administration, 2005.
20. Socidrogalcohol. Socidrogalcohol. Manejo clínico del paciente con patología dual. Recomendaciones de expertos. Socidrogalcohol, 2009 (available at socidrogalcohol.org).
21. Xunta de Galicia-Consellería de Sanidade. Plan estratégico de Saúde Mental. Galicia 2006-2011. Santiago de Compostela, 2007 (available at sergas.es).
22. Xunta de Galicia-Consellería de Sanidade. Plan de Galicia sobre Drogas: 2007-2009. Santiago de Compostela, 2009 (available at sergas.es).
23. Socidrogalcohol. Guía clínica de intervención psicológica en adicciones. Guías clínicas de Socidrogalcohol basadas en la evidencia científica. Socidrogalcohol, 2008 (available at socidrogalcohol.org).
24. Xunta de Galicia-Consellería de Sanidade. Programa de Incorporación Personalizado. Santiago de Compostela, 2004 (available at sergas.es).

CHAPTER 4

Care Approach for Dual Pathology Patients in Residential and Semi-residential Centers, Within the Framework of Care Provided by a General Hospital and Emergency Services, and in Specific Facilities

4.1 RESIDENTIAL CENTERS AND DUAL PATHOLOGY: THERAPEUTIC COMMUNITIES AND OTHER RESIDENTIAL CENTERS FOR THE MENTALLY ILL

J. Vitor Marques, J. M. Ramos, C. Pereiro Gómez, A. M. González López, M. A. Ortega Orozco, and G. A. Castaño Pérez

GENERAL

The approach and structure of treatment plans for addictive behaviors have undergone a remarkable process of development and specialization over time, with the aim of keeping pace with advances in knowledge in the field of addiction.

DOI: 10.4324/9781003786153-4

Thus, the treatment of addictive behaviors (with or without dual pathology) is currently structured within a specialized network that offers different types of care, provided by specialized, multidisciplinary technical teams:[1,2]

- **Outpatient modality**: In centers or care units specializing in the treatment of behaviors and addictions, and in mobile units or collaborating centers dependent on their outpatient referral centers
- **Semi-residential modality**: In centers, units, or day hospitals
- **Residential modality**: In therapeutic communities (TC) and in hospital units or services

Therapeutic Communities

Currently, the residential modality or regime is based primarily on TCs, which are perhaps the care resources that have evolved and specialized the most over time.

Heterogeneous therapeutic guidelines (not always supported by available scientific evidence), inadequate physical spaces, and technically unspecialized teams, among other characteristics, led the European Federation of Associations Involved in Drug Addiction to develop a "European Expert Group for the Study and Development of Quality in Therapeutic Communities" in 1996, which culminated in the formalization of the "Declaration on Quality Indicators in Therapeutic Communities."

TCs are currently conceived as medium/long-term residential facilities designed to provide inpatient treatment to individuals dependent on substances with and/or without other associated psychiatric disorders.[3–5] However, as has already been mentioned, TCs have not always represented this reality and are a constantly evolving resource.

TCs emerged in the 1950s in Great Britain with the aim of providing treatment to individuals with post-traumatic stress and other adverse experiences resulting from World War II, as structures that were inserted into the context of a psychiatric hospital.[6–8]

In the 1970s, after the Vietnam War, with the emergence of "new addicts," there was a need in the United States (US) to create and strengthen a series of care structures capable of responding to this new clinical demand. It was at this stage that we witnessed a veritable multiplication and proliferation of TCs for "these addicts," first in the US and later in Europe, which operated with specific care models, often in opposition to the medical model: Daytop Village, Phoenix House, Satori, and Portage, among others.[6,8]

Currently, TCs, regardless of the methodologies applied and their specific functional organization, are a care model whose objective is to achieve the biopsychosocial rehabilitation, based on a regime of hospitalization of the addicted patient, with or without dual pathology, when they are unable to consolidate and maintain abstinence in an outpatient or semi-residential setting, which has a major dysfunctional impact in psychopathological, organic, and/or social terms.

These organizations, through a specific and structured therapeutic program with different phases of intervention developed by multidisciplinary teams, aim to promote the rehabilitation of users, helping them to overcome their areas of difficulty and plan their future without substance use.[9,10]

Given that substance use does not end with the substance itself, but involves a whole lifestyle, admission to TCs is aimed at achieving a change in lifestyle, using the "community as a method" in a treatment environment that seeks to treat coexisting mental illness and psychological problems, improve social functioning, facilitate behavioral changes, and ultimately enable completion of a therapeutic program, integrating this new way of being into a lifestyle without resorting to the use of psychoactive substances.

The therapeutic approach in TCs is highly structured and autonomous, which distinguishes it from other types of residential rehabilitation, with clear expectations, consequences, roles, and schedules, in which residents progress through a hierarchy of increasing responsibilities.[10,11]

In terms of psychotherapeutic intervention, residents, under the supervision of the therapeutic team (made up of professionals from the health, social, and human sciences), may include in their composition "former drug addicts" in recovery and with specific training in the area of addiction. These individuals act as participatory agents, both in their own recovery and in the recovery of their peers through the interaction they establish with each other, becoming participatory agents throughout the process.[3]

In addition to the dynamics established between peers, TCs, to facilitate and enhance the biopsychosocial rehabilitation process of the hospitalized patient, must integrate effective medical/psychiatric, nursing, psychological, social service, and occupational therapy follow-up, with the aim of:

1. Creating a space for reflection with a view to developing the individual's personal history, allowing them to give new meaning and identify the necessary points of change.
2. Changing negative patterns of behavior, thinking, and feelings that predispose individuals to substance use in order to maintain consolidated abstinence.
3. Promoting autonomy and responsibility as pillars of adult life in society.
4. Developing the ability to establish and maintain healthy relationships, and breaking destructive patterns.
5. Promoting the acquisition of personal skills that enable individuals to find alternatives for a realistic life plan.
6. Promoting and enhancing social (re)integration through the development and contractualization of an individual reintegration plan.

In this context, TCs and other residential centers began a progressive therapeutic evolution, increasingly adapted to the new standard of users and new addiction problems. Today, they are an essential resource in a network of care for patients with dual pathology, highlighting the development of specific therapeutic programs for dual pathology with the aim of an intensive and comprehensive therapeutic approach (medical, psychotherapeutic, occupational, and socio-educational), with defined referral criteria and longer duration (on average 12 months or 6 months for treatment programs for addiction without dual diagnosis).[12]

However, the issue of the duration of in TC has always been quite controversial, and in this regard, the experience of cross-border TC in Coruña as a result of the COVID-19 pandemic must necessarily be a point of reflection. In this pandemic context, the Regional Ministry of Health of the Xunta de Galicia[13] established a series of conditions for the continuity of treatment in residential centers, which also included TC. With the aim of protecting the centers from possible outbreaks of COVID-19, the decision was made to cancel outings during patients' stays in residential programs and, therefore, to schedule their stays for three months. At the same time, it was decided to temporarily reduce the average number of places in these residential facilities (to half their usual capacity).

The experience of more than a year of care work under these conditions shows that, in addition to preventing the emergence of infectious outbreaks, the quality of the programs has clearly improved. the improvement in patient/professional ratios has enabled and enhanced:

- Better individual psychiatric, psychological, and socio-educational follow-up
- Optimization of physical spaces for TC activities, improving accommodation conditions
- Contrary to expectations, at the end of the year, lack of a decrease in the number of patients per year compared to the average number of patients in the "pre-COVID era," and lack of a decrease in the number of patients who completed their treatment with a "therapeutic discharge"

Given these results, we must rethink the duration of residential treatment in TC, since for dual patients, especially those with severe mental disorders, a six-month stay can be difficult to endure, even with a progressive release regime starting in the second month of hospitalization. We found that a three-month hospitalization regimen without outings was tolerated very well and had no impact on the final results of the TC program.

In similar circumstances are patients admitted to TC who are employed, either self-employed or employed by others, for whom long stays (6 months) create work difficulties, placing them before the dilemma of whether or not to enter TC. However, shortening their period of hospitalization has had clear advantages, since, in addition to enabling the necessary admission to TC for the stabilization of the patient, it has been possible to maintain previous working conditions for the vast majority of those affected.

On the other hand, the reduction in places, in addition to allowing for the optimization and improvement of the quality of TC treatment and patient satisfaction rates, has led to a clear reduction in conflict among inmates, facilitating their stay and avoiding forced and voluntary discharges.

The questioning of the TC model we maintained in our cross-border TCs in Coruña as a result of this experience in

"COVID times" has also made us reflect on whether the "traditional model of hospitalization in TC" is the most appropriate for a new type of dual patient, which is becoming increasingly common, namely one who presents a behavioral addiction as part of their dual diagnosis and who requires separation from the temporary living environment and more-intensive treatment for their addictive disorder in a residential treatment model.

The referral of users with dual pathology arises from the outpatient follow-up regime, with referral criteria focusing on the presence of:

- A high degree of psychopathological destructuring, taking into account not only the existence of substance use, but also the dual condition (substance use/simultaneous mental illness) with the consequent serious individual, family, and/or social repercussions
- A history of therapeutic failure in various outpatient approaches
- Unquestionable benefit from temporary isolation from their environment, not only in relation to cessation of substance use, but also considering their mental illness
- A problematic legal situation
- Motivation for lifestyle change and treatment
- Regardless of the treatment model adopted in TCs or other residential centers, treatment programs for users with dual pathology are equipped with the necessary specificity, aiming for a multidisciplinary, careful, and intensive approach, in which rapid stabilization and biopsychosocial rehabilitation are recommended, with the following general objectives:
    - Cessation of psychoactive substance use, preventing relapses
    - Raising awareness of the addictive problem and the simultaneous mental illness, promoting self-knowledge and self-control
    - Developing the ability to adapt to mental illness and adopting a healthy lifestyle
    - Reduction of problems arising from psychiatric disorders and psychoactive substance use
    - Monitoring of the patient's clinical condition
    - Facilitation and enhancement of the process of social (re)integration, promoting improvements in the family and social network
    - Developing habits and routines that promote improved functionality and autonomy in the patient
    - Promoting and enhancing therapeutic adherence

- Rehabilitation of cognitive, emotional, and behavioral skills that favor and/or improve the patient's personal and social development
- Exploration of the patient's areas of interest in order to increase motivation for treatment and improve their involvement in meaningful life activities to outline future goals
- Implement and consolidate the proper completion of appropriate medical-psychiatric treatment of concurrent pathologies
- In summary, this TC model for dual pathology patients adapts the classic principles and methods of TC intervention (patients learn through mutual support and affiliation with the peer community to stimulate change in themselves and others) to the circumstances of each resident, but with a series of adjustments that are considered essential:
  - Greater therapeutic flexibility and more-individualized treatments
  - Reduction in the intensity of the intervention regime, especially with regard to the conversion of the traditional encounter (confrontation) group into a highly structured, low-emotional-intensity conflict resolution (psychoeducational) group aimed at achieving greater self-understanding and personal autonomy, with behavioral changes aimed at a more favorable evolution of their problems.

Stages of Development

This entire treatment process must follow a guideline which, regardless of the therapeutic model adopted, can be divided into four phases (assessment, intervention, reevaluation, and conclusion):

- **Therapeutic assessment**: This consists of an initial comprehensive and multidisciplinary assessment, covering the areas of medicine and psychiatry, psychology and neuropsychology, occupational therapy, and social work, facilitating the collection of information and the development of guiding questions for an adequate conceptualization of objectives and therapeutic steps for the user.
- **Implementation and development of multidisciplinary intervention**: The need for temporary stages to reassess the care process initiated with the patient must always be taken into account, with the consequent (if necessary) restructuring and implementation of new objectives and new therapeutic stages, with the ultimate goal of completing and consolidating their recovery.
- **Conclusion**: At the end of the therapeutic program in TC, and after meeting the stipulated objectives, the user must be discharged and referred to their referral unit/outpatient center for outpatient follow-up, an essential step in maintaining and consolidating their stability, thus enhancing their process of social integration.

In summary, TCs (and other residential centers) are an essential therapeutic resource in a model of approach and follow-up for users with dual pathology, representing an indispensable complement to their outpatient and/or semi-residential follow-up, with the rehabilitative function being the one that determines the primacy of the therapeutic objectives to be achieved with the patient (dual or non-dual), rather than the care regime and the type of activities to be carried out (which must be adapted to the needs of each patient throughout their stay in these care facilities), avoiding the adoption of rigid approaches that only lead to a loss of contact with these patients, who are already difficult and have a high degree of biopsychosocial deterioration, contributing to further clouding their already unfavorable prognosis).[13]

REFERENCES

1. Socidrogalcohol. Manejo clínico del paciente con patología dual. Recomendaciones de expertos. Socidrogalcohol, 2009 (available at socidrogalcohol.org).
2. Haro G, Bobes J, Casas M, Didia J, Rubio G. Tratado sobre Patología Dual. Reintegrando la salud mental. Barcelona: MRA Ediciones, 2010.
3. Biel S, Plakun E. Therapeutic community then and now. Psychiatry. 2019;82(1):18–23. doi: 10.1080/00332747.2019.1565561.
4. Malivert M, Fatséas M, Denis C, Langlois E, Auria-combe M. Effectiveness of therapeutic communities: A systematic review. European Addiction Research. 2012;18(1):1–11. doi: 10.1159/000331007.
5. Kreager DA, Schaefer DR, Davidson KM, Zajac G, Haynie DL, De Leon G. Evaluating peer-influence processes in a prison-based therapeutic community: a dynamic network approach. Drug and Alcohol Dependence. 2019;203:13–18. doi: 10.1016/j.drugalcdep.2019.05.018.
6. Comas D. La Comunidad Terapéutica: Una Perspectiva Metodológica. En: D. Arnau (editor). La Metodología de la Comunidad Terapéutica. Spain: Fundación Atenea Grupo Gid, 2010.
7. Jones M. The concept of a therapeutic community. American Journal of Psychiatry. 1956:112(8):647–50. doi: 10.1176/ajp.112.8.647.
8. Lima P. Criação de Uma Comunidade Terapêutica Nos Açores: Viabilidade Política, Social e Económica (Master's thesis, Universidade Lusófona de Humanidades e Tecnologias - Faculdade de Ciências Sociais e Humanas, 2012.
9. Leon G, Unterrainer H. The therapeutic community: A unique social psychological approach to the treatment of addictions and related disorders. Frontiers in Psychiatry. 2020:11:786. doi: 10.3389/fpsyt.2020.00786.
10. Staiger P, Liknaitzky P, Lake A, Gruenert S. Longitudinal substance use and biopsychosocial outcomes following therapeutic community treatment for substance dependence. Journal of Clinical Medicine. 2020;9(1):118. doi: 10.3390/jcm9010118.
11. Bunt G, Muehlbach B, Moed C. The therapeutic community: An international perspective. Substance Abuse. 2008;29(3):81–87. doi: 10.1080/08897070802218844.
12. IDT. Linhas Orientadoras Para o Tratamento e Reabilitação em Comunidades Terapêuticas. IDT Department of Treatment and Reintegration. Lisbon, 2011.
13. Xunta de Galicia-Consellería de Sanidade (2003):. Catálogo de Programas Asistenciais do Plan de Galicia sobre Drogas. Santiago de Compostela, 2003 (available at sergas.es).

4.2 SEMI-RESIDENTIAL CENTERS (UNITS, CENTERS, AND/OR DAY HOSPITALS) AND DUAL PATHOLOGY

A. Piñón Blanco, F. Otero Lamas, M. T. Lage López, M. Villarino González, and M. S. Cardoso Carvalho

Day units (DU) constitute the semi-residential treatment modality for patients with substance-related disorders (SRD) and/or dual pathology. Among the different treatment modalities, they are a resource that expands the traditional offerings of outpatient centers (drug addiction treatment units) and residential centers (hospital detoxification units and therapeutic communities), providing psychosocial care based on keeping the patient in their community.[1]

In this sense, DUs are specialized resources for the treatment of people with SRD and/or dual pathology, on a day-care basis, offering a program of therapeutic, educational, and occupational activities aimed at the detoxification and rehabilitation of patients referred to them from the outpatient unit of reference. Patients are also returned to the DU after their therapeutic discharge for the necessary continuity of care until they achieve social reintegration, the true goal of any care process for addiction and dual pathology.[1]

The intervention strategy that characterizes this type of care, which allows patients to remain connected to their environment and promotes family involvement and the patient's social reintegration, is based on:[1]

- Prioritizing the psychotherapeutic component, primarily group interventions
- Promoting training, occupational, and educational aspects, prioritizing the inclusion of patients in the standard resources of the community of reference
- For full-time users, developing an intensive, daily therapeutic program; and accepting part-time users to work on specific therapeutic objectives of the individualized treatment plan through some of activities

We believe that the DU activity plan can and should be based on process-focused neuropsychological rehabilitation, which is the ideal DU model for a treatment network to improve the quality of care provided to users (with or without dual pathology). To this end, we will take as a reference the "Neuro-CEDRO" DU model (Vigo, Spain), which we will describe later.

Since addiction was conceptualized as a pathology of motivation and decision-making,[2,3] neuroscience has provided numerous pieces of evidence on the role of cognitive function alterations in addictive disorders,[4–6] neuropsychological alterations that are present even after prolonged periods of abstinence.[7] They have been shown not only to play a role in the etiopathogenesis of this pathology but also to be able to predict the evolution and clinical response of patients.[8,9]

The degree of cognitive impairment present at the time of receiving treatment can determine and/or mark the patient's progress throughout the treatment (the greater the number of relapses and dropouts, the worse the prognosis and the harder it is to integrate the information received in psychotherapeutic interventions, and the less awareness of the deficits).

For this reason, it is essential to establish neuropsychological profiles of functioning that allow us to develop treatment proposals adapted to the degree of impairment presented by our patients.

Advances in neuroscience have provided the scientific basis for the development of neurocognitive rehabilitation programs as a means of improving the therapeutic approach to drug addiction, and there is growing interest in improving neuropsychological rehabilitation procedures in their application to the treatment of addiction.[10–18]

In response to clinical needs and advances in the field of neuroscience, in recent years assessment techniques[10,19] and neuropsychological rehabilitation[11–13,15,20,21] have been incorporated into the care provided in day units for patients with SRD with/without dual pathology with the aim of providing effective treatments to address the neurocognitive deficits present in many of our patients. Specifically, it is important to note the significance that different studies attribute to specific working memory tasks as facilitators of important cognitive functions, such as learning, verbal comprehension, thinking, reasoning, and decision-making, and as generators of an efficient buffering effect against attentional bias toward salient stimuli related to substance use.[5,21,22]

In this sense, rehabilitation programs should be characterized as holistic programs, developed by specialized, interdisciplinary professionals and with ecological validity, making use of both quantitative and qualitative assessment.[23,24]

Following this idea, in a recent study conducted by our research group with DU patients, we found neuropsychological performance indicative of moderate cognitive impairment, reduced psychomotor, reading, and visuospatial processing speed, deficits in sustained, selective, and alternating attention subprocesses, and difficulties in the executive components of inhibition and cognitive flexibility. In terms of psychopathological symptoms, positive results were found on the clinical scales of obsession-compulsion, depression, anxiety, and psychoticism.[25]

Next, we will provide a brief description of the proposed model of DU "Neuro-CEDRO," a proposed intervention model based on process-based neuropsychological rehabilitation. Based on the neuropsychological rehabilitation work referenced in the literature and following the methodological principles of neuropsychological rehabilitation, the main rehabilitation techniques, and different theoretical reference models, the proposed model for the "Neuro-CEDRO" DU described below was developed.

Preliminary considerations:

- The use of psychoactive substances has been consistently associated with the presence of alterations in different neuropsychological processes: memory, attention, or executive functions.
- It is not possible to intervene in an altered process without adequate knowledge of how it works: hence the importance of theoretical reference models (advances in neuroscience).
- Process-based neuropsychological assessment is considered the first step in the rehabilitation process (profile of preserved and impaired abilities).

- With this in mind, process-based rehabilitation should be based on process-based neuropsychological assessment (theoretical reference models).
- Several studies have pointed out the usefulness of neuropsychological assessment in:
  - Choosing and adapting the most appropriate treatment program[26,27]
  - Better understanding the core clinical characteristics of addictive disorders[28,29]
  - Using an objective method to evaluate the effectiveness of treatments and the patient's situation in order to prevent relapse[26,30]

In short, the assessment of the neuropsychological profile of patients with SUDs and/or dual pathology is helping to better define their individual needs for each therapeutic intervention and to guide more efficient in achieving neurocognitive rehabilitation goals.

Table 4.1 details the cognitive-executive domains assessed and the neuropsychological instruments used in the neuropsychological assessment battery[19] used in the "Neuro-CEDRO" proposal.

Table 4.2 details the clinical assessment instruments, which are described below.

In order to interpret the results obtained in the assessment process (prior to the patient's admission to the DU), we used a structure based on a process analysis (processing speed processing speed, attentional subprocesses, and executive components).

TABLE 4.1 Cognitive-Executive Domains

Cognitive domain	Tests
Screening for mild cognitive impairment	Montreal Cognitive Assessment (MOCA)[31]
	WAIS-III[32]
Psychomotor processing speed and visuomotor coordination	Number key
Mental calculation and working memory	Arithmetic
Focused and sustained attention and working memory	Digits
Visual perception and psychomotor processing speed	Symbol search
Working memory	Letters and numbers
Psychomotor processing speed	Processing speed index (PSI)
Working memory	Working memory index (WMI)
	Stroop test[33]
Reading processing speed	Words
Selective attention	Color
Cognitive inhibition	Word-color
	Trail Making Test (TMT)[34]
Sustained attention, motor skills, and visuospatial visual search abilities	Part A
Alternating attention and cognitive flexibility	Part B
	Verbal Fluency Test
Frontal lobe functioning	Phonemic fluency[35]
Temporal lobe functioning	Semantic fluency

TABLE 4.2 Clinical Assessment Instruments

Psychopathological symptoms	SCL-90[36]
Frontal Systems Behavior Scale	FrSBe[37]
Anhedonia Scale	EAA[38]

To perform this analysis, we took into account different theoretical reference models, such as the factorial structure of care,[39] Sohlberg and Mateer's (1989) clinical model of attention and Miyake's (2000) factorial model of executive components.

To perform this analysis, we took into account different theoretical reference models, such as the factorial structure of care, Sohlberg and Mateer's (1989) clinical model of attention, and Miyake's (2000) factorial model of executive components. Figure 4.1 describes the process structure used.

Next, after interpreting the results based on theoretical reference models, we make a treatment proposal tailored to the profile of the patient with SRD and/or dual pathology.

In short, taking into account the degree of cognitive-executive impairment, clinical reports, and previous history, we make a proposal for intervention tailored to their impaired and preserved abilities.

Figure 4.2 describes the activities we offer to patients with SRD and/or dual pathology at the CEDRO-Vigo UAD, organized according to a series of cognitive-executive domains that have previously been evaluated. This intervention proposal is briefly described in the patient referral protocol to the DU and in detail in the neuropsychological assessment report.

The initial assessment will serve as a reference point for monitoring the patient's progress in treatment and the results of their individualized intervention plan, providing an objective method for evaluating the degree of patient deterioration and treatment effectiveness, with the aim of preventing relapses.

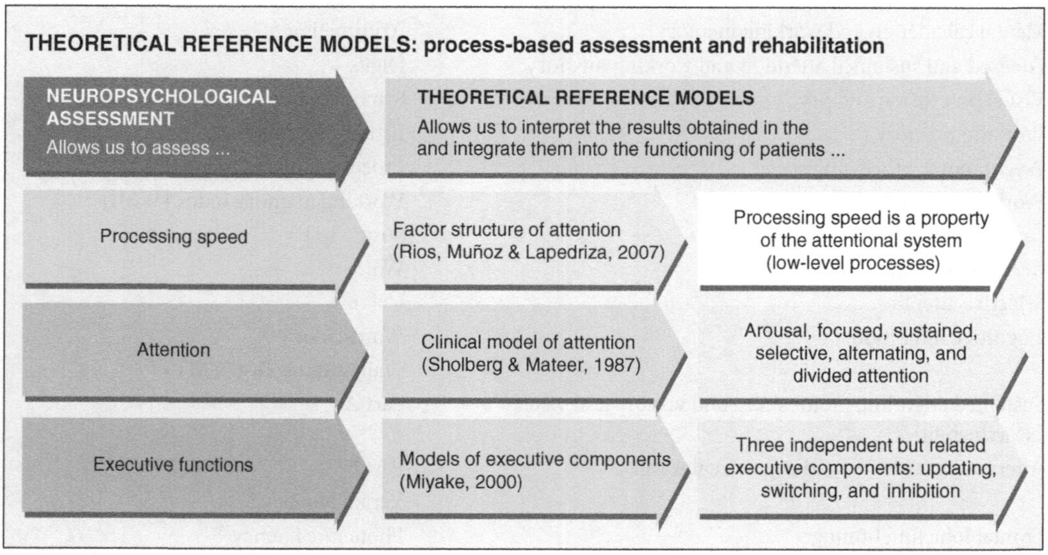

FIGURE 4.1 Structure diagram based on a process analysis.

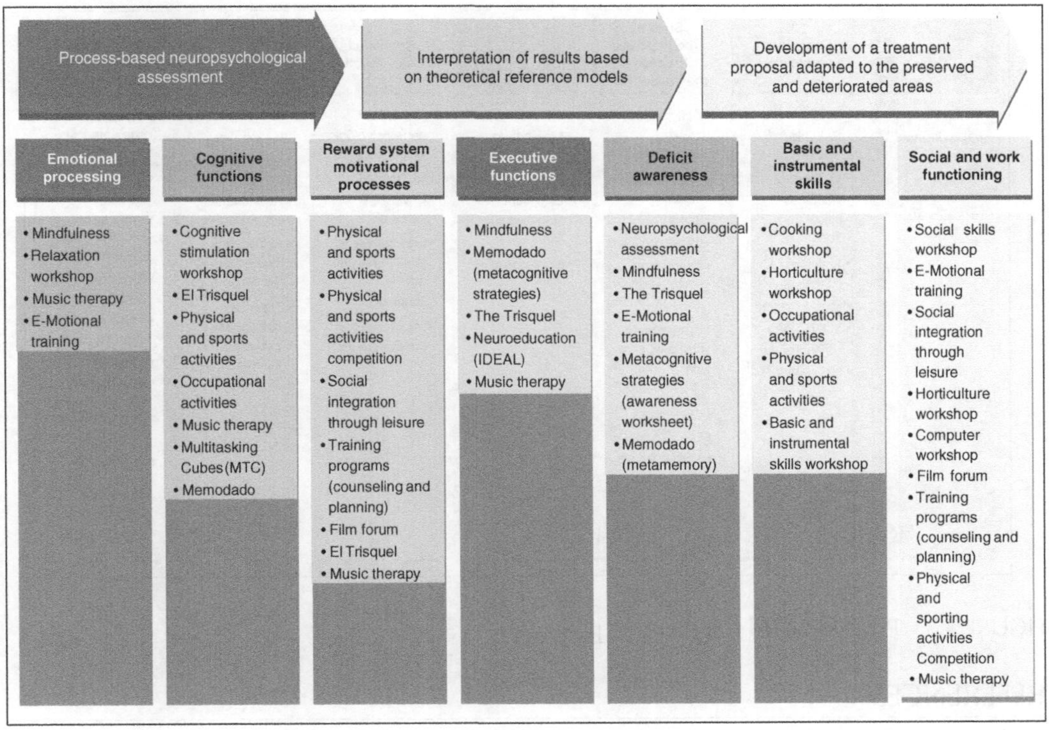

FIGURE 4.2 Domain diagram.

Following this intervention model, each patient is given an intervention plan tailored to their needs and abilities, which can help them become aware of their deficit, adjust their expectations for the future, and progress in their treatment. It provides clinicians with a structure that allows them to organize activities according to the main areas of intervention and to choose and adapt the most appropriate treatment program.

For example, a patient with mild neurocognitive disorder; with deficits in attentional subprocesses and in the executive components of updating (working memory), decision-making, and planning; and with difficulties in social cognition would be included in the following specific activities, which have been shown to be effective in improving cognitive-executive functioning in patients with SRD and/or different comorbid psychiatric disorders (see also Figures 4.2 and 4.3):

- Intervention program in the form of a board game, "El Trisquel"[40]
- Mindfulness-based relapse prevention program for addictive behaviors[41]
- "IDEAL" problem-solving strategy based on the reasoning of Burgues and Robertson
- "*E-Motional* training" program in social cognition, yielding beneficial results in all domains of social cognition.[42]

This day unit model is currently being implemented, and we hope eventually to conduct studies on its effectiveness.

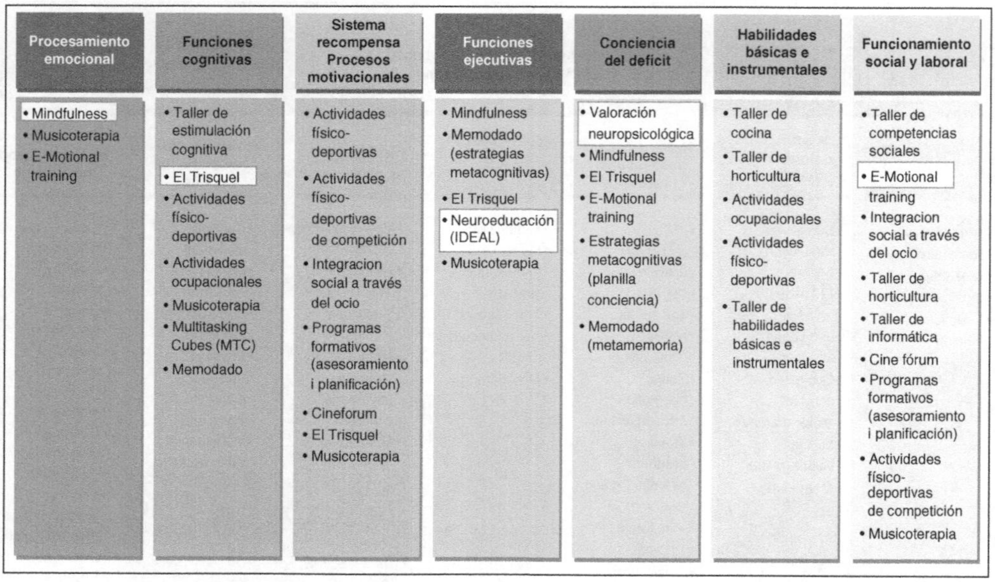

FIGURE 4.3 Process-based intervention proposal.

REFERENCES

1. Consellería de Sanidade C. Catálogo de programas asistenciais. Plan de Galicia sobre Drogas, 2003. Santiago de Compostela: Regional Government of Galicia. Ministry of Health (ENS)-Carlos III Health Institute. Ministry of Science and Innovation.
2. Kalivas PW, Volkow ND. The neural basis of addiction: A pathology of motivation and choice. American Journal of Psychiatry. 2005;162(8):1403–13.
3. Volkow ND, Koob GF McLellan AT. Neurobiological advances from the brain disease model of addiction. New England Journal of Medicine. 2016;374(4):363–71. http://dx.doi.org/10.1056/NEJMra1511480
4. Bickel WK, Moody LN, Eddy CR, Franck CT. Neuro-cognitive dysfunction in addiction: Testing hypotheses of diffuse versus selective phenotypical dysfunction with a classification-based approach. Experimental and Clinical Psychopharmacology. 2017;25(4):322.
5. Verdejo-García, A, García-Fernández G, Dom G. Cognition and addiction. Dialogues in Clinical Neuroscience. 2019;21(3):281–90.
6. Vergara-Moragues E, Acosta Barreto MR, Santiago-Ramajo S, Rivera D, Pardo Pachón JA, González-Saiz F, Arango-Lasprilla JC. Neuropsychological functioning of individuals with coca paste use disorder. Addiction Research & Theory. 2020;29:298–305. https://doi.org/10.1080/16066359.2020.1825692.
7. Fernández-Serrano MJ, Pérez-García M, Verdejo-García A. What are the specific vs. generalized effects of drugs of abuse on neuropsychological performance? Neuroscience and Biobehavioral Reviews. 2011;35(3):377–406.
8. Stevens L, Verdejo-García A, Goudriaan AE, Roeyers, H, Dom G, Vanderplasschen W. Impulsivity as a vulnerability factor for poor addiction treatment outcomes: A review of neurocognitive findings among individuals with substance use disorders. Journal of Substance Abuse Treatment. 2014;47(1):58–72.
9. Loughead J, Wileyto EP, Ruparel K, Falcone M, Hopson R, Gur R, Lerman, C. Working memory-related neural activity predicts future smoking relapse. Neuropsychopharmacology. 2015;40(6):1311–20.

10. Ruiz Sanchez de León JM, Pedrero-Pérez EJ, Rojo-Mota G, Llanero-Luque M, Puerta-García, C. Propuesta de un protocolo para la evaluación neuropsicológica de las adicciones. Revista de neurologia. 2011;53:483–93.
11. Piñón Blanco A, Otero-Lamas F, Vázquez-Justo E, Gui-llén-Gestoso C, Domínguez-González P, Cabrera-Riande J. Programa holístico de rehabilitación neuropsicológica para personas con déficits neuropsicológicos asociados al consumo de drogas (PHRN.DROG). Cádiz: Institute for Interdisciplinary Training (University of Cádiz), 2013. doi: 10.13140/RG.2.1.4936.6162
12. Piñón Blanco A. Juegos terapéuticos: El Trisquel. Adolfo Piñón Blanco (editor) Concello de Vigo (U.A.D CEDRO), 2014. ISBN 84-697-1941-6.
13. Rezapour T, Hatami J, Farhoudian A, Sofuoglu M, Noroozi A Daneshmand R, Samiei A, Ekhtiari, H. NEuro COgnitive REhabilitation for Disease of Addiction (NECOREDA) Program: From development to trial. Basic and Clinical Neuroscience. 2015;6(4):291.
14. Valls-Serrano C, Caracuel A, Verdejo-Garcia A. Goal Management Training and Mindfulness Meditation improve executive functions and transfer to ecological tasks of daily life in polysubstance users enrolled in the therapeutic community treatment. Drug and Alcohol Dependence. 2016;165:9–14. https://doi.org/10.1016/j.drugalcdep.2016.04.040.
15. Verdejo-García A. Cognitive training for substance use disorders: Neuroscientific mechanisms. Neuroscience and Biobehavioral Reviews. 2016;68:270–81.
16. García-Torres A, Vergara-Moragues E, Vergara-Moragues A. GALA Project. Proyecto GALA. Un estudio piloto de evaluación e intervención neuropsicológica en el Hogar GERASA. En; A. Piñón Blanco. Juegos Terapéuticos: El Trisquel. Vigo: Vigo City Council, 2014: 295–312.
17. García-Torres A, Vergara-Moragues E, Piñón Blanco A, Pérez-García M. Alteraciones neuropsicológicas en pacientes con VIH e historia previa de consumo de sustancias. Un estudio preliminar. Latin American Journal of Psychology. 2015;47(3):213–21.
18. Podzamczer PD, Muñoz-Moreno JA, Alcolea RD, Alonso VC, Antela LA, Blanch AJ, *et al.* Consensus statement on the clinical management of human immunodeficiency virus-associated neurocognitive disorders. Infectious Diseases and Clinical Microbiology. 2014;32(1):37–47.
19. Sieira-Valiño J, Iglesias-Fungueiriño M, Sánchez-Pérez M, Vázquez-Justo E, Guillén-Gestoso C, Domínguez-González P, *et al.* Batería neuropsicológica para la rehabilitación cognitiva en drogodependencia. Cádiz: Institute of Interdisciplinary Training (University of Cádiz), 2011. doi: 10.13140/RG.2.1.4750.5042.
20. Piñón Blanco A. Memodado. Cádiz: Institute of Interdisciplinary Training (University of Cádiz), 2010.
21. Verdejo-García A. Goal-based interventions for executive dysfunction in addiction treatment. In: Cognition and Addiction. Academic Press, 2020: 277–82.
22. Deldar Z, Ekhtiari H, Pouretemad HR, Khatibi A. Bias toward drug-related stimuli is affected by loading working memory in abstinent ex-methamphetamine users. Frontiers in Psychiatry. 2019;10:776.
23. León-Carrión J. Rehabilitation models for neurobehavioral disorders after brain injury. Brain Injury Sources. 1998;3:16–53.
24. Fernández-Guinea S. Estrategias a seguir en el diseño de los programas de rehabilitación neuropsicológica para personas con daño cerebral. Journal of Neurology. 2001;33(4):373–7.
25. Piñón A, Lage M, Carrera I, Vázquez M, Cerqueiro X, Bobadilla V, *et al.* Perfil neuropsicológico y sintomatología psicopatológica de pacientes con trastornos relacionaCapítulo 4 Abordaje asistencial del enfermo dual en centros residenciales 35 dos con sustancias a tratamiento en una unidad de día. Health Addictions/Salud y Drogas. 2019;19(1):70–9.
26. Aharonovich E, Nunes E, Hasin D. Cognitive impairment, retention and abstinence among cocaine abusers in cognitive-behavioral treatment. Drug and Alcohol Dependence. 2003;71(2):207–11.

27. Verdejo-García A, Bechara A. A somatic marker theory of addiction. Neuropharmacology. 2009;56:48–62.
28. Tirapu J, Landa N, Lorea I. Cerebro y adicción. Una guía comprensiva. Pamplona: Department of Health (Government of Navarra), 2004.
29. Yücel M, Lubman DI. Neurocognitive and neuroimaging evidence of behavioral dysregulation in human drug addiction: implications for diagnosis, treatment, and prevention. Drug and Alcohol Review. 2007;26(1):33–9.
30. Pace-Schott, E. F, Morgan, P. T, Malison, R. T, Hart, C. L, Edgar, C, Walker, M,Stickgold, R. Cocaine users differ from normals on cognitive tasks which show poorer performance during drug abstinence. The American Journal of Drug and Alcohol Abuse. 2008;34(1): 109–21.
31. Nasreddine ZS, Phillips NA, Bédirian V, Charbonneau, S, Whitehead V, Collin I, Cummings JL, Chertkow H. The Montreal Cognitive Assessment, MoCA: A brief screening tool for mild cognitive impairment. Journal of the American Geriatrics Society. 2005;53(4):695–9.
32. Weschler D. WAIS-III. Wechsler Adult Intelligence Scale. (3rd edition). Administration and Scoring Manual. Madrid: TEA, 2001.
33. Golden CJ. Stroop Manual: Color and Word Test. Madrid: TEA, 2020.
34. Reitan RM, Wolfson D. The Halstead-Reitan Neuropsychological Test Battery: Theory and Clinical Interpretation (2nd edition). Tucson: Neuropsychology Press, 1993.
35. Benton AL, Hamsher KD, Sivan A. Multilingual Aphasia Examination. Iowa City, IA: AJA Associates, 1989.
36. Derogatis LR. SCL-90-R (revised) version 24. Administration, scoring and procedures, manual I. Psychometric research. Baltimore: Johns Hopkins University School of Medicine, 1977.
37. Grace J, Malloy PF. Frontal systems behavior scale: FrSBe. Lutz, FL: Psychological Assessment Resources, 2001.
38. Olivares JM, Berrios GE, Bousoño M. The Self-Assessment Anhedonia Scale (SAAS). Neurology, Psychiatry, and Brain Research. 2005;12(3):121–33.
39. Ríos M, Muñoz JM. Attention and executive control after traumatic brain injury. Madrid: Editorial MAPFRE, DL, 2004.
40. Piñón Blanco A. El trisquel. A game as a cognitive stimulation tool for the treatment of drug addicts. University of Cádiz: Faculty of Labor Sciences, 2009.
41. Bowen S, Chawla N, Marlatt GA. Mindfulness-based relapse prevention in addictive behaviors. Clinical Guide. Bilbao: Desclée de Brouwer, 2011.
42. Vázquez-Campo M, Maroño Y, Lahera G, Mateos R, García-Caballero A. e-Motional Training®: Pilot study on a novel online training program on social cognition for patients with schizophrenia. Schizophrenia Research. Cognition. 2016;4:10–17.

4.3 THE DUAL PATIENT IN THE CONTEXT OF GENERAL HOSPITAL CARE: IN INPATIENT UNITS AND EMERGENCY DEPARTMENTS

T. Rodríguez Barca, J. Bello Porto, I. Fernández Baz, and B. Pérez Gálvez

Dual pathology can be defined as a disease that designates the simultaneous existence of an addictive disorder and another mental disorder or the intersection of the two.

The consequences of the coexistence of a psychiatric disorder and a substance dependence/abuse disorder include a higher number of hospital admissions, more-frequent visits to emergency departments, greater family instability and social marginalization, a higher incidence of violent behavior and suicidal ideation or behavior, and poorer medication compliance and response to treatment.

Drug-dependent patients may present with any type of associated psychiatric disorder, the most common being personality disorders (37–65%), depressive disorders (17–60%), and anxiety disorders (11–28%).[1]

A study conducted in Madrid[2] with patients undergoing treatment in mental health and drug addiction care networks found that 77% of patients with psychosis had a diagnosis of associated substance abuse disorder.

It is well known that patients with dual pathology suffer from greater psychopathological severity, higher relapse rates, poorer adherence to treatment, greater complexity in consumption, higher risk of suicide, and poorer physical health. For all these reasons, it is to be expected that such patients' profiles will have higher rates of hospital admission and readmission.

DUAL PATHOLOGY IN HOSPITAL UNITS

Some studies from the last century[3] indicated that one-third of patients admitted to psychiatric hospitals exhibited dual pathology. Already in this century, and in psychiatric hospitalization units in general hospitals, there are studies that put this prevalence at 17.3%, and lifetime prevalence at 24%.[4–6] The most commonly used substance in hospitalized patients (excluding nicotine) is alcohol, followed by cannabis and cocaine.[5]

It is not uncommon for patients with dual pathology to be admitted to medical specialties other than psychiatry, either because of symptoms directly related to substance use or for other reasons. Therefore, other specialists must have a basic understanding of how to identify and manage the particularities of these patients. Below, we list several factors that should be taken into account in patients during hospitalization:

- It is not uncommon for patients to consume substances during hospitalization, so urine toxicology tests should be performed, especially if the patient receives visitors or goes on outings.[4]
- It is not always possible to make an immediate diagnosis during hospitalization. Identifying the psychiatric condition or its coexistence with substance abuse disorder is sometimes complicated, as the substance mimics the underlying condition, and on other occasions, it is the substance itself that causes symptoms similar to those

produced by different psychiatric illnesses. The latter disappear when consumption is stopped, so it is recommended to allow a window period after cessation of consumption to make a definitive diagnosis.[5]

- Therefore, we must be cautious when assigning "psychiatric labels" to patients admitted to the hospital. When in doubt, it is better to wait and see how the patient progresses and monitor them. We must work with the patient to help them tolerate the uncertainty that the absence of a diagnosis may cause.[7]
- It is also recommended that, while there is doubt as to whether substance use is involved or whether the symptoms are induced by substances, the patient should be kept off antipsychotic medication in order to assess the condition. However, it is common for symptoms of psychomotor agitation, auto- or heteroaggressiveness, severe depression, or suicide risk to appear, preventing us from keeping the patient off treatment.
- It is common for dual patients to be perceived as difficult or confrontational by healthcare professionals because they are frequent users of healthcare services (emergency care, readmissions, etc.), have poor adherence to treatment, are aggressive, etc., especially if they have a comorbid personality disorder.
- Their presence can be perceived negatively by the healthcare team, but some studies report that the more experienced the physician is, the less frequently they consider the patient to be difficult.
- It is common for prescribed medications to fail or not have the expected results in dual pathology patients. This is due to poor therapeutic adherence or the simultaneous use of drugs—as witness the loss of efficacy of antipsychotics when cocaine is used at the same time.
- Another aspect that should be taken into account in these patients is their tendency to continuously demand more medication than prescribed during hospitalization (not exclusively psychotropic drugs). Sometimes, these patients do not openly acknowledge their consumption, or try to hide it, further complicating diagnosis and treatment, but there are a number of clues that should make us suspect substance use:
    - Continuous absences from medical appointments.
    - Frequent conflicts in the family, personal, work, or legal spheres
    - Changes in behavior during different medical visits depending on consumption
    - Failure of prescribed treatments
    - Requests for increased treatment

All admitted patients (regardless of medical specialty) should undergo a thorough medical history review regarding their use of legal and illegal drugs in order to prevent possible withdrawal syndromes, make an accurate diagnosis, and understand why previous treatments have failed.[6]

We must learn to differentiate whether the symptoms presented by a patient are caused by the substance itself, by withdrawal from it, or by a psychiatric illness. Sometimes this differentiation is complicated.

Take benzodiazepine withdrawal, for example: the clinical picture can range from sensory hypersensitivity, nausea, diaphoresis, myoclonus, dysphoria, and anxiety to thought distortions, mistrust, and interpersonal hostility, which can be misinterpreted as the onset of a psychotic episode. Symptoms may persist for weeks or months, appearing and disappearing in waves, which further complicates diagnosis.

Therefore, we must also take into account the presence of prolonged withdrawal syndromes, which can appear weeks or even months after the cessation of substance use, such as alcohol, benzodiazepines, or cocaine, and which can produce symptoms of anxiety, depression, insomnia, and irritability, among others, and which are easily confused with a mood or anxiety disorder.[5,6]

In these situations, it would be advisable to explain to patients that these are temporary symptoms resulting from chronic consumption and not to carry out pharmacological interventions, unless the intensity of the symptoms requires it or the symptoms are prolonged (some authors refer to a duration of more than six weeks).

DUAL PATHOLOGY IN EMERGENCY SERVICES

In the emergency setting, it is necessary to establish an accurate diagnosis as quickly as possible in order to offer the patient the appropriate treatment as quickly as possible, but there are two determining factors we will encounter:

- The characteristics of these patients
- The context of the emergency

The approach to a dual patient in the emergency department is multidisciplinary.

Steps to Follow for the Assessment of a Dual Patient in the Emergency Department

1. There should be appropriate triage upon arrival at the emergency department.
2. If the patient presents with psychomotor agitation (frequent), the priority will be to ensure both their safety and that of others, by means of:
   - Verbal restraint measures: This is always the first measure to be implemented and only if this proves ineffective should the next step be taken.
   - Pharmacological and/or physical restraint measures. It should be remembered that physical/mechanical restraint measures require the application of strict protocols that each center must have approved and that the professionals involved in these clinical situations must be aware of.
3. Medical assessment with a complete medical history, obtaining information from the patient (often not possible), family, and electronic resources regarding previous history

4. A systematic physical examination using equipment, taking vital signs, assessing nutritional status, and performing relevant additional tests:
    - Urinalysis for toxins: essential
    - Blood tests: complete blood count, biochemistry with ions, coagulation, and liver profile
5. After the patient has been stabilized and the symptoms of intoxication and/or withdrawal have been resolved, a comprehensive psychopathological examination to determine the presence of psychopathological decompensation of the underlying psychiatric disorder
6. Determination of the appropriate diagnosis and therapeutic intervention:
    - Discharge from hospital with referral to a specialized drug addiction center in your community and, if at all possible, a brief motivational intervention.
    - Hospital admission to the Psychiatric Hospitalization Unit[6,7]

In addition to these general considerations, let us analyze some clinical situations in greater detail.

Dual Psychosis in Hospital Emergency Rooms

Dual psychosis is one of the most common diagnoses in substance users and, at the same time, one of the most complex in emergency departments.

The rates of substance abuse are significantly higher among psychotic patients than in the general population, including the consequences of such abuse, greater vulnerability to this disorder, earlier onset of symptoms, and poorer clinical and psychosocial outcomes.

One of the main challenges with these patients is distinguishing between psychosis induced by substances and primary psychotic disorder:

- **Substance-induced psychotic disorder**: A transient condition that usually resolves within 24 to 48 hours. If we observe a decrease in the intensity of psychotic symptoms over time, we are likely dealing with an induced condition.
    - The clinical picture observed in the emergency room may vary depending on the type of substance consumed: paranoid ideation, referentiality, various types of sensory phenomena (visual, auditory, tactile), psychotic distress, or manic symptoms.
    - The duration of psychotic symptoms is limited to periods of intoxication or withdrawal, but because withdrawal syndrome for some drugs appears relatively late, the onset of these symptoms may occur up to four weeks after discontinuing the substance.

- **Schizophrenia and addictive disorder**:
  - Cannabis, cocaine, and amphetamines: More abrupt onset of symptoms with more intense positive symptoms, greater motor disturbances, and visits to the emergency department
  - Alcohol: More hostile and threatening behavior; higher risk of suicide; more non-compliance with treatment and physical illnesses

Dual Affective and Anxiety Disorders in Hospital Emergency Departments[6,7]

Patients with mood or anxiety disorders who use substances and attend an emergency department show clinical worsening with more intense symptoms, a higher risk of suicide, and a lower response rate to treatment.

Alcohol produces an immediate decrease in anxiety, encouraging consumption. And that consumption and its withdrawal induce anxiety, reinforcing consumption. Alcohol-dependent individuals with mood or anxiety disorders present more frequent emergency care and a higher risk of parasuicidal behaviors and psychomotor agitation.

Dual Disorders That Include Personality Disorders in Hospital Emergency Departments[6,7]

It is known that substance abuse is often associated with a personality disorder, the most common being antisocial disorder and emotional instability.

The admission of these patients to hospital emergency departments often leads to tense clinical situations with episodes of psychomotor agitation or aggression, which can cause a certain degree of "rejection" on the part of healthcare professionals. It is therefore essential to acquire management strategies that avoid confrontation or criticism.

REFERENCES

1. Pereiro C, Fernández J. Guía de adicciones para especialistas en formación. Valencia: Socidrogalcohol, 2018.
2. Arias F, Szerman N, Vega P, Mesias B, Basurte I, Morant C, *et al.* Estudio Madrid sobre prevalencia y características de los pacientes con patología dual en tratamiento en las redes de salud mental y de atención al drogodependiente. Addictions. 2013;25(1):118–27.
3. Chinchilla A. Manual de Urgencias Psiquiátricas. Elsevier Manson, 2015.
4. Crowley TJ, Chesluk D, Dilts S. Drug and alcohol abuse among psychiatric admissions. A multidrug clinical toxicologic study. Archives of General Psychiatry. 1974;30(1):13–20.
5. Katz G, Durst R, Shufman E, Bar-Hamburger R, Grunhaus L. Substance abuse in hospitalized psychiatric patients. The Israel Medical Association Journal: IMAJ.2008;10(10):672–5.
6. Pascual F, Fernandez J. TUS + TM: concepto, epidemiología, diagnóstico. Marco general de tratamiento. Socidrogalcohol, 2017.
7. Vallejo Ruiloba J. Introducción a la Psicopatología y la Psiquiatría. Dirigido por Juan Vallejo Ruiloba (8ª edición). Barcelona: Elsevier, 2015.

4.4 SPECIFIC DEVICES FOR THE CARE OF DUAL PATIENTS: SPECIFIC DUAL PATHOLOGY UNITS

M. Torrens Melich, A. M. Coratu, R. B. Sauras Quetcuti, D. García Fuentes, C. M. Sousa Franco, I. Vieira Murta, J. Teixeira, G. Mateu Codina, and F. Fonseca Casals

According to the review carried out by the teams from the dual pathology units in Lisbon and in Coimbra, they agree that this model is the ideal one to apply, provided it is located in an area with a sufficient critical mass of population, as is the case of the Dual Pathology Unit of the Institut de Salut Mental del Hospital del Mar in Barcelona, which we will describe below.

DUAL PATHOLOGY UNIT—INAD MODEL

Introduction

The World Health Organization (WHO) defines "dual diagnosis" as "the co-occurrence in the same individual of a substance use disorder (SUD) and another psychiatric disorder."[1] Other terms applied to these patients are "dual pathology," "dual disorders," "concurrent disorder," and "comorbid disorder." In recent years, there has been a considerable increase in concern about the detection and treatment of other simultaneous psychiatric disorders in individuals with drug abuse/dependence, also known as dual pathology. These "dual patients" or "dual-diagnosis patients" constitute a high-risk group both from a health perspective (more severe clinical pictures, higher number of hospital admissions, greater use of general emergency services, and higher risk of infections such as HIV and HCV) and from a social standpoint (more violent behavior, greater marginalization, and more illegal behavior) if the two pathologies are not diagnosed and treated correctly and jointly.[2,3]

However, one of the main problems these patients present is the difficulty in evaluating and establishing a diagnosis and designing an appropriate treatment plan that addresses the dual pathology as a whole. Patients with dual pathology pose a therapeutic challenge not only as individuals but also as a group of patients, who often do not fit into standard treatment policies.[4,5]

Background

In Spain, as in most EU countries, there are three healthcare networks: the General Health Network, the Mental Health Network, and the Addiction Care Network.[2]

- The **General Health Network** involves general outpatient primary care (e.g., basic health areas), regional hospitals, and university or tertiary hospitals that house more-specialized and subspecialized units and services.
- The **Mental Health Network** is a specialized network that was created later, following the restructuring of mental health care from the former psychiatric institutions to a network with resources for outpatients (mental health centers), hospitals (units for

psychiatric patients), and medium- to long-term care facilities (residential psychiatric centers, day centers, etc.).

- The **Addiction Care Network** is the most recent network, developed since the mid-1980s in response to the heroin epidemic. Since then, this network has been consolidated and, although with

There are differences depending on the autonomous community, but in general it consists of primary addiction care centers, hospital units (detoxification units), and medium-stay centers (therapeutic communities, day centers, etc.).

INSTITUTE OF NEUROPSYCHIATRY AND ADDICTIONS OF THE PARC DE SALUT MAR

The Institute of Neuropsychiatry and Addictions (INAD), within Parc de Salut MAR (PS-MAR) treats mental health and addiction problems in an urban area of around 800,000 people, some 500,000 of whom live in the coastal area of the city of Barcelona and the rest in the Barcelonès Nord area.

In both areas, there are various specialized mental health and addiction care facilities, both outpatient and inpatient. In mental health, there are adult mental health centers and child and adolescent mental health centers, as well as inpatient units for acute patients, located in a general university hospital and a specialized hospital. In addiction, there are treatment centers and hospital detoxification units, located in a general university hospital.

In 2007, the first Dual Pathology Unit (DPU) with 11 beds was created for the Litoral area, and in 2010, the second Dual Pathology Unit with 13 beds was created for the Barcelonès Nord area. These two units respond to the needs of patients with acute decompensated dual pathology who, due to their clinical characteristics, require intensive treatment on a 24-hour hospitalization basis.

DUAL PATHOLOGY UNIT-PSMAR

The main characteristics of these Dual Pathology-PSMAR units are described below.

Mission

The mission of the DPU-INAD focuses on:

- Developing a multidisciplinary team specializing in dual pathology that enables complex diagnostic assessment, as well as multimodal treatment with pharmacological, psychological, family, and social interventions
- Advising professionals from different mental health and addiction care facilities on diagnostic problems or difficulties in treating patients with mental disorders and substance abuse
- Participating in the training and teaching of dual pathology to future mental health specialists (internal medicine residents, psychology residents, and nursing residents)

- Encouraging, promoting, and developing high-quality research activities in the field of dual pathology
- Participating in the dissemination of knowledge in specific areas of expertise

Objectives

The main objective of the DPU-INAD is to offer specific and integrated treatment for dual pathology, with an emphasis on diagnosis and therapeutic approach.

Therapeutic Program

DPU-PSMARs are differential care units within the detoxification unit and the acute unit of conventional general psychiatry, and their objective is to offer a comprehensive, highly specialized approach, particularly in diagnosis and joint therapeutic treatment. Table 4.3 describes the main differential characteristics between the Hospital Detoxification Unit (HDU), the Dual Pathology Unit (DPU), and the Acute Psychiatric Hospitalization Unit (APHU).

TABLE 4.3 Differences Between DPU-PSMAR Units: HDU, DPU, and APHU

	HDU	DPU	APHU
Admission characteristics	Scheduled. Voluntary. Partial environmental isolation (no visits or permits, but calls and cell phones allowed).	Urgent/Scheduled. Voluntary/Involuntary. Partial environmental isolation (no visits or leave, but phone calls and cell phones are allowed).	Urgent/Scheduled. Voluntary/Involuntary. Environmental isolation only if necessary.
Purpose of admission	Diagnosis and treatment of severe SUD that cannot be treated on an outpatient basis. Preliminary step to relapse prevention (e.g., therapeutic community, day hospital) or rehabilitation.	Joint diagnosis and treatment of SUD and non-SUD (dual pathology).	Diagnosis and treatment of non-SUD psychiatric disorders.
Intervention	• Detoxification. • Relapse prevention. • Psychoeducation. • Study and treatment of medical comorbidity. • Study and treatment of non-decompensated psychopathological comorbidity. • Social intervention (if necessary).	• Detoxification. • Relapse prevention. • Psychoeducation. • Study and treatment of decompensated psychopathological comorbidity. • Social intervention (if necessary). • Occupational therapy.	• Study and treatment of uncompensated psychopathological comorbidity. • Psychoeducation. • Social intervention (if necessary).
Referrals	Mainly addiction network services.	Addiction network and mental health network services.	Mainly mental health network services.

SUD: Substance Use Disorder. HDU: Hospital Detoxification Unit. APHU: Acute Psychiatric Hospitalization Unit. DPU: Dual Pathology Unit.

Admission Requirements

Admission Indications and Admission Process

The indications for admission to the DPU-PS-MAR are the simultaneous presence of a disorder due to psychoactive substance use and a severe mental disorder which, due to its clinical characteristics or the presence of severe behavioral disturbances, requires integrated treatment on an inpatient basis.

Inclusion Criteria

- Be of legal age.
- Presence of a severe psychopathological disorder requiring hospitalization due to acute decompensation and a substance use disorder.

Exclusion Criteria

- Acute decompensation or severity of comorbid organic pathology that makes admission to a general hospital ward more appropriate (e.g., Infectious Diseases, Gastroenterology, etc.)
- Presence of a substance use disorder, without any other psychiatric pathology (either axis I or axis II) requiring immediate hospitalization in a unit
- Cognitive disorders in patients with substance abuse in the absence of psychopathological decompensation requiring psychiatric admission

In order to take on patients with more severe psychopathology and at greater risk of social exclusion, admissions are prioritized through the psychiatric emergency service.

Intervention

Given the severity of the patients' condition and the difficulties involved in evaluating them on an outpatient basis, one of the most distinctive features of the DPU-INAD program is that it focuses on the diagnosis of dual pathology. In this regard, psychodiagnostics are performed through interviews specially designed for the diagnosis of psychiatric comorbidity in drug-using patients, in which the therapeutic team is specially trained and is a teaching reference in Spanish, personality diagnosis, and neuropsychological evaluation. In addition, a study of the patient's physical condition is carried out, with special emphasis on infectious diseases (HIV infection, HCV, etc.). An assessment of social needs is also carried out in order to establish a comprehensive and multidimensional diagnosis that facilitates the design of a comprehensive therapeutic plan.

The treatment offered is also comprehensive (for both pathologies at once) and multiple, having pharmacological, psychological, and social approaches.

Human Resources

To carry out the program, a multidisciplinary therapeutic team is available, made up of professionals in psychiatry, psychology, internal medicine, social work, occupational therapy, social education, and nursing.

Referral and Discharge

Once the condition that led to admission has been stabilized, patients are referred to different care resources (outpatient or for longer stays) within the mental health network, the addiction network, and the social services network in the region.

CONCLUSIONS

Dual Pathology Units-PSMAR have proven effective in the acute treatment of patients with uncompensated dual diagnosis, avoiding the "wrong door" phenomenon and facilitating a comprehensive approach to patient care.

This chapter has been partially funded by the Carlos III Institute (ISCIII)-FIS-FEDER Primary Care Addiction Research Network (RIAPAD-RICORS), grant no. RD21/0009/0001.

REFERENCES

1. World Health Organization (2010). Lexicon of alcohol and drug terms published by the World Health Organization.
2. Torrens M, Mestre-Pintó JJ, Domingo-Salvany A. Comorbidity of Substance Use and Mental Disorders in Europe. Luxembourg: Publications Office of the European Union, 2015.
3. Volkow ND, Torrens M, Poznyak V, Sáenz E, Busse A, Kashino W, *et al.* Managing dual disorders: A statement by the Informal Scientific Network, UN Commission on Narcotic Drugs. World Psychiatry. 2020;19(3):396–7.
4. Torrens M, Martin-Santos R, Samet S. Importance of clinical diagnoses for comorbidity studies in substance use disorders. Neurotox Res. 2006;10(3–4):253–61.
5. Torrens M, Rossi PC, Martinez-Riera R, Martinez-Sanvi-sens D, Bulbena A. Psychiatric co-morbidity: treatment in complementary systems or in one system? Substance Use and Misuse. 2012;47(8–9):1005–14.

CHAPTER 5

Pharmacological Treatment

Criteria for Quality Prescribing in the Treatment of Dual Pathology Patients

S. J. Ferreira da Silva Alexandre, C. Gama Elías, B. Salazar Laya, M. A. Celdrán Hernández, and E. Echarri Arrieta

QUALITY PRESCRIPTION IN PATIENTS WITH DUAL PATHOLOGY

Definition

The WHO defines prescription quality in terms of the rational use of medicines.[1] That is, when patients receive:

- Medication appropriate to their clinical needs
- In doses corresponding to their individual requirements
- For an appropriate period of time and
- At the lowest possible cost to the patient and the community

It is well known that prescribing medication is a complex act, influenced by multiple factors. We can say that the concept of a quality prescription must be developed, making the best use of the medication, but we must also take into account other aspects, such as diagnosis, suitability for the corresponding therapeutic indication, and the patients' perspective, since today they have more information and come with more demanding health requirements; consequently, greater rigor is needed when prescribing.

Quality prescribing is a process that includes:

- Appropriate prescribing of medications (effectiveness)
- Availability of effective, safe, and quality-proven medications
- Optimal cost-benefit ratio
- Proper conditions for preservation, storage, dispensing, and administration
- Agreement with the patient

DOI: 10.4324/9781003786153-5

Taking this starting point into account, can we guarantee that it will be met in patients with dual pathology (DP)?

Effectiveness

The first premise refers to the effectiveness[2] of medications, i.e., that the prescription is appropriate for the clinical needs of patients.

It is important to start with the difference between effectiveness and efficacy. When we talk about efficacy, we are talking about the response to a drug, demonstrated through high-quality clinical trials—studies whose methodology includes at least the following characteristics:

- Defined objective
- Comparator
- Tools for measuring response
- Clinically and statistically significant results

It is a complicated process that can take years, but it is a necessary process for marketing and authorizing a drug.

Information on efficacy obtained from clinical trials (CTs) is expanded over time with the results of effectiveness studies, which are the results of the use of a drug (efficacy) in routine clinical practice.

This information comes from independent studies in clinical practice. This is what we call *evidence-based medicine.* If we extrapolate these definitions to the field of mental health (MH) and, more specifically, to DP, when talking about appropriate and effective prescribing as a quality term,[3] we encounter an additional problem: most of the drugs used in clinical practice are *off-label*, i.e., they are used for purposes other than those indicated in the summary of product characteristics. This is due, among many other reasons, to the fact that the diagnosis of DP is not codified as such by the main disease classification entities.[4,43]

When using off-label drugs,[5] we generally encounter two common scenarios:

- They are used within a safety framework, supported by scientific evidence, i.e., there are studies on the therapeutic effect of a drug for an indication for which it is not approved.
- They are used within a framework with less scientific support.

In both cases, off-label use must always be based on the clinician's experience and on the consensus among the various clinical guidelines and expert committees.

In the specific case of DP, we more frequently encounter this second situation.[6] There are few studies with good evidence, which makes it particularly important that prescriptions be agreed upon and assessed on an individual basis, depending on the clinical case.

In DP, there is an absolute need for clinical practice guidelines (CPGs) and treatment consensus in patients with DP. These guidelines should include drugs, off-label indications, doses, and duration.[7]

Availability of Effective, Safe, and Quality-Proven Medications—Off-Label Use

Off-label use should be exceptional and limited to situations in which there are no authorized therapeutic alternatives. However, off-label use has become increasingly common in recent years.

Why? It is a common and generally uncontrolled practice,[8] which includes not only prescribing outside the indication for which its use has been authorized, but also prescribing outside the authorized doses or duration not recommended by regulatory agencies (in the EU, the European Medicines Agency [EMA])[9]

The origin of off-label use lies in the fact that there is clinical data supporting a particular therapeutic use for an already authorized drug, but this data is not included in the drug's summary of product characteristics.

Three circumstances in which uses outside the summary of product characteristics are particularly relevant:

1. Therapeutic areas in which research activity is very intense and the pace of scientific knowledge may precede the procedures necessary to incorporate these changes into the drug's summary of product characteristics.
2. Lack of commercial interest in conducting the studies necessary to obtain authorization from agencies, especially when the patent expires and generics appear. A widespread example is the use of quetiapine for behavioral disorders in patients with dementia.
3. Lack of agreement between agencies. The indications approved in the EMA summary of product characteristics do not necessarily coincide with those approved by the FDA (U.S. Food and Drug Administration). Often, a clinical trial conducted in the US cannot be extrapolated to Europe and vice versa in order to obtain authorization for an indication (e.g., asenapine is authorized in the European Union only for the treatment of bipolar disorder, while the FDA also authorizes it for schizophrenia).

In psychiatry, the lack of indications for many diagnoses makes this a necessary practice.[10]

Reasons for off-label prescribing:

- Diagnoses without indication (personality disorders, dual pathology, mental retardation, addictions, eating disorders, etc.)
- Age range
- At-risk population not being included in clinical trials

- Lack of response to treatments indicated in the package insert, dosage, and duration
- Association/potentiation or minimization of adverse effects

In general, off-label use is estimated at around 20%; however, in specialties such as oncology,[11] they rise to 50–75%, and if we focus on psychiatry, this percentage rises to 23.3% for antidepressants, 60.7% for neuroleptics, and 50.2% for mood stabilizers. Of these, about 80% of off-label uses have little scientific evidence. And if we focus on DP, off-label use is the norm: lack of EC and the concept of DP as an unrecognized diagnosis.

Safety and Cost-Benefit

Off-label prescribing seeks a beneficial therapeutic effect, but it has many drawbacks, such as the risk of undocumented side effects and toxicity[12] and increased pharmaceutical spending.

Furthermore, it should be noted that, on occasion, the lack of scientific evidence to support such prescriptions puts extra responsibility on the prescribing physician. In addition, these prescriptions, being off-label, generate doubt and confusion among professionals and patients alike, given the difficulty of coordination between the different healthcare network providers.

Off-label uses can be considered a prescription with a possible risk for patients:

- If patients are outside the age range or have not been included in clinical trials, we have no evidence or safety data.
- If doses usually exceed those authorized and tested in pivotal studies, the risk of adverse effects increases.
- Potentiation and/or association may occur in the management of adverse effects (therapeutic cascade):
  - Increased potential risk of toxicity
  - Increased interactions
  - Increased costs

In other specialties such as oncology, where off-label use is very common (50–75%), it is standard practice to request written authorization, with bibliography based on scientific evidence.

Why Is This Done in Oncology but Not in DP?

Among the most plausible explanations are: the extremely high cost of cancer treatments, the rapid pace of therapeutic advances with dozens of new molecules each year, the hospital use of drugs, the safety profile, etc.

There are certain situations in which it is advisable for regulatory agencies to issue a recommendation based on the available evidence regarding efficacy and safety. However, most off-label uses occur within clinical practice, so case-by-case authorization is not required.

It is therefore left to the centers to propose therapeutic care protocols.[13] These protocols, approved by the center and based on CPGs, can include clear recommendations on when to issue an off-label prescription with scientific evidence, which supports and streamlines care within the regulatory framework.

Patients' Perspective

We must bear in mind that in today's society, a change in the doctor–patient relationship is taking hold,[14] largely due to a change in the latter. Today, patients are better educated, more aware, and more sensitive to disease and medication use. Health has become a demand. This means that when prescribing, we must do so more rigorously, taking into account the needs of patients, but also involving them in decision-making. Following the Good Clinical Practice Guidelines (ICH [International Conference on Harmonization] Tripartite Harmonized Guideline),[15] the physician must adequately justify the need for the use of the medication in the medical record; inform the patient of the possible benefits and risks and obtain their consent, on the basis of that patient's right to decide freely after receiving adequate information about the available clinical options.[16]

Where Are We Headed?

Considering the situation we are starting from—the common practice of off-label use, the speed with which scientific information is disseminated, and the lack of clinical trials to obtain new conditions of use authorized by drug agencies—there has been controversy for years over the lack of a significant connection between the nomenclature of psychotropic drugs and their use.[17]

In 2018, the European College of Neuropsychopharmacology (ECNP) decided to publish an annual classification of psychotropic drugs according to their mechanism of action and pharmacology (*Neuroscience-based Nomenclature* [NbN]).[18] This publication (which is also available as an app for electronic devices) is updated every year, with the aim of helping clinicians apply treatments in their day-to-day work.

The main objectives of this publication are:

- To move from a disease-based classification (antidepressants, antipsychotics, anxiolytics) to a classification based on pharmacology.
- To open the door to contemporary knowledge in neuroscience and incorporate recent findings in central nervous system research into the classification of drugs used to treat psychiatric disorders.
- To replace an outdated (sixty-year-old) nomenclature of psychotropic drugs with a contemporary nomenclature based on neuroscience.
- Provide an educational tool that reflects the breadth of available psychotropic drugs.

In summary, when we talk about prescription quality, we are referring to prescriptions that are appropriate for patients' clinical needs, a concept that encompasses effectiveness, safety, cost-benefit, and patient perception. However, when we refer to patients with DP, we encounter the barrier of indications authorized by regulatory agencies for the use of drugs. Off-label uses are the norm in DP, but we should see this as an area for improvement, and not as an insurmountable problem.

Given that legislation recognizes this situation, we must view these off-label uses as part of innovation in clinical practice and, in many cases, the only possible treatment for certain conditions. We must identify these situations as starting points for future research and incorporate the indications supported by studies into CPGs and treatment protocols, without waiting for authorization from the relevant agencies, which is unlikely to be granted due to a lack of commercial interest in conducting clinical trials for the approval of new indications.

Last but not least, we must not forget to always inform patients and obtain their consent, especially in these times when patient empowerment is more prevalent than ever.

CONTEXT

The difficulty of intervening in dual pathology is related to the lack of knowledge about its prevalence, the complexity of its diagnosis, and the scarcity of clinical data, which is directly related to the complexity of the users. They demonstrate greater psychopathological severity than non-comorbid patients, higher rates of risky behavior, more psychosocial problems, and, sometimes, criminal behavior.[19]

Acute or chronic substance use can induce symptoms that mimic mental illness, making it difficult to differentiate between mental illness and symptoms of intoxication and/or withdrawal. On the other hand, mental illness can have a negative impact on addiction. These interactions make diagnosis and decision-making about the best available treatment difficult. The type of addiction (heroin, cocaine, cannabis, amphetamines, tobacco, alcohol, and gambling, among others) must be taken into account, on the one hand, and the type of mental illness (anxiety, depression, personality changes, schizophrenia and bipolar disorder, attention deficit hyperactivity disorder, personality changes, and eating disorders, among others), on the other.

There are multiple combinations between mental illness and addiction, and the fact that the patient might also have multiple addictions considerably complicates the interpretation of the case and its diagnosis. Unfortunately, there are no biomarkers, as there are for other non-psychiatric diseases (e.g., blood sugar in diabetes and blood pressure in hypertension) to support the diagnosis.[19,20]

In patients, comorbidity manifests itself in terms of clinical severity, psychosocial dysfunction, and poorer quality of life, and only a good response to their needs will have a positive impact and, consequently, reduce harm.

From the point of view of the available evidence, mental illness and addiction should be addressed simultaneously and in an integrated manner (not fragmented across different services) by an interdisciplinary team, including pharmacological and non-pharmacological therapies (motivational, behavioral, cognitive, and contingency management).[20–22] Both interventions demonstrate efficacy and synergy when applied simultaneously rather than in isolation. Professionals in integrated teams are better adapted to the needs of users, have more experience in managing situations, and are able to provide more organized and structured support.[21]

Furthermore, we must not forget that there exist populations with special needs, such as homeless people, prisoners, active users who do not seek help, and adolescents.[19–21]

On the other hand, psychiatric disorders in children and adolescents appear to be associated with higher levels of substance addiction throughout life compared to young people without such disorders.[23] Adolescence is a developmental period that predisposes individuals to experiment with new social activities outside the family and school environment, which allow for the consolidation of identity and the transition to adulthood. This period is also highly vulnerable to the onset of first episodes of mental illness. It is not always easy to distinguish which of the two types of disorders arises first, whether they develop independently or influence each other. However, at these ages, symptoms of mental illness are more frequently described before the onset of substance use.[24] Some studies report that comorbid patients will have less adherence to pharmacological and non-pharmacological treatments, will more easily abandon intervention programs, and will more readily accept healthcare support after hospitalization, compared to patients with psychiatric pathology alone or addiction alone. These users are characterized by more relapses, worse clinical evolution and response, and greater use of health resources, such as emergency room visits, agencies and other services.[25]

The pharmacological monitoring of these users should be more comprehensive and the therapeutic objectives to be achieved should be well structured, involving the following:[26]

- Establishing and maintaining a therapeutic relationship
- Encouraging adherence to therapy
- Achieving stabilization of mental illness
- Reducing consumption and maintaining abstinence.
- Working with the user to raise awareness about the illness
- Preventing relapses
- Informing and educating the user, family members, and/or caregivers about comorbidity and alternative therapies
- Rehabilitating psychosocial life in the community

However, some limitations have been identified that may render the clinical results of pharmacological intervention unfeasible. These include the lack of effectiveness of therapeutic regimens associated with the difficulty of diagnosis, their high complexity, the use of potentially addictive drugs (benzodiazepines), the route of administration and the number of daily administrations, side effects, and drug interactions.[25]

When prescribing, special attention should be paid to the efficacy, interactions, and side effects of medications, as these are fundamental for adherence and for users with a history of or mental illness, who, if known, may be more likely to self-medicate.[27]

The consequences of non-adherence to pharmacological and non-pharmacological interventions will predict the worsening of comorbidities and psychopathological symptoms, with a significant impact on social and family relationships and quality of life.[25]

Psychiatric disorders associated with addiction have different prevalences depending on the combinations that can be made between mental illness and addiction or multiple addictions. Although complex, the best diagnosis must be obtained in order to implement personalized, effective, and safe treatment for each user. There are not many published studies that have a maximum level of evidence and consensus on therapeutic regimens; however, as already mentioned, a quality prescription can be made, in the treatment of psychiatric illnesses and/or addictions.

PSYCHIATRIC DISORDERS OF MAJOR RELEVANCE IN THE APPROACH OF THE DUAL PATHOLOGY PATIENT

Schizophrenia

Schizophrenia is a serious psychiatric disorder that affects approximately 1% of the world's population.[28] Patients with this disorder are highly vulnerable to substance addiction, which is estimated to be present in 40–70% of them, a percentage considerably higher than that of the general population.[29] The most common addictions identified in several studies are tobacco, with a prevalence of 70–80%, alcohol (21–86%), cannabis (17–83%), and more recently cocaine (15–50%).[29] Some studies suggest that cannabis during adolescence is associated with an increased risk of developing psychosis in the future, with estimates that these users may develop schizophrenia within 2 to 5 years.[30]

The instability, disorganization, and lack of knowledge about the disease on the part of the patient will be reflected in a lack of adherence to therapy and, consequently, in higher relapse rates and greater use of health services. The approach to schizophrenic patients with addiction should include psychosocial and pharmacological therapy accompanied by a multidisciplinary comprehensive care team.

Atypical antipsychotics are preferred in the treatment of schizophrenia because they have fewer extrapyramidal effects, reduce compulsive behaviors, and have a better withdrawal profile.[10,20] The choice of medication should take into account the patient's preferences, possible side effects, the type of formulation, and interactions with other drugs and substances of abuse.[27,31,32]

As for tobacco, both nicotine patches and bupropion have good results in smoking cessation and abstinence without aggravating psychotic episodes. Varenicline, on the other hand, although it can be used, appears to aggravate psychiatric symptoms.[29] In the treatment of alcoholism, naltrexone, disulfiram, acamprosate, or desipramine can be used, the latter drug not being marketed in Spain.[29]

Bipolar Disorder

Bipolar disorder often occurs alongside other psychiatric conditions, such as anxiety, personality disorders, obsessive-compulsive disorders, and addictions.[33] It is estimated that 42% of these patients abuse alcohol and 20% abuse cannabis, followed by other illicit substances. The smoking rate in this population is very high, around 68%.[34] Patients in the manic phase are 14 times more likely to develop an addiction to a substance of abuse and 6 times more likely to develop an addiction to alcohol.[33] In both the manic and depressive phases, patterns of substance abuse are repeated, masking symptoms and making diagnosis difficult.[6,20]

Substance abuse, in addition to aggravating the normal course of the disease, has a negative impact on treatment adherence, reducing its effectiveness and requiring higher doses. Comorbidity is associated with an increase in episodes and hospitalizations.[34] The treatment of comorbid bipolar disorder should include a pharmacological component (mood stabilizers and/or anticonvulsants, antipsychotics, and specific therapy for addictions) and a psychosocial component (to prevent/treat episodes of mania and depression, minimize adverse effects, and recognize trigger factors).[35]

Lithium is the most widely used mood stabilizer, with positive effects in preventing or reducing manic episodes and treating depression.[35,36] In the absence of a clinical response, other mood stabilizers, such as anticonvulsants, can be added to the treatment, which will play an important role in reducing and decreasing the severity of depressive episodes.[35,36] The most commonly used are valproate, lamotrigine, carbamazepine, and topiramate. To minimize episodes of delirium, erratic mood, and severe behavioral disorders, which are more characteristic of the manic phase, some antipsychotics, such as quetiapine, risperidone, aripiprazole, and olanzapine, are used with good results.[35,36] Quetiapine can even be used during very prolonged periods of depression.[35]

Addiction treatment is very important in the context of bipolar disorder, but it is often only possible after mood stabilization.[34] Some anticonvulsants, such as valproate and carbamazepine, appear to be useful in both bipolar disorder and reducing alcohol abuse, as well as in alcohol and cocaine abuse in patients without psychiatric illness.[33] Valproate and quetiapine are also an option in cases of comorbidity of alcohol abuse and bipolar disorder. Acamprosate and naltrexone are another option for treating alcohol abuse.[33,34]

Depression

Depression and anxiety are the two most commonly diagnosed psychiatric problems in people seeking help for addiction problems.[37]

Worldwide, the prevalence of major depression is twice as high in women and manifests early during adolescence.[38,39] For cultural, social, biological, and behavioral reasons, women tend to experience feelings of sadness, worthlessness, and guilt, while men are more likely to report fatigue, irritability, insomnia, and loss of interest in activities previously associated with pleasure.[38,39]

Major depression is often associated with other conditions, such as anxiety, post-traumatic stress, substance addiction, and pain,[38] and studies have described the association of major depression with alcohol abuse (in 24% of men) and with opioids and nicotine (in 49% of women).[27,29,40,41]

Comorbidity is associated with poorer health outcomes, greater illicit substance use, more severe courses of illness, higher rates of suicide, and fatal overdoses.[42]

The treatment of this comorbidity involves psychosocial and pharmacotherapeutic intervention for depression and addiction. Antidepressants should be chosen individually, taking into account tolerability, possible interactions, and comorbidities. It has been observed that some antidepressants, such as imipramine,[13] desipramine (not marketed in Spain or Portugal), work well in the treatment of depression when alcohol abuse is present, but have little impact on maintaining abstinence, suggesting the need for effective intervention in substance abuse.[20] Methadone or buprenorphine can be used for opioid dependence, and naltrexone and acamprosate for alcohol abuse.[27]

Personality Disorders

A personality disorder (PD) is a persistent pattern of internal experience and behavior that deviates dramatically from the expectations of the individual's culture. It is a diffuse and inflexible pattern that begins in adolescence or early adulthood, is stable over time, and causes distress or impairment. The DSM-5 describes ten types of PD: paranoid, schizoid, schizotypal, antisocial, borderline, histrionic, narcissistic, avoidant, dependent, and obsessive-compulsive.[43]

Comorbidity between PD and dependencies is common.[44–46] The prevalence of PD is estimated to vary between 10 and 15% in the general population and between 50 and 70% in patients treated for addiction.[44–48]

Borderline and antisocial PDs are the PDs most commonly associated with addictions.[44–51]

Dependencies and PDs are pathologies characterized by their long duration, and over time, their association worsens the prognosis of both: PDs have a negative impact on the evolution of dependencies, with more severe cases and a more unfavorable prognosis.[44,45] Dependencies seem to negatively affect the evolution and functioning of patients with PDs.[47]

The treatment of addiction does not lead to remission of PD, which in itself has little impact on the course of PD. It is therefore also necessary to focus on the treatment of PD, incorporating it into the treatment of substance use.[44,52] The exclusive treatment of substance use disorder does not contribute to therapeutic success in addressing the dual diagnosis, as substance abuse is likely to be promoted and exacerbated by the symptoms of PD.[44,52]

Although psychotherapy is the most common treatment for personality disorders, with a greater evidence base for dialectical behavioral therapy, pharmacotherapy is mainly indicated for symptom management, acute crises, or the treatment of other concomitant conditions, such as anxiety, psychosis, and depression. In these cases, antipsychotics, antidepressants, and anticonvulsants or mood stabilizers are used; the latter can also reduce withdrawal symptoms.[44,52,53]

Attention Deficit Hyperactivity Disorder (ADHD)

Patients with ADHD are associated with an increased risk of developing a substance use disorder (SUD), regardless of age, gender, ethnicity, and setting (outpatient/inpatient).[54–59]

The risk also appears to be independent of the diagnostic procedure, the primary substance of abuse,[59] including addiction to gaming (video games) and the Internet.[57]

However, in the scientific literature, prevalence values vary with the substance(s) of abuse, age, the diagnostic instrument used, and the timing of the ADHD diagnosis, and are easily skewed because withdrawal and abstinence symptoms (during the detoxification phase) can easily distort the picture.[56]

ADHD comorbid with SUD has a negative effect on the course of addiction:

- Patients become addicted earlier, consume more substances, and are hospitalized more frequently than patients without ADHD.[56,57] ADHD is also associated with higher rates of relapse after successful treatment for addiction.[56]
- There seems to be consensus that nearly one in four patients with SUD also meets the criteria for ADHD diagnosis.
- For this reason, it is important to implement appropriate screening procedures in clinical practice to identify these dual-diagnosis patients as early as possible.[56,57,59]
    - SUD predicts poorer treatment outcomes for ADHD, and early detection plays a crucial role in the prevention and treatment of both disorders in psychiatric and addiction settings.[54,57]

The therapeutic approach should consider a combination of psychotherapy and pharmacotherapy.[69–71]

The severity of addiction is an important factor to consider, as it may be necessary to stabilize the addictive aspect of the dual diagnosis before beginning to treat ADHD, but there is general consensus on the advisability of requiring abstinence before initiating pharmacotherapy for ADHD.[61]

Stimulant treatment is the pharmacological treatment of choice.[54,58–60] Even in adolescents with coexisting ADHD and SUD, pharmacological treatment of ADHD is recommended, especially with psychostimulants.[54]

There is concern about the potential for abuse in treatment, mitigated by the emergence of long-acting formulations, particularly oral osmotic release system formulations of methylphenidate (OROS-MPH) and lisdexamfetamine, with significantly lower rates of misuse and diversion than immediate-release preparations.[54,58–60] Treatment requires careful titration and monitoring of clinical effectiveness and adverse effects. Higher doses of psychostimulants may be needed in patients with concurrent ADHD + SUD than in those without SUD to achieve a favorable effect.[54,55,58]

Studies in patients with ADHD + SUD have provided some evidence on the effectiveness of methylphenidate, lisdexamfetamine in the short and long term and, to a lesser extent, bupropion, pemoline (not marketed in Spain or Portugal) and atomoxetine, but all show that these drugs are only moderately effective, especially in reducing substance use, and are associated with a higher frequency of adverse effects that cause treatment discontinuation. Pharmacological treatment appears to have more positive effects when combined with psychotherapy.[54,59]

Anxiety Disorders

Anxiety disorders (particularly panic and post-traumatic stress) are often associated with substance use, with an estimated prevalence of anxiety in the order of 35%.[6,20] Panic and post-traumatic stress are the most common types of anxiety in patients with addictions, with a prevalence of 1% to 10% and 30%, respectively.

Cannabis users, from an early age, often present symptoms of anxiety, which is a risk factor.[62]

The prevalence of anxiety among opioid users is estimated to be between 26% and 35%.[20]

Psychotherapy and pharmacotherapy are the most commonly used methods to address this highly prevalent comorbidity, although their combination or the use of one to the detriment of the other is not evident: intervention can begin with the problem for which the patient shows greater availability, and if the expected results are not achieved, the two therapeutic strategies can be replaced or combined.[63–65]

Antidepressants are the drugs of choice for treating anxiety, and among these, SSRIs and SNRIs offer the best tolerability profile.[63,66] They are effective in treating generalized anxiety in the short and long term, and venlafaxine has also been shown to be effective in acute treatment and in preventing panic attacks.[66]

Anticonvulsants and atypical antipsychotics have shown some efficacy in anxiety, but due to their side effects and lack of clinical data, they are relegated to second-line treatment or considered adjunctive therapies[63]: For example, pregabalin has been shown to be effective in preventing relapse in generalized anxiety and social phobia, and quetiapine has been shown to be effective in generalized anxiety.[66]

Benzodiazepines can also be used as adjunctive therapy for a short time in these comorbidities. However, given that they can promote sedation, cause cognitive impairment, and lead to abusive behavior, their use should be reserved for acute crises of anxiety/agitation and while waiting for antidepressants to take effect.[20,63,66]

Eating Disorders (EDs)

Eating disorders are mental illnesses related to abnormal eating habits, which can range from binge eating (bulimia) to refusing to eat (anorexia), with significant repercussions on both the physical and mental health of those who suffer from them. The literature indicates that patients with EDs who abuse substances have more severe symptoms and worse outcomes than those with EDs alone, including more medical complications and psychopathological, longer recovery times, poorer functional outcomes, higher relapse rates, higher rates of suicide/suicide attempts, and higher mortality rates.[67,68]

EDs mainly affect young women, and most cases are diagnosed in adolescence. The most common EDs are bulimia nervosa (BN), anorexia nervosa (AN), and binge eating disorder (BED).[69]

The association between EDs and SUDs is strong, apparently bidirectional, and certainly complicates the diagnosis, treatment, and prognosis of both.[67–72]

Scientific literature shows that, worldwide, the estimated comorbidity of EDs and SUDs ranges from 3% to 50% and that approximately 25% of young people with eating disorders have patterns of substance abuse; as they get older, they are more likely to consume alcohol and cannabis. Bulimia nervosa seems to be a better predictor of substance abuse than anorexia nervosa or other eating disorder diagnoses.

From the opposite perspective, 35% of alcohol or illicit substance users have an eating disorder, whereas the prevalence of eating disorders in the general population is 3%.[67,69,72]

Addictive behavior is diverse: substances (caffeine, tobacco), insulin, thyroid medications, stimulants, or over-the-counter medications (laxatives, diuretics) may be used as energy boosters or for weight loss; and alcohol or psychoactive substances may be used for emotional regulation or as part of a pattern of impulsive behavior.[67]

The literature indicates that ED and SUD should be addressed simultaneously with a multidisciplinary approach and that, depending on the medical and psychiatric evaluation, hospitalization may be necessary for stabilization.[67,72]

Considering the neurobiological theory of etiology, some authors suggest that pharmacological treatment should target the dopamine, glutamate, and opioid neurotransmitter systems, also used in the treatment of SUD. However, when addressing this dual disorder, pharmacotherapy should not be the primary treatment in itself, but it may be indicated in combination with other therapeutic interventions, including psychoeducation about the etiological similarities, risks, and consequences of behaviors and substance abuse; dietary education and planning; cognitive challenging of eating disorder attitudes and beliefs; and building skills and mechanisms for resilience to obstacles and relapse prevention.[67,72]

REFERENCES

1. De Vries TPGM, Henning RH, Hogerzeil HV, Fresle DA. WHO Action Programme on Essential Drugs). Guide to good prescribing: a practical manual/TPGM. WHO (1998), accessed at: https://apps.who.int/iris/handle/10665/66661.
2. Martínez Nieto C. Ensayos clínicos en España. Ética, normativa, metodología y aspectos prácticos (1ª edición). May 2017. ISBN: 978-84-697-3116-1.
3. Comité Permanente de Médicos Europeos. Resolución sobre la calidad de la prescripción. Spanish Medical Association. General Council of Medical Associations, Brussels, August 30, 2003. December 15, 2003.
4. World Health Organization (WHO). CIE-10-ES Diagnósticos (3ª edición-enero 2020). Actualización Julio 2020. Clasificación Internacional de Enfermedades (10ª revisión), Modificación clínica. Spanish edition © Ministry of Health, Consumer Affairs, and Social Welfare. Directorate-General for Public Health, Quality, and Innovation. Subdirectorate General for Health Information.
5. Arocas Casañ V. Prescripción Hospitalaria de Medicamentos fuera de Ficha Técnica. Department of Pharmacology. University of Murcia, 2016.
6. Barral C, Ros-Cucurull E, Roncero E. Prescripción "Off-Label" en 19 Patología Dual. J Dual Pathol. 2014;1(3):10.
7. Dorado M. Uso de Fármacos Fuera de Indicación en Patología Dual, Necesidad Clínica. Grupo de trabajo sobre fármacos de fuera de indicación. J Dual Pathol. 2014;1(3):11.
8. Gillick MR. Controlling Off-Label Medication Use. Ann Intern Med. 2009;150:344–7.
9. European Medicines Agency. Regulating off-label use of medicines in Europe. Policy brief, 2018; accessed at: https://www.acpjournals.org/doi/10.7326/0003-4819-150-5-200903030-00108.

10. Murthy P, Chand P. Treatment of dual diagnosis disorders. Curr Opin Psychiatry. 2012;25:194–200.
11. Abernethy AP, Raman G, Balk EM, Hammond JM, Orlando LA, Wheeler JL, *et al.* Reliability of compendia Methods-Label Oncology Indications. Ann Intern Med. 2009;150:336–43.
12. Ansani N, Siro C, Smitherman T, Smitherman T, Fedu-tes-Henderson B, Skledar S, *et al.* Strategy to promote safe, innovative off-label use of medications. Am J Med Quality. 2006;21(4):225–61.
13. Gazarian M, Kelly M, McPhee JR, Graudins LV, Ward RL, Campbell TJ. Off-label use of medicines: consensus recommendations for evaluating appropriateness. MJA. 2006;185(10):5448.
14. Calleja-Hernández MA, Morillo Verdugo R. El modelo CMO en consultas externas de Farmacia Hospitalaria. Spanish Society of Hospital Pharmacy (SEFH). 2016. ISBN: 978-84-608-6548-3.
15. ICH. Guía Tripartita armonizada de ICH. Normas de buena práctica clínica. 1997. https://ichgcp.net/es
16. Álvarez FJ. La prescripción de fármacos fuera de indicación en patología dual: hoja de información al paciente y consentimiento. Journal of Dual Pathology. 2014;1(3):12.
17. Pellicer C. Investigación y aspectos éticos en medicamentos huérfanos. Curso de Desarrollo Profesional. Spanish Society of Hospital Pharmacy, 2018.
18. Neuroscience-based Nomenclature (NbN). European College of Neuropsychopharmacology (ECNP). https://www.ecnp.eu/research/neuroscience-based-nomenclature-nbn/. 2018.
19. European Monitoring Center for Drugs and Drug Addiction. Perspectives on drugs: Comorbidity of substance use and mental health disorders in Europe, 2016.
20. Torrens M, Mestre-Pintó JI, Domingo-Salvany A. Comorbidity of substance use and mental disorders in Europe. European Monitoring Centre for Drugs and Drug Addiction, 2016.
21. Mancheño-Barba JJ, Navas-León S, Gutiérrez-Lopez ML, de la Rosa-Cáceres A, Cáceres-Pachón P, Lozano, OM. Perfiles de pacientes con patología dual: ¿qué diferencias existen entre los que acuden a las unidades de salud mental comunitaria y a los centros de tratamiento de drogodependencias? Ann Psychol. 2019;35(2):233–41.
22. San L, Arranz B, Bernardo M. Why a Dual Pathology Clinical Guideline? Analysis of the evidence. Por qué la necesidad de una Guía de Práctica Clínica de Patología Dual? Análisis de la evidencia. Rev Psiquiatr Salud Ment (Barc.). 2016;9(2):67–9.
23. Groenman AP, Janssen TWP, Oosterlaan J. Childhood Psychiatric Disorders as Risk Factors for Subsequent Substance Abuse: A Meta-Analysis. J Am Acad Child Adolesc Psychiatry. 2017;56(7):556–9.
24. Elejalde JD, Hurtado RD, Arango C. Protocolos de intervención: Adolescentes y patología dual. Spanish Society of Dual Pathology-SEPD, 2016.
25. Roncero C, Gómez-Baeza S, Vázquez JM, Terán A, Szerman N, Casas M, *et al.* Perception of Spanish Professionals on Therapeutic Adherence of Dual Diagnosis Patients. Actas Esp Psiquiatr. 2013;41(6):319–29.
26. Torres GN, Cristobal JP, Rosa Martin J. Dual Diagnosis: An Integrated Approach to Treatment: Evidence-based Clinical Practice Guidelines. J Drug Abuse. 2019;5(2):4.
27. Lingford-Hughes AR, Welch S, Peters L, Nutt DJ; British Association for Psychopharmacology, Expert Reviewers Group. BAP updated guidelines: evidence-based guidelines for the pharmacological management of Substance abuse, harmful use, addiction, and comorbidity: recommendations from BAP. J Psychopharmacol. 2012;26(7):899–952.
28. Khokhar JY, Dwiel LL, Henricks AM, Doucette WT, Green AI. The Link Between Schizophrenia and Substance Use Disorder: A Unifying Hypothesis. Schizophr Res. 2018;194:78–85.
29. National Institute on Drug Abuse (NIDA): Common Comorbidities with Substance Use Disorders NIH Research Report, 2020.

30. Chaudhury S, Krishna ST, Kumar AB. Impact of Substance Use Disorder on Presentation of Schizophrenia. Dual Diagn: Open Acc. 2016:1(2).
31. Keepers GA, Fochtmann LJ, Anzia JM, Menjamin S, Ly-ness JM, Mojtabai R, *et al.* The American Psychiatric Association practice guideline for the treatment of patients with schizophrenia. American Psychiatric Association, 2021.
32. Kelly TM, Daley DC, Douaihy AB. Treatment of substance abusing patients with comorbid psychiatric disorders. Addict Behav. 2012;37:11–24.
33. Hunt GE, Malhi GS, Cleary M, Lai HM, Sitharthan T. Prevalence of Comorbid Bipolar and Substance Use Disorders in Clinical Settings, 1990-2015: Systematic Review and Meta-Analysis. J Affect Disord. 2016;206:331–49.
34. Salloum IM, Brown ES. Management of Comorbid Bipolar Disorder and Substance Use Disorders. Am J Drug Alcohol Abuse. 2017;43(4):366–76.
35. National Health Service (NHS). Bipolar Disorder Guideline, accessed at: https://www.nhs.uk/mental-health/conditions/bipolar-disorder/. Last updated March 14, 2019.
36. American Addiction Center: treating addiction with severe Bipolar Disorder, accessed at: https://americanaddictioncenters.org/co-occurring-disorders/bipolar. Last updated February 2020.
37. Mohamed II, Ahmad HEK, Hassaan SH. Assessment of Anxiety and Depression Among Substance Use Disorder Patients: A Case-Control Study. Middle East Current Psychiatry, 2020;27:22.
38. McQuaid R. Clinical Practice Guideline for the Treatment of Depression Across Three Age Cohorts. American Psychological Association, 2019.
39. Anxiety and Depression Association of America (ADAA). Clinical practical review for major depressive disorder.
40. Lydecker KP, Tate SR, Cummins KM, McQuaid J, Granholm E, Brown SA. Clinical Outcomes of an Integrated Treatment for Depression and Substance Use Disorders. Psychol Addict Behav. 2010;24(3):453–65.
41. Conner KR, Pinquart M, Gamble SA. Meta-Analysis of Depression and Substance Use Among Individuals with Alcohol Use Disorders. J Substance Abuse Treatment. 2009;37(2):127–37.
42. Coughlin LN, Pfeiffer P, Ganoczy D, Lin LA. Quality of Outpatient Depression Treatment in Patients with Substance Use Disorder. The American Journal of Psychiatry. Published Online: Oct. 29, 2020.
43. American Psychiatric Association. DSM 5. Manual Diagnóstico y Estadístico de los Trastornos Mentales (5ª edición). Editorial Médica Panamericana, 2017.
44. Parmar A, Kaloiya G. Comorbidity of Personality Disorder among Substance Use Disorder Patients: A Narrative Review. Indian J Psychol Med. 2018;40(6):517–27.
45. Korsgaard HO, Torgersen S, Wentzel-Larsen T, Ulberg R. Substance Abuse and Personality Disorder Comorbidity in Adolescent Outpatients: Are Girls More Severely Ill Than Boys? Child Adolesc Psychiatry Ment Health. 2016;10:8. Doi: 10.1186/s13034-016-0096-5.
46. Krieger DM, Benzano D, Reppold CT, Fialho PO, Pires GB, Terra MB. Personality Disorder and Substance Related Disorders: A Six-Month Follow-up Study with a Brazilian Sample. Jornal Brasileiro de Psiquiatria. 2016;65(2):127–34.
47. Hasin D, Fenton MC, Skodol A, Krueger R, Keyes K, Geier T, *et al.* Personality Disorders and the 3-Year Course of Alcohol, Drug, and Nicotine Use Disorders, Arch Gen Psychiatry. 2011; 68(11):1158–67. Doi:10.1001/archgenpsychiatry.2011.136
48. Fridell M, Bäckström M, Hesse M, Krantz P, Perrin S, Nyhlén A. Prediction of Psychiatric Comorbidity on Premature Death in a Cohort of Patients with Substance Use Disorders: A 42-Year Follow-Up, BMC Psychiatry. 2019;19:150.
49. Boog M, van Hest KM, Drescher T, Verschuur MJ, Franken IHA. Schema Modes and Personality Disorder Symptoms in Alcohol-Dependent and Cocaine-Dependent Patients. Eur Addict Res. 2018;24:226–33.

50. Belcher AM, Volkow ND, Moeller FG, Ferré S. Personality Traits and Vulnerability or Resilience to Substance Use Disorders. Trends Cogn Sci. 2014;18(4):211–7. Doi: 10.1016/j.tics.2014.01.010
51. Tomko RL, Trull TJ, Wood PK, Sher KJ. Characteristics of borderline personality disorder in a community sample: comorbidity, treatment utilization, and general functioning. J Pers Disord. 2014; 28(5):734–50. Doi: 10.1521/pedi_2012_26_093.
52. Pinacle Treatment Centers. Comorbid borderline personality and substance use disorder: https://pinnacletreatment.com/blog/comorbid-borderline-personality-disorder-and-substance-use-disorder/. Updated June 2019.
53. Gianoli MO. Treatment for comorbid borderline personality disorder and alcohol use disorders: A review of the evidence and future recommendations. Exp Clin Psychopharmacol. 2012;20(4):333–44. Doi: 10.1037/a0027999
54. Özgen H, Spijkerman R, Noack M, Holtmann M, Schellekens ASA, van de Glind G, *et al.* International Consensus Statement for the Screening, Diagnosis, and Treatment of Adolescents with Concurrent Attention-Deficit/Hyperactivity Disorder and Substance Use Disorder. Eur Addict Res. 2020;26:223–32. Doi: 10.1159/000508385
55. Van Emmerik-van Oortmerssen K, van de Glind G, van den Brink W, Smit F, Crunelle CL, Swets M, *et al.* Prevalence of Attention-Deficit Hyperactivity Disorder in Substance Use Disorder Patients: A Meta-Analysis and Meta-Regression Analysis. Drug Alcohol Depend. 2012;122(1-2):11–9.
56. Groenman AP, Oosterlaan J, Rommelse N, Franke B, Roeyers H, Oades RD, *et al.* Substance Use Disorders in Adolescents with Attention Deficit Hyperactivity Disorder: A 4-Year Follow-Up Study. Addiction. 2013;108(8):1503–11. Doi: 10.1111/add.12188.
57. Schoenmacker GH et al. Role of Conduct Problems in the Relation Between Attention-Deficit Hyperactivity Disorder, Substance Use, and Gaming. European Neuropsychopharmacol. 2020;30:102–13.
58. Groenman AP, Oosterlaan J, Rommelse NN, Franke B, Greven CU, Hoekstra PJ, *et al.* Stimulant Treatment Profiles Predicting SUP. Br J Psychiatry. 2013;203(2):112–9. Doi: 10.1192/bjp.bp.112.124784
59. Crunelle CL, van den Brink W, Moggi F, Konstenius M, Franck J, Levin FR, *et al.* International Consensus Statement on Screening, Diagnosis and Treatment of Substance Use Disorder Patients with Comorbid Attention Deficit/Hyperactivity Disorder. Eur Addict Res. 2018;24(1):43–51. Doi: 10.1159/000487767.
60. Harstad E, Wisk LE, Ziemnik R, Huang Q, Salimian P, Weitzman ER, *et al.* Substance Use among Adolescents with ADHD: Reasons for Use, Knowledge of Risks, and Provider Messaging/Education. J Dev Behav Pediatr. 2017;38(6):417–23.
61. Crunelle CL, Matthys F. Good Clinical Practice in the recognition and treatment of ADHD in adults with substance use dependence. Guide For Clinical Practice. Update 2016. Vereniging voor Alcohol en andere Drug problemen vzw (VAD). Forum voor Verslavingsgeneeskunde. Vrije Universiteit Brussel (VUB), 2916.
62. Marmorstein NR. Anxiety Disorders and Substance Use Disorders: Different Associations by Anxiety Disorder. J Anxiety Disord. 2012;26(1):88–94.
63. Katzman MA, Bleau P, Blier P, Chokka P, Kjernisted K, Van Ameringen M; Canadian Anxiety Guidelines Initiative Group on behalf of the Anxiety Disorders Association of Canada/Association Canadienne des troubles anxieux and McGill University, Antony MM, Bouchard S, Brunet A, Flament M, Grigoriadis S, Mendlowitz S, O'Connor K, Rabheru K, Richter PM, Robichaud M, Walker JR. Canadian Clinical Practice Guidelines for the Management of Anxiety, Posttraumatic Stress and Obsessive-Compulsive Disorders. BMC Psychiatry. 2014:14(Suppl 1):S1.

64. Smith JP, Book SW. Anxiety and Substance Use Disorders: A Review. Psychiatric Times. 2008;25(10):19–23.
65. Ströhle A, Gensichen J, Domschke K. The Diagnosis and Treatment of Anxiety Disorders. Dtsch Arztebl Int. 2018;155(37):611–20.
66. Baldwin DS, Anderson IM, Nutt DJ, Allgulander C, Bandelow B, den Boer JA, *et al.* Evidence-Based Pharmacological Treatment of Anxiety Disorders, Post-Traumatic Stress Disorder, and Obsessive-Compulsive Disorder: A Revision of the 2005 Guidelines from the British Association for Psychopharmacology. J Psychopharmacol. 2014;28(5):403–39.
67. Gregorowski C, Seedat S, Jordaan GP. A Clinical Approach to the Assessment and Management of Co-Morbid Eating Disorders and Substance Use Disorders. BMC Psychiatry. 2013;13:289.
68. Keshishian AC, Tabri N, Becker KR, Franko DL, Herzog DB, Thomas JJ, *et al.* Eating Disorder Recovery is Associated with Absence of Major Depressive Disorder and Substance Use Disorders at 22-year Longitudinal Follow-Up. Compr Psychiatry. 2019;90:49–51.
69. Eskander N, Chakrapani S, Ghani MR. The Risk of Substance Use Among Adolescents and Adults with Eating Disorders. Cureus. 2020;12(9):e10309.
70. Bahji A, Mazhar MN, Hudson CC, Nadkarni P, MacNeil BA, Hawken E. Prevalence of Substance Use Disorder Comorbidity Among Individuals with Eating Disorders: A Systematic Review and Meta-Analysis. Psychiatry Research. 2019;273:58–66.
71. Flores Fresco MJ, Blanco Gandía, MC, Rodríguez Arias M. Alteraciones de la Conducta Alimentaria en Pacientes con Trastorno por Abuso de Sustancias. Clinical and Health. 2018;29(3):125–32.
72. Wiss DA. The Role of Nutrition in Addiction Recovery: What We Know and What We Don't. Chapter 2. The Assessment and Treatment of Addiction–Best Practices and New Frontiers. 2019, accessed at: https://doi.org/10.1016/B978-0-323-54856-4.00002-X.

CHAPTER 6

Nursing and the Dual Pathology Approach

M. J. Álvarez Alonso, C. Carballal Balsa, M. L. Bugallo Pardo, F. C. Pessoa Esteves, and M. C. Vallejo Curto

Over the years, it has been necessary to evolve nursing practices and interventions in order to provide care and effective responses to problems associated with substance use, whether this is the cause or consequence of a psychiatric disorder in the same individual, which has been agreed to be called *dual pathology* (DP).

What began in Spain back in the 1980s, in drug addiction units, on an outpatient basis and providing basic care to alleviate withdrawal symptoms and dispensing pharmacological treatments, has now become a nursing practice specializing in the care of people with DP and the development of specific care plans, as part of an interdisciplinary team and a basic element in the patient's interaction with the unit.

The concept of dual pathology is not defined in the *Diagnostic and Statistical Manual of Mental Disorders* (DSM-5) or in the International Classification of Diseases and Injuries (ICD). There are no clear diagnostic criteria, which means that a large number of patients cannot be diagnosed early on. International and national epidemiological studies determine that 70% of these patients with substance use disorder have another mental disorder simultaneously or sequentially. Some authors consider that this reality is underestimated, as it could cover 100% of these patients, but current instruments that diagnose categories rather than symptoms do not allow it to be detected. In fact, this "comorbidity" is not optimally detected when diagnostic categories are used instead of symptomatic dimensions that may not reach the diagnostic threshold.

Integrated treatment has been recommended as the most effective care alternative for addressing this pathology, since mental illness and addiction are treated in the same center and by the same interdisciplinary team.

Currently, in most cases, these types of patients are treated in *addiction units*, as there are not enough *dual pathology units* (DPU) or national facilities where they can be treated.

These centers must be staffed by an interdisciplinary team that offers comprehensive care, providing the most appropriate treatment at all times and facilitating rehabilitation and reintegration.

DOI: 10.4324/9781003786153-6

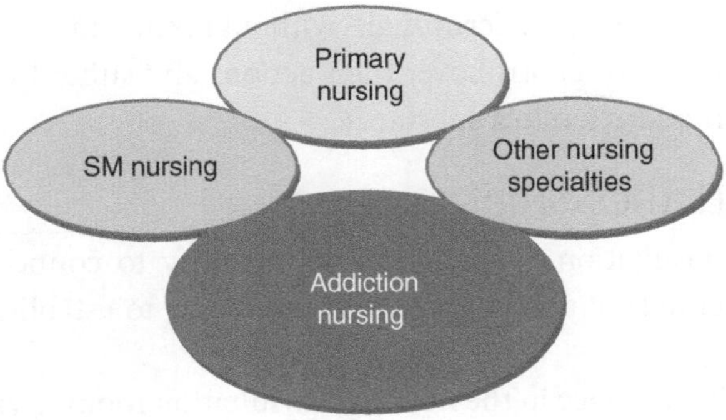

FIGURE 6.1 Functions related to the nursing profession. Álvarez MJ, Garabán MJ. Nursing management of patients with Dual Pathology (DP) (2020).

DP individuals are particularly important users of the healthcare system, from both a health and a social perspective. In addition, it should be noted that they have more relapses, longer stays in different health services, problems with adherence to treatment, increased suicidal ideation, higher rates of risky behavior and associated infections (acquired immunodeficiency virus, hepatitis C virus, sexually transmitted diseases, etc.), loss of family and social relationships, and higher rates of unemployment and marginalization.

People diagnosed with dual pathology require specific and comprehensive care, with nursing professionals playing a fundamental role in their holistic assessment.

The functions related to the nursing profession are care, management, teaching, and research at all the levels of health care: primary, secondary, and tertiary (Figure 6.1).

Similarly, nursing involves social integration activities, coordinating with different drug addiction or mental health (MH) services and with primary and specialized care centers, prisons, community agents, and social services.

The Nursing Care Process (NCP) is a method applied to nursing practice on a theoretical basis. It is an approach to problem-solving based on reflection and requires interpersonal cognitive skills in order to meet the needs of the user and their family.

When planning care, we must take into account the points discussed below.

ABSENCE OF PREJUDICE

A multidisciplinary and comprehensive assessment, adaptation to the real needs of the dual patient, and not prejudging their behavior, consumption, or attitude allows us to offer them the best care and responses, as there are many difficult situations for their families, for professionals, and even for themselves. Society tends to negatively label those who suffer from an addictive and/or mental disorder, highlighting the negative aspects and emphasizing their condition as an important part of who they are, even though that might not be true in their case.

The consumption of alcohol and other drugs causes individuals to develop behaviors that are inappropriate for social constructs. They may suffer from physical and/or mental illnesses that distance them from the context of normality. Sometimes, they engage in criminal behavior and are associated with accidents, abuse, or crime, causing people to label them "vicious," "apathic," or "criminal," without taking into account their condition as individuals who have lost control over their actions and suffer from an urgent need to consume due to their addiction to a substance.

THERAPEUTIC RELATIONSHIP

The first nursing consultation gives us the opportunity to connect and communicate with the patient, if clinical circumstances allow, in order to establish a good therapeutic relationship.

The interview will take place in the nursing consultation room, giving it the importance and confidentiality it requires. We will introduce ourselves, showing empathy and accessibility, without forgetting that we are healthcare professionals. It is very important to take into account and care for all the aspects of patient reception, our environment, and our verbal and nonverbal attitude.

Our attention must be focused on the user, showing interest and avoiding distractions such as the telephone or computer. We must maintain an upright posture, our body leaning forward, not crossing our arms, and showing an attitude of active listening. We must establish a dialogue in which the interviewee can express concerns without feeling interrogated or pressured, making them feel that we are there to help them. Appropriate language should be used, avoiding technical terms. Our tone of voice should be soft but firm, and we should look them in the eye, showing interest without being inquisitive.

The interview will be personalized and semi-structured, adapted to the characteristics of the DP user and in a biopsychosocial context, enabling the initial approach to be established. It will be carried out during the assessment phase, which will be addressed later more comprehensively and specifically.

However, we can improve this process by conducting a series of self-administered questionnaires (https://bi.cibersam.es/busqueda-de-instrumentos), such as:

- Salamanca Questionnaire for *screening* personality disorders (Antonio Pérez Urdániz, Vicente Rubio Larrosa, M. Esperanza Gómez Gazol)
- Self-reported questionnaire for screening ADHD in adults (ASRS-V1.1, WHO Composite International Diagnostic Interview)
- Barratt Scale
- AUDIT (Alcohol Use Disorders Identification Test)
- Suicide Ideation Scale
- Side Effects Scale (Udvalg for Kliniske Undersøgelser, UKU)
- Motivational Interviewing (MI): designed by Miller and Rollnick in 1991; based on the basic principles of "client-centered therapy" applied to Prochaska and DiClemente's stages of change
- DiClemente (1983): the therapist selecting the most appropriate intervention strategies based on the stage of change the patient is in

TABLE 6.1 Vulnerable Personality Variants

Internalizer (egodystonic)	Externalizer	Self-Absorbed (egosyntonic)
Cluster C prototype	Cluster B prototype	Cluster A prototype
Treatment seeker	Demanding and manipulative	Indifferent and suspicious
Appropriate and/or submissive behavior	Seductive, intimidating, impulsive, or unstable behavior	Reserved, passive behavior with little expressiveness
Primarily a user of depressant or sedative substances	User of all types of substances	Mainly consumes THC and stimulants
Good prognosis	Poor prognosis	Variable prognosis

- Brief exploration of the Galician Forum for the Study of Personality (Foro Galego de Estudos da Personalidade, FGEP): allows the three variants of vulnerable personality to be differentiated, the most pronounced characteristics of which are shown below (Table 6.1).

The data provided by this assessment lay the foundations for the development of interventions and clinical reasoning that improve care, showing us the way to carry out nursing diagnoses, following the NANDA-I taxonomy.

All these aspects will facilitate the approach, relationship, and therapeutic adherence.

THERAPEUTIC ADHERENCE

To achieve this, we must take four factors into account:

1. Those related to the disease itself, as it is often the clinical symptoms of the disorders that make it difficult to comply with guidelines or lead to abandonment
2. Those related to the environment: aspects related to family or the absence thereof, economic factors, social factors, legal factors, and available resources
3. Those related to low effectiveness or the presence of side effects, which often lead to a deterioration in quality of life
4. Those related to the therapeutic team, highlighting their ability to establish a bond and foster a therapeutic alliance

In addition to these four factors, the following will help maintain and increase adherence:

- Interventions tailored to the patient's circumstances: clinical, cognitive, and/or social (harm reduction, change of appointments, change from scheduled intervention to brief intervention, crisis care)
- Health education
- Counseling interventions
- Motivational interviewing
- Prevention of risk situations and relapses

PATIENT APPROACH

Nursing staff must possess a series of skills to approach and treat patients with DP:

- Cognitive or intellectual skills: problem analysis and solving, critical thinking, management of psychoeducational and cognitive-behavioral interventions; maintain ongoing training in psychiatric, addictive, and comorbid pathologies and their different pharmacological treatments; identify current and potential health problems through observation, assessment of user needs, and correct decision-making
- Interpersonal skills: ease of communication with patients, active listening, observation skills, and trust-building
- Technical skills: administration of medications, vaccines, and injections; collection of blood and urine samples; and performance of various procedures to assess health parameters

CRISIS CARE

Throughout life, crises occur that abruptly interrupt the normal course of people's lives. A crisis situation can also arise during a rehabilitation process.

A crisis can be defined as a temporary state of disorder and disorganization, characterized mainly by the individual's inability to deal with particular situations using the usual methods of problem-solving, and by the potential for a radically positive or negative outcome.

Crises can be evolutionary, i.e., predictable or inherent in the passage of time and the attainment of life stages, or circumstantialaccidental, sudden, and unexpected. What they have in common is that they interrupt the course of life, causing changes in emotional balance.

How these crises are overcome will determine whether emotional balance is restored in a healthy way or whether deterioration occurs, preventing progress and causing stagnation at this point in life or rehabilitation.

How a crisis is dealt with will depend on a number of variables:

- **Personal variables**: Biology, age, gender, ethnic group, personal style, socioeconomic status, learning history, beliefs, previous experiences, personal life situation, stage of life at which the crisis occurs, subjective sense of coping ability, previous pathologies, availability, and education of social support networks.
- **Situation variables**: Type of event, origin, magnitude, degree of exposure, available resources for help, etc.
- **Consequences**: Personal, meaning of the losses experienced, intensity of the symptoms caused, subjective importance, and subsequent stressors

The following will facilitate our care in crisis situations for patients diagnosed with DP and help us make the most appropriate decision at that time:

- Having conducted an interdisciplinary assessment and knowing the patient's history and background
- Rapid assessment, through observation of nonverbal language and listening to their demands, of possible intoxication, withdrawal, psychotic episode, anxiety attack, etc.
- Trying to create a calm atmosphere that the patient does not perceive as hostile
- Being aware that confrontation and rigidity are not appropriate strategies

Despite all of the above, the desired objective is not always fully achieved. Each intervention should contribute to laying the foundations of trust through motivation, avoiding directive interventions. Patience and flexibility are required, remembering that habits, behaviors, and conduct do not always respond to preserved intellectual and volitional capacities, but rather that the pathology itself and factors related to emotional development, attachment, and insight, among others, are elements that can alter them.

NURSING INTERVENTION PROTOCOL FOR IMPROVING THE QUALITY OF CARE FOR DUAL PATHOLOGY PATIENTS

The **nursing care process** (NCP) is a system of interventions for the health care of individuals, families, and communities that uses the scientific method to identify needs and as to support problem-solving. The NCP consists of five phases: assessment, diagnosis, planning, implementation, and evaluation.

ASSESSMENT

This involves gathering as much information as possible, both objectively and subjectively, from the patient themself and their family or companions, and from a thorough review of their medical history. The NANDA-I domain assessment provides us with an overview of the person.

Following these domains, we will describe what we should assess in each of them and the most frequent NANDA-I (2021–2023) diagnoses in patients diagnosed with DP, but always bearing in mind that they are variable, as all patients are different, come for different circumstances and/or situations, and have very different objectives.

DIAGNOSIS

The NANDA-I taxonomy is the tool used to name, order, and classify nursing diagnoses. Using this universal taxonomy makes it possible to standardize nursing records. The diagnoses in this type of patient can be many and varied. In addition, it should be noted that the NANDA-I taxonomy is revised every two years, and changes may be made.

PLANNING

This is the phase in which the actions to be taken by the nurse to resolve the problems identified in the nursing diagnosis are determined through a care plan, planning the outcomes to be achieved (NOC) and the interventions to be performed (NIC).

Domain 1: Health promotion

Assessment	**Most frequent NANDA diagnoses**
Measurement of health parameters Drug allergies Medical and surgical history Prescribed and/or on-demand treatments Recent blood tests and serology Hygiene and clothing STDs/pregnancy/Abortion Current consumption: route, quantity, and frequency Family and personal history of drug addiction, alcoholism, and/or SM Insight/knowledge of your condition Adherence to treatment	00293 Willingness to improve self-management of health 00276 Ineffective self-management of health 00188 Tendency to engage in health risk behaviors 00292 Ineffective behaviors for maintaining health

Domain 2: Nutrition

Assessment	**Most frequent NANDA diagnoses**
Nutritional status Appetite, intake, and diet Food allergies/intolerances Meal times Psychotic behaviors, presence of rituals, and/or restrictions due to delirium Difficulty chewing/swallowing Missing teeth Condition of skin and mucous membranes	00002 Nutritional imbalance 00178 Risk of impaired liver function 00197 Risk of intestinal motility 00296 Risk of metabolic syndrome 00234 Risk of overweight

Domain 3: Elimination and exchange

Assessment	**Most frequent NANDA diagnoses**
Excretory functions of the body and their disorders: gastrointestinal, urinary, and skin Incontinence Substance use	00011 Constipation 00013 Diarrhea 00197 Risk of dysfunctional gastrointestinal motility

Domain 4: Activity/Rest

Assessment	Most frequent NANDA diagnoses
Mobility problems Performance of activities of daily living (ADL) Leisure and free time Lifestyle assessment Facial expression, tics, and extrapyramidal side effects caused by neuroleptics Hygiene and clothing Presence of hyperactivity or states of psychomotor agitation State of inhibition/catatonia Rest habits Alterations in the sleep–wake cycle Use of addictive substances Use of drugs such as hypnotics and sedatives	00032 Ineffective breathing pattern 00088 Impaired ambulation 00102 Self-care deficit: feeding 00108 Self-care deficit: bathing 00109 Self-care deficit: dressing 00154 Wandering 00198 Sleep pattern disturbance 00095 Insomnia 00168 Sedentary lifestyle

Domain 5: Perception-cognition

Assessment	Most frequent NANDA diagnoses
Sensory-perceptual and cognitive abilities Judgment and decision-making Level of awareness and attitude towards the environment Orientation (space-time and person) Presence of hallucinations, delusions, suicidal ideation, obsessions, etc.	00131 Impaired memory 00251 Unstable emotional control 00128 Acute confusion 00222 Ineffective impulse control 00279 Thought process disorder

Domain 6: Self-perception

Assessment	Most frequent NANDA diagnoses
Self-esteem Mood and affect Body image perception	00119 Chronic low self-esteem 00124 Hopelessness 00225 Risk of personal identity disorder

Domain 7: Role-relationships

Assessment	Most frequent NANDA diagnoses
Roles and responsibilities Availability of support networks Family structure Family reaction to illness	00052 Impaired social interaction 00058 Risk of impaired bonding 00063 Dysfunctional family processes 00229 Risk of ineffective relationships

Domain 8: Sexuality

Assessment	Most frequent NANDA diagnoses
Satisfaction with sexual activity	00059 Sexual dysfunction
Problems related to sexual identity	00065 Ineffective sexuality pattern
Loss or alterations in reproductive capacity	
Side effects of neuroleptics	00227 Risk of ineffective mothering process
Use of protective measures during sexual intercourse	00305 Risk of delayed child development
STDs/pregnancy/abortion	

Domain 9: Coping-stress tolerance

Assessment	Most frequent NANDA diagnoses
Tolerance-adaptation capacity	00069 Ineffective coping
Ability to cope with everyday events	00071 Defensive coping
Coping mechanisms	
Fears, phobias, ideas, or thoughts	00072 Ineffective denial
Poisoning: opiates, alcohol, and BZD	00141 Post-traumatic syndrome
	00210 Impaired resilience
	00146 Anxiety
	00241 Impaired mood regulation
	00259 Risk of acute withdrawal syndrome
	00226 Risk of ineffective activity planning

Domain 10: Vital signs

Assessment	Most common NANDA diagnoses
Values and feelings	00083 Decision conflict
Religious beliefs	00244 Risk of impaired independent decision making
	00175 Moral distress
	00066 Spiritual distress

Domain 11: Safety/protection

Assessment	Most frequent NANDA diagnoses
Risk of suicide	00037 Risk of intoxication
Route of substance use	00004 Risk of infection
Substance poisoning	00289 Risk of suicidal behavior
	00035 Risk of injury
	00140 Risk of self-directed violence
	00138 Risk of violence directed at others

Domain 12: Comfort

Assessment	**Most frequent NANDA diagnoses**
Social skills	00214 Discomfort
Awareness of illness	00053 Social isolation
Family support	00054 Risk of loneliness

Domain 13: Growth/development

Assessment	**Most frequent NANDA diagnoses**
Childhood illnesses	00314 Delayed child development
Learning disorders	
Abuse	

It should be noted that it is necessary to:

- Set priorities
- Set objectives
- Determine actions or interventions
- Record the plan

IMPLEMENTATION

In this phase of the nursing process, the activities that constitute the specific nursing actions necessary to carry out the nursing interventions (NIC) will be applied and recorded.

EVALUATION

Assess the patient's current situation and compare it with the results (NOC) that had been set. The conclusions drawn will determine whether the nursing interventions have produced the desired results and this will give us the information we need in order to know whether they should be: terminated if the objectives have been met; extended if the objectives have only been partially met and more time is needed; or modified if they have not been met, or achieved, in which case we must reconsider the nursing interventions.

REFERENCES

1. Casas LA, Conde AM, Fernández HJL, Flórez MG, Forti BMA, Forti SL, *et al.* Personalidad: exploración, diagnóstico y tratamiento. Foro Gallego de Estudio de la Personalidad (FGEP). Forti Sampietro L (coordinator). Personalidad: exploración, diagnóstico y tratamiento. Madrid: Docta Ediciones, 2015.
2. De las Cuevas C, Sanz EJ. Métodos de valoración de la adherencia al tratamiento psiquiátrico en la práctica clínica. Rev Iberoam Psicol Salud (online journal) 2016 (Apr 28, 2020);7(1):25–30. doi:10.1016/j.rips.2015.10.001.

3. Fornés VJ, Carballal BMC. Enfermería de Salud Mental y Psiquiátrica. Guía práctica de valoración y estrategias de intervención. Madrid: Editorial Médica Panamericana, 2001.
4. Ibarra Barrueta O, Morillo Verdugo R (coordinators). Lo que debes saber sobre la adherencia al tratamiento. Badalona: Euromedice Vivactis, 2017.
5. North American Nursing Diagnosis Association. Diagnósticos Enfermeros. Definiciones y Clasificación 2021-2023 (12ª edición). Editorial Elsevier.
6. Pagès Puigdemont N, Valverde Merino MI. Métodos para medir la adherencia terapéutica. Ars Pharm [online journal] 2018 [2020 Apr 29];59(3):163–72. doi: 10.30827/ars.v59i3.7387.
7. Pascual Mollá M, Pascual Pastor F. El estigma en la persona adicta. Adicciones. 2017;29(4): 223–226.

CHAPTER 7

Recommendations for an Effective Approach to the Social Integration of Dual-Pathology Patients

The Importance of the Process of "Social Destigmatization"

A. Mariño Blanco, A. J. De Jesús Roque,
and C. A. Pinto da Rocha

People suffering from **dual disorders** (the coexistence of an addictive disorder and another mental disorder in the same individual) continue to be steeped in a stigmatizing social mindset, as there are still sectors of the population that consider drug addiction to be a personal choice rather than an illness. This leads to this group of patients being left unprotected and/or socially excluded, which will further hinder their already difficult process of social reintegration, the true goal of any intervention framework for addiction and dual pathology.

Social exclusion affects a multitude of areas of life (personal, health, family, environment, economy, education, employment, and legal problems), so these individuals will require a rehabilitation plan with comprehensive interventions.

In facilitating and promoting the social integration of these patients, it is essential to maintain positive interactions with society, which involves (re)establishing links between individuals and their social context in order to create or repair their social ties—ties established between citizens and social systems and in this case conditioned by the process of social stigmatization already mentioned.

The paths to social integration for citizens with dual pathology are often slow and winding, as they require comprehensive and systemic interventions. It is a process that affects society and citizens in an interactive way and aims to create conditions that allow the latter to freely choose to fully exercise their citizenship.

DOI: 10.4324/9781003786153-7

In recent years, integrated intervention models have been advocated, focusing on the real needs of citizens at risk of disintegration.[1–3]

Promoting the exercise of citizenship in populations with dual pathology involves developing responses that, on the one hand, are backed by the specificity and scope necessary to address the different vulnerabilities of these citizens and, on the other hand, operate in an integrated manner in order to take into account the complexity of the associated biopsychosocial problems.[1–3]

The most frequent problems for a significant segment of this group are as follows:

- The unemployment rate in Spain remains very high, and this has led to an increase in the number of people who need assistance to meet basic needs (housing, food, etc.), thus increasing the number of people living marginal lifestyles ("homeless").[4,5]
- We also find a significant percentage of people who suffer from social isolation, as well as a lack of a stable living space.[6]
- A large number of patients also have a low level of education and lack job training to compete in a critical job market.
- In addition, there has been a high percentage of patients with criminal records and periods in prison, which contributes to increasing this process of social stigmatization.

Nor can we forget the continuous increase in the number of people born outside Spain and in an irregular situation, who add other risk factors: family dysfunction, overcrowding, disruption of cultural habits and difficulties in adapting, employment and legal obstacles, and, in many cases, lack of knowledge of the language.

In a study carried out in the center of Coruña in 2010, these people already accounted for 12% of the patients treated, and that number has continued to grow.

Having another comorbid mental disorder adds to the problems caused by drug use. Here, social work interventions must be geared toward comprehensive responses to achieve the necessary and full social integration that will enable them to live as citizens with duties and rights.

ROLE OF SOCIAL WORK IN THE APPROACH TO THE DUAL PATHOLOGY PATIENT

Social work involves not only providing resources or benefits, but also offering assistance and support in the form of *accompaniment/mentoring* during the "process of social reintegration" in order to achieve the necessary changes that will lead to real integration into the community. Social integration is a continuous process, and support is provided throughout the patient's therapeutic program at the center where they are treated.[7,8]

In the European Union, health and social responses to problems arising from addiction and related issues, including dual pathology, are developed within the context of national and local legal and policy frameworks, according to which certain principles, methodologies, and essential phases must be followed:[9]

- Identify the nature of the problem to be addressed in each individual.
- Select possible effective interventions to address these problems.
- Implement, monitor, and evaluate the impact of these personalized intervention plans.

Social integration/inclusion involves carrying out different actions tailored to the needs of each individual, with varying degrees of integration and variables at each stage of the process.[9]

Given that each person starts from a particular situation, this means that interventions are personalized and flexible, tailored to each person and their circumstances, and must take into account their needs, interests, abilities, particular situation, etc., in order to develop a personalized intervention plan.

The following indicators will help us measure the degree of integration of the person: [1,3,10–12]

- Maintaining a stable daily routine (sleeping, eating, dressing, working, studying, having free time, etc.)
- Making a positive assessment of each of their own life stages
- Ensuring economic self-sufficiency in order to be able to undertake and sustain daily activities
- Maintain adequate social and personal relationships that strengthen their support network to facilitate their integration process
- Possess a clear self-awareness of the social role being played, translated into sufficient social competence, a defined social image, social participation, and/or an attitude favorable to breaking out of circles of exclusion

Likewise, there are a number of factors involved in the processes of social incorporation:

- Social network
- Income
- Prestige—derived from job or activity performance
- Formal and informal learning
- Maintaining curiosity and an active attitude
- Socio-family situation

- Health
- Use of leisure and free time
- Subjective perception of the degree of satisfaction with all of the above

PROPOSAL FOR PROTOCOLIZATION OF THE INTERVENTION OF THE SOCIAL WORKER TO IMPROVE THE QUALITY OF CARE FOR THE DUAL PATIENT

Support as a social work methodology in the social integration processes of people admitted to treatment in the centers of the Galician addiction network is based on a personalized model of social integration intervention that can be extrapolated to other countries.[1,11–14]

What Does This Intervention Model Consist Of?

To explain this intervention model, we will first explain what we mean by "social integration": a personalized and flexible socialization process consisting of actions and interventions that aim to actively involve, empower, promote, and facilitate people's autonomy, development, social well-being, participation, and critical thinking skills in their environment.

The personalized incorporation program (PIP) is a technical procedure that integrates an open and dynamic personalized process of actions, activated by the social work professional, and which has three **key elements of intervention**:

- **Intervention with the user**: The aim is for interventions to be directed at alleviating the psychosocial deficits presented by the individual through a process of professional interventions that seek to support, but also to empower the patient in the development of strategies and skills and in the use and search for resources, prioritizing standardized ones.
- **Community intervention**: PIP focuses both (1) on promoting the structured use of existing resources through the guidance of social workers and optimizing resources through coordination and continuity and (2) on the commitment and shared responsibility of the different social agents in the social incorporation processes of this group of patients.
- **Evaluation**: This is a guide for decision-making and for systematizing and evaluating the methodologies used in the process and evaluating its results (in Galicia, this task is carried out through a computer application of the PIP itself).

The PIP model defines **areas of intervention** to facilitate computerized data collection and subsequent analysis of the results of this process:

- **Social support and assistance area**: This includes, not only interventions aimed at alleviating subsistence situations through benefits and the use of social resources, but also interventions that serve to develop the individual's abilities in order to achieve autonomy and full participation as a citizen.

- **Employment area**: Interventions here focus on the acquisition of habits and skills specific to the world of work.
- **Training area**: This includes interventions aimed at achieving basic formal training, encouraging motivation for continuing education, and providing occupational and professional training for those who need it.
- **Judicial area**: The aim is to ensure that people with convictions and/or pending cases have the necessary resources and support to continue their rehabilitation plan and thus achieve full social integration.
- **Therapeutic area**: This type of intervention focuses on the treatment and resolution of psychological and biological problems related to addiction/DP, as a fundamental part of the social integration process.

Bases Underpinning the PIP Intervention Methodology for PIP Intervention in Dual Pathology

In order to enable the development of the PIP and respond to user demands, we have:

- **The social worker**: The social worker will accompany the user throughout the process of social reintegration; their duties include selecting candidates for the program, conducting a social assessment (including an organized proposal for interventions), and **working with the patient to define** their integration plan and social itinerary. The aim is to encourage the user's active participation throughout the process and to act as an intermediary with the different social mechanisms and agents in the community.[2,8] Likewise, this person applies the Program and Project registration system (a specific computer application in Galicia), evaluating and reformulating the development of the PIP to better suit the needs of patients, which often change throughout their therapeutic process.
- **Social diagnosis**: This is the fundamental tool of the social worker and is the result of the analysis and interpretation of the data collected, which relates to the person's abilities, limitations, deficits, motivations, and interests, in order to allow us to personalize the objectives.[1,2,15,16]

The social diagnosis should answer the following questions:

- What are the main areas and specific objectives of the intervention?
- What aspects will it focus on?
- What are the main supports and capabilities available?
- What will the intervention methodology be?
- How will the most suitable integration activities be planned and implemented?
- How long is the intervention or the activities to be carried out in the PIP expected to last?

THE INTEGRATION PROJECT

This is the set of specific interventions carried out jointly with the patient, which identifies and selects priorities, and must include the objectives, actions, and resources that we are going to use.

Objectives and Itineraries

The insertion project is strategically based on the definition of reintegration itineraries.

The Project also establishes the accompanying and mentoring measures, a framework within which to place the commitments and relationships between the professional and the patient. Accordingly, it is made up of *objectives* actions and resources that make up the *itineraries*, as follows:

- **Objectives**: These are the result of the diagnostic assessment and the user's participation, which will lead to their personalization and the search for intervention strategies to achieve them.
- The objectives will depend on the characteristics, situation, needs, potential, motivation, and interests of each person.
- We will start with low-level objectives and, if the process allows, move on to more ambitious goals in order to achieve greater responsibility and control of the patient's own life.
- **Itineraries**: These are structured processes based on defined objectives, through mutually committed participation between the tutor, the user, and their immediate environment.

Itineraries are developed through a "continuum" of *actions* and use of *resources* (prioritizing standardized ones), seeking to promote and/or facilitate the most normalized and integrated socialization possible for users in their reference environment.

The set of **interventions** that will define this personalized itinerary must follow, among others, the following principles:

- Joint responsibility and active participation of the user in their social integration project
- Individuality and flexibility in actions, ensuring, as far as possible, that they are tailored to the needs of each person
- Systematic motivation and support from the social worker throughout the process
- Follow-up with defined monitoring of actions, thus ensuring a process of continuous evaluation

Resources: Management and Coordination

Social reintegration processes are usually supported by both general and specific resources, although prioritizing the use of standardized/general resources is essential in the integration project.

Among the most requested resources at present are those related to access to basic needs (housing, financial assistance, pensions, soup kitchens, shelters), but resources related to leisure and free time activities are also necessary.

Coordination with these resources is one of the tasks that must be undertaken in the design and implementation of individualized social incorporation itineraries.

The establishment of social support networks, which hold society as a whole accountable and committed to solving existing problems related to the integration of dual diagnosis patients, is a fundamental part of this program.

Follow-Up

Once the social integration project has been defined, the social worker carries out a continuous evaluation of that project. Follow-up is one of the important aspects of support in the social integration process. Thus, in this phase, assessment is made of achievements and/or setbacks that occur along the established path, including sessions, interventions, actions taken, changes in attitude, tasks completed or omitted, mediation interventions with resources, etc., in order to enable continuous evaluation for better adjustment to the patient's needs.

Supporting the social integration itinerary also involves supporting the acquisition and development of tools for self-esteem. For example, the enhancement of personal, social, and professional skills and competencies reduces feelings of insecurity and social marginalization and promotes behaviors and attitudes that lead to a progressive increase in self-confidence and trust in others. This contributes to their empowerment as citizens with rights and duties, strengthening their capacities, confidence, vision, and leadership as members of a social group, in order to promote positive changes in the situations in which they live.

Users should find in this follow-up work support, guidance, and motivation for change, acceptance, and realistic comparison of expectations, which entails a reformulation of hypotheses, objectives, and actions, and an assessment of whether to remain in or leave the PIP.

Evaluation

As already mentioned, this program has a computer application in Galicia that collects data in a structured way on the social integration processes of addicted patients and those with dual pathology treated in the network centers, thus allowing for the following to be known and evaluated:

- **The structure**: It relates costs to objectives, reporting on the efficiency of the PIP.
- **The processes**: It relates activities to objectives, reporting on the effectiveness of the PIP.
- **The results**: It focuses on efficiency and analyzes the effects of the PIP and its benefits.

Through the computer application that manages this PIP program in Galicia, we can know the user's profile, sociodemographic data, health, and social variables; by recording actions/resources, we can obtain information about the areas where intervention has taken place (educational, occupational, social, and/or legal) and measure the effectiveness of the program by evaluating the reasons/causes for leaving the program (number of therapeutic discharges, dropouts, referrals, force majeure, etc.).

PIP METHODOLOGY

The social integration process is not subject to any specific treatment phase or care modality, meaning that individuals can be referred from different programs and/or services within the drug addiction care network and/or, where appropriate, from other care providers in coordination with the network's centers.

The program is strategically based on the demarcation of itineraries and the tutoring of follow-up through sequences, the **fundamental axes** of which are:

- The implementation of the objectives defined in the social diagnosis
- The establishment of a framework for tutoring and, where appropriate, "accompaniment," which can facilitate the efficient channeling of the itineraries to be followed
- The gradual, coherent, and synergistic deployment of actions, timed to coincide with the course of the patient's itinerary
- Continuous analysis and evaluation of the personalized social integration process

CRITERIA FOR ACCESSING THE PIP PROGRAM

Patients accessing a PIP must meet certain basic requirements:

- Presence of social deficits (socio-family, work, training, legal, etc.)
- Motivation and commitment to change in the areas and conditions agreed upon, with their participation
- Not be in a period of psychopathological, psychoemotional, and/or incapacitating substance use destabilization that prevents them from continuing the process

Achieving social integration through this rehabilitation process is the goal of us professionals who work with these individuals. However, we must accept that each individual needs a different social project, appropriate to their current situation, and that *it is they who decide how far they want to go* in their search for well-being, interaction, and integration into their environment.

Social incorporation should facilitate and empower individuals to achieve balance in their lives, where they can feel satisfied with their chosen level of well-being/integration.

REFERENCES

1. SICAD (Service for Intervention in Addictive Behaviors and Dependencies) 2014. Linhas Orientadoras para a Mediação Social e Comunitária no âmbito de Reinserção de Pessoas com Comportamentos Aditivos e Dependências. Lisbon: SICAD.
2. Xunta de Galicia. Programa de incorporación personalizado. Colección drogodependencias. Department of Health, 2003.
3. Left J, Warner Richard. Inclusão Social de Pessoas com Doenças Mentais. Coimbra: Almedina, 2008.
4. Capucha Luís. Exclusão social e acesso ao emprego: paralelas que podem convergir. Society and Work. 1998;3:60–69.
5. Capucha Luís. Grupos Desfavorecidos Face ao Emprego – Tipologia e Quadro Básico de Medidas Recomendáveis. Lisbon: IEFP, 1999.
6. Bruto da Costa A. Exclusões Sociais (5ª Edição). Lisbon: Gradiva, 2005.
7. Carvalho M. Ética Aplicada ao Serviço Social – Dilemase Práticas Profissionais. Lisbon: Pactor, 2016.
8. Carvalho M. Ser Assistente Social - Retrato(s) da Profissão. Lisbon: Pactor, 2020.
9. European Monitoring Centre for Drugs and Drug Addiction. Respuestas sanitarias y sociales a los problemas relacionados con las drogas. Una guía europea. EMCDDA, 2017.
10. Comas D. Los Programas de Integración socio-laboral de Drogodependientes. GID Group, 1995.
11. Funes and Artiaga J. Drogodependencias e Incorporación Social. "Propuestas para pensar y actuar." Madrid: Ed. National Plan on Drugs, 1991.
12. Mariño A. La Incorporación Social en Drogodependencias ¿una cuestión pendiente? Official Association of Diplomates in Social Work of Galicia, 1996.
13. Ituarte A. Procedimiento y proceso en trabajo social clíniCapítulo 7 Recomendaciones para una aproximación eficaz a la incorporación social 75 co. Colección Trabajo Social. Series Textos Universitarios.. Madrid: Editorial Siglo XXI, 1992.
14. Ló A. Contextos de Trabalho e Processos de Integração de Toxicodependentes, Lisbon: IDT, 2007.
15. Ander-Egg E. Investigación y Diagnóstico para el Trabajo Social. Humanitas, 1987.
16. Aguilar Ma J, Ander-Egg E. Evaluación de Servicios y Programas sociales. Madrid: Editorial Siglo XXI, 1992.

CHAPTER 8

Addressing the Legal and Ethical Aspects of Dual Pathology

8.1 MEDICAL-LEGAL ISSUES AND THEIR APPROACH IN DUAL PATHOLOGY: MEDICAL-LEGAL ASPECTS OF THE APPROACH TO DUAL PATIENTS

J. L. Fernández Hierro and M. J. Veiga Candán

In this chapter, we do not intend to conduct an exhaustive analysis of the legal problems that may arise from dual pathology, but simply to make some notes on the most frequent ones or to provide some new insights into what is already well known. We will also offer some reflections on advances in neuroscience and the possible influence they may have on our legal view of dual pathology. It is important to note that a diagnostic label is not particularly relevant from a psychiatric-legal point of view (even successive editions of the DSM warn in their introductory pages of the risk of using the manual in legal contexts). In assessing the criminal responsibility of an offender, it is not so much the diagnosis they receive that matters, but rather how the symptoms they suffer influenced the commission of the crime, i.e., how they altered their understanding of the circumstances surrounding it and whether the defendant had the capacity to choose another course of action in accordance with that understanding. For example, partial or complete diminished responsibility might be accepted in a patient with schizophrenia who commits an assault to defend themselves from those he delusionally believes are persecuting him to harm him. However, it is unlikely that mitigating or exonerating circumstances would apply if the same patient were to devise a complex financial engineering scheme to defraud investors. Nevertheless, in serious psychotic cases, it is common to consider their lack of criminal responsibility, but there are fewer cases of other types of disorders in which some degree of diminished responsibility is applied, and it is exceptional for them to be considered criminally irresponsible.

DOI: 10.4324/9781003786153-8

CRIMINAL CAPACITY OF MENTAL DISORDERS

Although highly criticized, categorical diagnoses allow us to quickly intuit which disorders most frequently generate criminal behavior and, therefore, are of greater psychiatric-legal interest.

It is well known (among professionals, not the general population) that people with mental illness are no more likely to commit violent acts or other crimes than those without mental illness. However, it should be noted that drug use significantly increases the likelihood that those who use drugs will exhibit some degree of violence. Unfortunately, the prevalence of substance abuse among our patients is higher than in the general population, which contributes to the perception that people with mental illness can be violent.

Psychotic Disorders

Schizophrenia is the most representative disease of what is popularly known as "insanity" and, in legal language, as "alienation," terms that emphasize the subject's inability to judge reality and conduct themselves appropriately. The (widely held) idea about the "dangerousness" of schizophrenic patients does not correspond to reality (see below, section "Assessment of the Risk of Violence"). However, schizophrenics sometimes develop violent behaviors characterized by their strangeness, apparent lack of logic and motivation, the way they are committed, and even their extreme violence. The peculiarities and striking nature of psychotic behaviors make their crimes rare, but they inevitably appear in the media, reinforcing the stigma of mental illness. Regarding the lack of motivation, criminology reminds us that there are no "unmotivated crimes," but rather crimes whose motives we do not know. These motives are sometimes delusional. Only on some occasions do we learn after the crime has been committed about the delusional content that allows us to understand what happened. These behaviors occur only during severe decompensations. That is why adequate treatment, patient adherence to it, and the collaboration of those around them are essential in order to provide early warning in the event of medication abandonment or relapse into drug use and, even more so, the reappearance of symptoms.

The criminal characteristics of patients with persistent delusional disorder are very different, given their irrefutable conviction about the delusional theme and the preservation of the rest of their lives. It is worth noting their sense of justice to the point that they place their moral standards above the law and even commit crimes (including murder) convinced that they are doing the right thing (given the seriousness of the affronts they believe they have suffered and their belief that exemplary punishment for their aggressors is necessary). For the professional, the crime of the jealous person who kills their partner may be "understandable" (we emphasize the quotation marks) in terms of illness. However, judges are unlikely to perceive as not criminally responsible someone who leads an otherwise perfectly orderly lifestyle.

In addition, some psychoactive substances are capable of inducing paranoid delusions that extend beyond the period of intoxication and after clarity of consciousness has been regained (e.g., jealous delusions in alcoholics, other paranoid content in cocaine users, etc.).

Affective Disorders

Crimes caused by depression are rare, especially when it comes to serious crimes. One exception is so-called extended suicide, in which the individual first kills a loved one, usually a son or daughter, and then commits suicide. These are usually severely depressed individuals who kill their loved ones with the intention of saving them from a future they believe will be full of suffering. It is, so to speak, a compassionate or altruistic homicide. However, depression of this nature is unlikely to be part of a dual disorder.

More likely is the commission of crimes and the influence of drugs during the manic phase of bipolar disorder: these range from assaults due to "manic rage" to financial crimes due to the financial risks they take, sexual crimes due to heightened libido, and even usurpation of titles or personalities (due to the delusional belief that they are in possession of them). These behaviors are usually not premeditated, and once recovered from the manic phase, the patient does not usually makes excuses and tends to show remorse (and even intense feelings of guilt after a shift to the depressive phase). These manic phases and symptoms can easily be precipitated by substance abuse. Doubts about criminal responsibility usually arise from situations in which the imbalance is not apparent (between critical periods, bipolar patients are as likely to commit crimes as the general population).

In manic episodes, "prodigality" is also of psychiatric-legal interest: the patient squanders their money or assets, which can lead to legal repercussions and a modification of their civil capacity (e.g., guardianship). This can in turn lead to litigation in which it is necessary to determine whether the alteration of their mental state was apparent when a financial transaction was carried out, from which it might be inferred that a third party maliciously took advantage of their vulnerability.

Organic Mental Disorders

Drug use is more likely to trigger a confusional syndrome in patients with traumatic brain damage. Injuries sometimes cause an apathetic syndrome that does not usually lead to legal problems. However, in many cases, the sequela is an orbitofrontal or "disinhibited" syndrome that often leads to illegal behavior.

Personality Disorders

The correlation between violence and psychoactive substance use is particularly evident in personality disorders. This close relationship manifests itself in several ways:

1. The use of psychoactive substances increases the likelihood of violent behavior, especially in unstable individuals, such as most people with personality disorders.
2. Violent behavior is often used to obtain drugs.
3. The use of violence is more frequent in certain environments where drugs proliferate.
4. The abuse of psychoactive substances and violent behavior may share some causal factors.

The cluster to which the patient belongs may modify these interactions: Cluster A patients tend to lead deficient and unsatisfactory lives, but it is not common for them to behaviors have significant legal repercussions, except in cases where comorbid substance use triggers transient psychotic symptoms, which can disinhibit them and even induce aggressive responses. The criminal profile of Cluster C patients ("Anxious/Fearful Subjects") is usually very low.

In short, most patients with personality disorders whose behavior has legal repercussions belong to Cluster B. Their clinical characteristics, especially with regard to interpersonal relationships, disregard for norms, lack of empathy, and, in general, their "predatory" style (especially in the case of psychopathy) explain much of their difficulties with the law. However, it is fair to recognize that the diagnostic criteria of categorical classifications put more emphasis on behavior and criminality than on these traits.

WHAT PERSONALITY TRAITS UNDERLIE THE GENESIS OF LEGAL PROBLEMS?

The previous section referred to categorical models. Dimensional diagnosis in personality disorders is based on the concept of "traits" and models based on factor analysis to isolate correlations between various traits. A trait is defined as a disposition to exhibit patterns of behavior and respond in a certain way to certain types of situations, and it involves a more or less stable way of behaving in real life. From this approach, *personality* is a set of traits that combine in a stable way in different situations, while *personality disorders* would be maladaptive variants that overlap imperceptibly with each other and with normality. We must begin by remembering that there is no consensus among authors on the specific name or content of the dimensions or factors, let alone the multiple facets that make up personality. Nevertheless, the reader will have no problem identifying which factors underlie each theory in the aspects discussed below.

Impulsivity

Impulsivity has been defined as a diminished ability to resist acting on impulses. This is often accompanied by a great difficulty in anticipating the repercussions of one's behavior and learning from "repeated negative consequences" (an aspect that will be fundamental in the psychiatric-legal field). Impulsivity is associated with a tendency to act without thinking, quick responses, impatience, and low tolerance for frustration. Even as a child, impulsive individuals will attract negative attention: poor school performance, difficulty sticking with a job they find boring (they spend as little time and effort as possible on it), and difficulty persisting in activities whose rewards are long-term. Impulsivity can also lead to accidents and other dangerous situations due to a lack of consideration of the associated risks.

Impulsivity is a common trait in various personality disorders, especially those in the former DSM Cluster B. Lack of impulse control is also associated with an increased risk of excessive consumption of legal or illegal psychoactive substances, as well as difficulties in managing money. On the other hand, drug use increases this impulsivity. Functional neuroimaging studies suggest that impulsive individuals have lower serotonergic activity in the prefrontal cortex, which translates into a decrease in inhibitory capacity over limbic structures, such as the amygdala.

However, to approach their legal consequences, a psychodynamic perspective may be useful. Psychoanalysis does not consider the drive without considering its object: the impulse is always directed at something or someone; a neutral drive is impossible.

Thus, if it is a represented **internal object**, impulsivity can lead to a "neurotic cascade" that puts one's own fortune at risk (with gambling addiction, legal conflicts of an economic nature may arise, or guardianship may even be sought); it attacks the pleasure principle (self-harm), physical integrity (reckless actions that in some cases could even be considered equivalent to suicide), or even life (suicide).

If the defect lies in the control of impulses directed at **external objects**, this neurotic cascade becomes a "psychopathic cascade," with much more obvious legal ramifications: attack on the property (kleptomania, theft) or on the sexual freedom of others; or posing a risk to health (drug trafficking), physical integrity (reckless driving), or even life (homicide).

Psychiatrists and psychologists often use the term *impulsivity*, but we know little about it. Our contribution in the legal field is limited. Even if we assert that a patient suffers from a serious impulse control deficit, this usually has little impact on exempting them from responsibility. Impulsivity is more likely to be considered an exculpatory factor, or at least a mitigating factor, when it accompanies a major psychiatric disorder (schizophrenia, bipolar disorder, or even full-blown drug intoxication). Impulsivity is rarely considered as an isolated character trait or as part of a personality disorder. There is a well-known anecdote about a judge who, when the psychiatric expert described a patient's criminal behavior as an "irresistible impulse," asked the expert, "And if there had been a police officer right behind him at that moment, would that impulse have been just as irresistible?"

We have numerous scales for assessing impulse control deficit: Barrat Impulsivity Scale (BIS-11), Buss-Durkee Hostility Inventory (BDHI), Impulsivity Rating Scale (IRS), Plutchik Impulsivity Scale (EI), Ramón y Cajal Impulse Control Scale (ECIRyC), etc. However, these are self-administered scales and their usefulness for expert assessment is questionable given the obviousness of the items and the absence of validity indices.

In the field of expert opinion, it is important to contrast this impulsivity in a wide range of current and past situations, especially if the impulsive reactions have been clearly maladaptive and harmful to the subject. For impulse control deficit to mitigate a person's criminal responsibility, two requirements must be met: (1) that high impulsivity explains why and how the unlawful conduct was carried out; and (2) that this is the patient's usual way of functioning and the person generally acts to their detriment. Therefore, before assessing the defendant, experts must have extensive knowledge of the ongoing legal proceedings, the subject's biography, and passages from it in which their impulsive reactions have clearly harmed them.

Aggression/Violence

Depending on what or who it is directed against, we divide **aggression** into:

- **Self-aggression**: This comprises suicidal and parasuicidal behaviors and self-harm. These are common reasons for admission to psychiatric hospitalization units, but they rarely have other legal repercussions.

- **Heteroaggression**: This encompasses a wide range of behaviors: against objects (hitting walls, doors, etc.); destructive acts (breaking objects, throwing them on the floor or out the window); or against people: verbal (insults, sarcastic comments) or physical actions (beatings, rape, murder).

(Because self-aggression has fewer legal repercussions, we will focus on heteroaggression.)

The WHO defined **violence** as: "the deliberate use of physical force or power, whether threatened or actual, against oneself, another person, a group, or a community, that either results in or has a high likelihood of resulting in injury, death, psychological harm, developmental disorders, or deprivation." This definition is somewhat contrived and artificial, and is the result of seeking to be both "politically correct" and to bring together aseptically nuances that are difficult to capture without referring to examples. We differentiate between:

- **Predatory violence**: Characterized by premeditation and the absence of motives (in the sense of a threat to one's own integrity). Remember that there are always motives; "there are no unmotivated crimes, only crimes whose motives we do not know." The motivations for a person to engage in violent behavior can be the desire for power, sex, revenge, or domination. People who exhibit predatory violence tend to carry it out in a cold manner and show only a minimal vegetative alert reaction. It is common in psychopaths.
- **Irritative or affective violence**: there is an increase in reactions of alertness, anger, or fear, lack of planning, and an imminent threat or the presumption of one, even when it is false. The goal of affective violence is to confront threats in order to improve survival. Human behavior is often compared to animal behavior to illustrate the differences between aggression and violence. In animals, "aggressive behavior" is an evolutionary requirement; it is necessary for the preservation of the species, that is, it is adaptive. Therefore, we do not always speak of aggression in a negative sense. In contrast, the term "violence" is often used pejoratively: violent is aggressive behavior that receives a negative social judgment. Only humans are capable of cruelty and malice, which is not only non-adaptive for the species, but also destructive. In other words, the term "violence" would apply to forms of aggression that have no biological utility, where adaptive value has been lost.

From a dimensional perspective, the personality traits most prone to violence are impulsivity, poor affective regulation, narcissism, and paranoia. With regard to the DSM-5 alternative model for PDs, the domains most implicated in violent behavior are negative affectivity (facets: emotional lability and distrust), detachment (facet: restricted affectivity), antagonism (insensitivity), and disinhibition.

Violent behavior often leads to requests for psychiatric assessment/reports. The most common type of assessment is a retrospective assessment (expert assessment: establishing imputability = "capacity to be guilty") or a current assessment (establishing the framework for serving a sentence or the suitability of security measures), also with a view to analyzing certain psychological elements related to the process (gender violence, sexual abuse, and assault).

Assessment of the Risk of Violence

It is increasingly common for judges to ask clinicians to give their opinion on an expert matter, i.e., to help them define the appropriate safety measures for the patient, given the violent behavior for which they have been tried. In other words, we are asked to assess the risk of that person exhibiting violent behavior again and what the best strategies are for controlling it—although the question is often phrased in terms of the patient's "dangerousness."

The term **dangerousness** is a legal concept, but it also forms part of everyday language. It refers to an individual's propensity to commit violent and dangerous acts, reflecting the future probability of violent behavior. It emerged in criminology during the Lombroso era (the concept of *temibilitá* proposed by Rafaelle Garofalo). Dangerousness is rooted in the psychological characteristics of the subject ("constant and active perversity") that explain their propensity for violence. Dangerousness was considered a pathological mental state of constitutional origin. Lombroso was representative of those who believed that criminals are born, not made. This would have notable repercussions on the criminal responsibility of criminals: to the extent that (in Lombroso's opinion) they are carriers of a birth defect, they would not be responsible for their acts. This implied a very deterministic position: if dangerousness could be accurately detected, recidivism could be prevented as long as those with this attribute were kept in confinement ("kidnapped" forever, in cases where they were "incorrigible," or "suppressed" when their incorrigibility made them "too dangerous," to use terms used by Lombroso). But it proved to be flawed, as the concept was very unspecific and led to many errors, both false positives and false negatives. Although he went down in history for his physiognomist theories, Lombroso deserves more credit for other achievements: while fighting with the Piedmontese army in the battles of Magenta and Solferino, he discovered the antiseptic properties of alcohol, a much more important and yet lesser-known contribution.

Today, we have changed our paradigm. We have moved from a model based on dangerousness to a model based on *assessing the risk of violence*. Predicting future violent behavior is not methodologically very different from predicting whether it will rain at the weekend in a certain place, whether interest rates will rise, or whether a patient with high blood pressure and diabetes will suffer a myocardial infarction. Our limitations in terms of prediction are considerable, but economists and meteorologists do not seem to be particularly effective in their long-term predictions, and yet we listen to them attentively. A storm, an AMI, or a violent act are uncertain events, the result of the interaction of various variables and difficult to predict. The possibility of making prediction a rigorous task will depend on the correct definition of the criterion to be predicted, in this case violence.

Violence includes cognitive, attitudinal, emotional, and motivational components that are interrelated. Furthermore, we can subdivide it according to the way it is exercised (psychological, physical, sexual, economic), and also according to the characteristics and context of the relationship between aggressor and victim. Each type of violence has specific risk and protective factors. Unlike dangerousness (a discrete, static, and generic variable that leads to decisions "all or nothing"), the risk of violence is a variable and specific *continuum* that allows for graduated decisions to be made about the future prognosis of violence. Dangerousness only allowed for two strategies: control (committal) or "nothing." Risk assessment broadens the possibilities for intervention because it allows procedures to be adjusted at the individual and contextual levels, thereby generating many more possibilities for intervention. Research today offers a wealth of data on these risk factors for violence.

The MacArthur Violence Risk Assessment Study

The *MacArthur Violence Risk Assessment Study* (Monahan *et al.*, 2001), conducted in the United States, is one of the most renowned studies on the risk of violence in the psychiatric population. John Monahan summarized the existing literature at the time of its publication. It is an excellent source of information on the main risk factors for violence in this population. It is a large-scale, prospective, multicenter study. To this end, a cohort of 1,136 psychiatric patients of both sexes aged 18–40 years, discharged from three hospitals in the US with a diagnosis of thought or affective disorder, substance abuse, or personality disorder, were followed for one year, regardless of whether or not they had a history of violence. While hospitalized, they were assessed for more than 130 potential risk factors for violence, the main criterion to be studied and predicted. Certain background information and biographical data were also explored prior to the patients' discharge. Some important conclusions drawn were as follows:

- In terms of violence, gender differences are quantitatively insignificant. The main differences are qualitative. Male violence is more frequently related to substance abuse and is more serious. Female violence is less serious and limited to the family environment, but it is not much less frequent.
- There are no differences regarding race or educational level, although violent subcultures do exist.
- Among people with a history of hospitalization for mental disorders, the prevalence of serious violent incidents over a one-year period is close to 30% (28%).
- Most violence occurs at home, and the victims are family members and friends.
- In hospitalized patients, the risk accumulates in the first few days of admission.
- Drug use is a more significant cause of violence than mental disorders themselves. Drug abuse increases the risk of violence in both patients with mental disorders and people without disorders, but substance use is more prevalent in people with mental disorders, which contributes to the false perception that violence is inherent to mental disorders.

- No mental disorder is directly associated with an increased risk of violence in the absence of drug use.
- Schizophrenia is less associated with violence than personality disorders, and among these psychopathy is most associated.
- Hallucinations do not have excessive influence, except for those of the "harmful" type.
- Delusional thinking does not seem to have a significant influence either.
- A suspicious attitude does increase the risk of violence somewhat.
- Violent fantasies about causing harm do have an influence.
- There is a highly predictive association with violence: history of previous violence + violent fantasies + substance use + having been a victim of physical abuse in childhood.
- The PCL-SV is one of the best predictors of violence in both the general population and the psychiatric population, especially when associated with substance use.

Emotional Instability

Emotional instability characterizes many Cluster B patients and can lead them to be both victims and aggressors. Logically, the risk will be greater in one direction or the other depending on the accompanying personality traits that define the specific personality disorder in question: **psychopaths** account for the highest proportion of aggressors, while **histrionic disorders** account for a large proportion of people whose emotional instability makes them prone to becoming victims of aggression. In **borderline disorder**, the outcome will be highly variable. Millon's clinical subtypes may be useful in guiding risk assessment:

- **Discouraged subtype**: Shares characteristics with dependent and avoidant patterns. They form submissive relationships, although their feelings of emptiness and fear of abandonment lead them to parasitic relationships and masochistic subordination. Therefore, they will be victims, and rarely aggressors.
- **Petulant subtype**: Combines characteristics of borderline personality disorder with those of negative or passive-aggressive personality disorder. This makes them impatient, unpredictable, pessimistic, complaining, resentful, envious, bitter, and dissatisfied. However, they tend to alternate their verbal attacks on those they consider do not love them enough with the introjection of their hostility.
- **Self-destructive subtype**: In addition to borderline characteristics, this subtype combines depressive or masochistic traits. It is systematically self-punitive. Individuals either isolate themselves from others or become extremely dependent and needy. Negative feelings tend to become self-destructive.

- **Impulsive subtype**: Combines borderline traits with those of histrionic and antisocial patterns. If they do not get constant attention, they intensify their strategies of seduction, irresponsibility, and impulsivity. They are capricious, superficial, and appear frivolous. Fear of loss causes them great distress, followed by despondency and irritability. They are potentially suicidal, but also potentially heteroaggressive.

Patients with striking emotional instability often generate a variety of legal problems: from determining whether or not an admission is considered involuntary (even if requested by the patient themselves) to trials to modify their civil capacity, including the patient's parental capacity with respect to a minor child, assessments of patients who have been victims of some type of abuse (unstable patients are often very vulnerable in this regard), and so on.

Lack of Responsibility

Failure to assume certain legal responsibilities may result in the patient becoming involved in legal proceedings about which we will probably have to report, either as clinicians (witnesses) or as experts. It is not uncommon to see abandonment of family obligations (neglect in the care of minors or the elderly, failure to pay alimony); of work obligations (civil or even criminal liability for damages caused by leaving one's job or failing to perform one's duties); of financial obligations (failure to pay taxes, fines, etc.); or of legal obligations (failure to appear in court, failure to return to prison after a furlough). However, we must be careful not to apply this trait only to marginalized individuals who do not assume responsibilities of various kinds. The worlds of business and politics are full of successful psychopaths. Only sometimes is their irresponsible behavior detected, and they rarely have problems with the law.

It is likely that the judicial authority will ask us to report about a patient we have treated who has evaded their responsibilities (we are often asked to do so at the request of their lawyer, who will fervently defend the causal relationship between a mental disorder and irresponsible behavior); but it should be remembered that if we are aware of a crime, even if it is a crime of omission of responsibility, we have an obligation to report it ex officio.

IMPUTABILITY AND CONTRIBUTIONS FROM NEUROSCIENCE: NEUROETHICS

Concept of Accountability

A **crime** is a "typically unlawful and culpable act for which the law prescribes a penalty." However, under certain circumstances, the judge may determine that a person is not criminally responsible for the crime they have committed. **Criminal responsibility** is the ability of human beings to understand that their behavior harms the interests of their fellow human beings and to adapt their actions to that understanding. It means attributing to someone the consequences of their actions, for which the act must be carried out with discernment, intention, and freedom. It is an exclusively legal concept on which the concepts of responsibility and guilt depend.

Those who lack these capacities, due to insufficient maturity (minors) or serious mental disorders, cannot be found guilty or held criminally responsible for their actions. According to another definition, criminal responsibility is the "ability to act culpably" (and without guilt there is no crime). "A person acts culpably if, according to the legal system, they could have acted differently from how they did" (Rodríguez Devesa). This "ability of a person to be held accountable for their actions" has its origins in Aristotelian thinking. It depends on the sum of: capacity to understand + volitional freedom. That is, the capacity to understand the illegality of an act (understands what they are doing) + capacity to direct their actions in accordance with that understanding (knows what they are doing and is free to choose to perform the act, i.e., "wants" to do it). Psychiatry can be useful in no other legal concept.

Our penal code does not define criminal responsibility. It merely lists causes that restrict or nullify it: (1) mental abnormalities or disorders (a mere psychiatric diagnosis is not sufficient; it is necessary to determine the influence of the symptoms on the subject's ability to understand the situation and on their freedom to choose their actions); (2) temporary mental disorder; (3) complete intoxication by alcohol or drugs and withdrawal syndrome (provided that they were not sought for the purpose of committing a crime); (4) a state of necessity or insurmountable fear; (5) acting in a state of rage, blindness, or passion; and (6) serious alterations in perception that severely alter the awareness of reality.

In the case of drug use, the intoxication requirement involves three elements: a biological or psychiatric component (a state of "full" intoxication at the time of committing the crime), a psychological component (that intoxication makes it impossible to understand the unlawful nature of the conduct or to act in accordance with that knowledge), and a negative requirement (that intoxication was not caused for the purpose of committing the crime).

It is not always easy to determine whether a criminal act is symptomatic of a mental disorder. As we have already seen, substance abuse precipitates decompensation and increases the risk of violence and criminality in most mental disorders. However, the interaction is particularly relevant in personality disorders. The latter are not usually considered "insanity," as conceived by the previous penal code to consider a reduction in criminal responsibility. The "doctrine of free will" prevailed, from which it is difficult to justify that those suffering from a personality disorder lacked free will when their criminal behavior occurred. The "new" code, instead of insanity, uses the more open concepts of "alteration" or "anomaly." This, together with the inclusion of personality disorders in psychiatric classifications and the growing knowledge of the neurobiology underlying them, has led to the questioning of the aphorism that personality disorders are almost always imputable.

The current penal code allows for the possibility that any trait, anomaly, alteration, or personality disorder might be grounds for a reduction or even exemption from criminal responsibility. However, for this to apply, the trait, anomaly, alteration, or disorder must be sufficiently severe that the person who committed the act did not understand the illegality of the act or found it impossible to act in accordance with that understanding.

It is generally assumed that patients with personality disorders do not suffer from sensory perception disorders, nor from disorders of thought form or content, nor from severe cognitive impairments or isolated impairments of functions such as attention, concentration, and memory. They are people who understand and reason correctly, with full awareness of reality. Therefore (we repeat, *a priori*), their symptoms do not affect their ability to understand the scope of their actions.

Another question is whether their symptoms allow them to act in accordance with this understanding, taking into account the characteristics of their actions, which are often impulsive and "irresistible." It can be really difficult to determine whether a particular behavior was uncontrollable as a result of the personality disorder ("irresistible impulse," subject to a reduction in criminal responsibility) or whether the person, even taking into account their personality traits, was capable of inhibiting their behavior and behaving differently than they did ("unresisted impulse," criminally responsible). Case law assumes that personality disorders do not diminish criminal responsibility unless they coexist with other mental disorders that cause significant cognitive or volitional alterations.

The small proportion of judgments recognizing diminished criminal responsibility, as well as the exceptional cases involving total exemption from criminal responsibility have occurred in cases with comorbid diagnoses of mental retardation, organic mental disorder, and drug use. It is accepted that a diagnosis of personality disorder facilitates more impulsive and thoughtless behavior; but, for purposes of assessing accountability, a mere diagnosis of personality disorder can be considered of little relevance. This low consideration is based on a pragmatic argument already echoed by Kurt Schneider: given the high prevalence of these disorders and their poor prognosis (especially in relation to psychopathy and almost certain therapeutic failure), it would be dangerous for the sake of social welfare to leave the door open to their non-imputability. This is reflected, for instance, in the wording of the Supreme Court ruling of November 23, 1996 (the *Boixos nois* case):

> In psychopathy, the dilemma between guilt and prevention is evident in a paradigmatic way. From the point of view of guilt, the abnormality of the psychopath could lead to a reduction in punishment. From the point of view of prevention, however, certain psychopathic personalities are particularly frightening and call for strong security measures. It is therefore necessary to exercise an option which, in a state governed by the rule of law, can only be the strict maintenance of the principle of guilt.

In other words, personality disorders are no longer classified under axis II; but, in terms of their impact on criminal responsibility, they remain "second-class" disorders. Furthermore, lawyers are wary of the lack of agreement among professionals regarding diagnoses, as well as the modification of criteria over the course of a few years. This is especially true given that some of those criteria are often seen by them as "normal" variations in human thinking and behavior. Perhaps they themselves have identified to some degree with certain diagnostic symptoms and criteria, with the added difficulty of determining at what point on *the continuum* these common traits can be considered pathological.

Neuroethics

Neuroscience is providing more and more data on brain function and how it is altered in some mental disorders.

When it comes to criminal responsibility, most studies have focused on personality disorders, especially psychopathy. However, contributions from neuroscience might call into question an idea repeated so often it has become an aphorism: that psychopaths are criminally responsible because they understand the illegality of their actions and have chosen to act in that way ("free will"). But if psychopaths suffer from abnormalities in brain function that prevent them from feeling empathy, they might not be entirely free when it comes to engaging in certain behaviors that we consider unlawful, even cruel.

Knowledge of the brain mechanisms in relation to human behavior has led to the emergence of a new discipline, **neuroethics**, described in 2002 as "the study of ethical, legal, and social issues that arise when scientific findings about the brain are applied to medical practice, legal interpretations, and health policy." I propose a little game: in the above definition, replace "the brain" with "medicine"... and you will have a good definition of "bioethics."

For Professor Adela Cortina, neuroethics has two meanings:

- The **ethics of neuroscience**, which seeks to develop an ethical framework to regulate neuroscientific research and the application of knowledge in this field to human beings
- The **neuroscience of ethics**, which refers to the impact of neuroscientific knowledge on our understanding of ethics itself, i.e., the neural basis of morality and ethical reasoning—e.g., the substrate of free will

Let's review some of the lessons neuroscience has taught us in recent years.

Kevin Dutton's thesis (*The Wisdom of Psychopaths: What Saints, Spies, and Serial Killers Can Teach Us About Success*) is that being a psychopath, someone who lacks the empathy, compassion, and self-awareness that blocks ordinary people in difficult situations, is not a bad thing. Psychopaths are fearless, cold-blooded, and capable of making decisions in high-pressure situations where others collapse. Dutton invites us to think of psychopathic traits as dials on a mixing board. If we turn all the equalizers up to the max, the noise is unbearable, but if we adjust the mixer with a few touches of boldness, ability to concentrate in extreme situations, lack of empathy, and mental toughness, we can get, for example … a good surgeon.

This reminds us of **Joshua Green**'s famous *trolley* moral dilemmas: the possibility of preventing a train from running over five people by diverting it to a track where there is only one person (case 1) or by throwing another person onto the track (case 2). Almost everyone would pull the switch in case 1, but only those with psychopathic traits would throw someone onto the track (case 2). This suggests that there are two kinds of empathy, a "cold" kind (case 1) involving the prefrontal cortex and posterior parietal cortex, and a "warm" kind (case 2) involving emotional centers of the brain such as the amygdala.

Psychopaths continue to judge case 2 in an impersonal and cold manner—using their prefrontal cortex. There is an evolutionary explanation: throughout human evolution, direct violence against other members of the clan was inhibited. Throwing a person under a train triggers these aversive emotional responses, but moving the tracks and derailing it does not, because it bears no resemblance to circumstances that we or our ancestors have experienced. Another practical example occurred during the Holocaust: if genocide was carried out by very direct methods (e.g., shootings), Nazi soldiers suffered. When they switched to using gas chambers and had no contact with the victims, these atrocities ceased to affect the perpetrators.

In another famous experiment, by **Stanley Milgram**, a "subject" (actually an actor) supposedly received electric shocks, following instructions from "teachers" ("ordinary citizens" who are the real test subjects) with the aim of improving the subject's memory. Upon hearing the subject's screams, many participants refused to continue, but others went on to administer the shocks. According to Milgram, the conditions necessary to achieve this harmful behavior are: presenting some rational justification for the undesirable action, having an "authority" indicate it, manipulating language (it is not about "harming" other people, but "helping" them), and facilitating the dilution of responsibility so that it is never attributable to a single individual.

Another well-known experiment from some time ago is the "Stanford Prison Experiment." **P. Zimbardo** wondered what would happen if a "good" person were placed in a "bad" environment. Would good people dominate and change the evil of the environment, or would it corrupt even the good? He selected 75 psychologically "stable" students from Stanford University and randomly assigned them to be either prisoners or prison guards. Very soon, some prisoners rebelled … and the guards began to repress them and commit abuses that escalated. The experiment, which was supposed to last two months, lasted only six days. Zimbardo believes that, unlike the Milgram experiment, in his there is no authority figure to obey; subjects simply get carried away by what the group is doing, by intense emotional states, or by situational cues that incite violence. In Zimbardo's words, "The evil situation triumphed over good people."

The motor cortex, responsible for the precise control of our own movements, is activated simply by observing the movements of another person. **Iacoboni** found that mirror neurons are activated to a greater degree when the motor actions we see are not isolated, but are framed in a specific context, which means that these neurons have the ability to interpret the intentions of the other person. This constitutes the biological basis of what is now known as the **theory of mind** or **mentalization**. The actions performed by a subject are accompanied by the perception of the intentions that drive them. Thus, the action itself is associated with the intention that set it in motion, and when another person performs the same action, the mirror neurons evoke in the observer the intention associated with it. The ability to interpret the intentions of others is essential for successful social interaction.

The theory of mind or mentalization is defined as the psychological ability we possess to represent in our minds the mental states of others (thoughts, desires, beliefs, intentions, knowledge) and, through this psychological representation, to explain and predict their behavior. Theory of mind enables individuals to act without difficulty in their interpersonal relationships and allows them to anticipate or predict the emotional reactions of others, which is essential in the mating process. The proper development of the theory allows us to use metaphors and recognize sarcasm or irony in others. Patients with neuropsychiatric disorders, such as schizophrenia, autism, Asperger's syndrome, or personality disorders, have difficulty perceiving the emotions of others, which is why they behave rudely, lack subtlety, lack compassion (or empathy), or are egocentric or aggressive.

Empathy, compassion, and understanding are necessary to raise awareness. It is an emotional response that is more appropriate to the situation experienced by the other person than to one's own situation; it is putting oneself in the other person's place. "I can feel what you feel, even though I realize that it is not my feeling." We are born with mechanisms that allow us to be empathetic, but we do not know why some people are more empathetic than others. It might have an evolutionary purpose. For example, parents need to realize if their children are suffering in order to help them. But there are cases, such as in war, where it is necessary to be able to detach oneself. So we need a balance, and in certain contexts too much empathy can be negative. According to some studies, when a person with autism observes emotional expressions, certain areas of the brain are more activated than in people without autism. without autism: autistic people are "overwhelmed" by the emotions of others (the opposite of the view that used to be held of people with autism). At the other end of the continuum, patients with schizophrenia show less activation of these brain areas, making them more indifferent to the emotions of others.

Theory of Mind and Psychopathy

Psychopaths are emotionally cold and superficially charming and irresponsible, traits that are present from childhood. One might assume that these individuals would be incapable of empathy because they have "innate" alterations in the development of their ability to "mentalize." But some studies suggest that psychopaths develop theory of mind skills in such a way that allows them to understand the emotional states of others in a purely instrumental way, avoiding empathy; psychopaths decide when to be empathetic. **Christian Keysers**, using functional magnetic resonance imaging, observed that when viewing certain scenes, psychopaths showed activation of specific brain regions, but to a lesser extent than the control group. When expressly asked to be empathetic, the psychopaths achieved the same levels of empathy in the test as the control group. The author interprets this as meaning that "psychopathy may not be so much an inability to be empathetic, but rather a reduced propensity to do so spontaneously." The results of this study suggest that the charming yet cruel personality typical of psychopaths may be due to this ability to be empathetic "only when they want to be." In other words, they have no problem perceiving the feelings of others (the "recognition" phase of empathy), but they can choose whether their behavior is empathetic in accordance with that perception (the "response" phase of empathy).

This leads us to reflect on the **accountability of psychopaths**. For someone to be accountable, they must have the empathy necessary to understand that by breaking the law, they cause harm to another. Psychopaths understand the law, but do not feel it as their own. Therefore, given these alterations in the functioning of certain areas of the brain, it can be argued that psychopaths are not free to choose their behavior. Let's take a closer look:

- As **Baron-Cohen** (*Zero Empathy*) states, the concept of evil is difficult to explain if we do not relate it to the concept of empathy. We can all "switch off" our empathy, for example, in order to work while a beggar asks for money at the door of our office. This slight and temporary disconnection is possible even in "empathetic" people. However, empathy is not actually a binary operation (on/off). It is not like a light switch, but rather like a potentiometer that regulates the intensity of the light. It is a dimensional quality, whose variability in the population can be expressed by a normal distribution (Gaussian bell curve): some people are permanently at the lower end of this dimension and we consider them "evil" or cruel. In Baron-Cohen's opinion, this can be observed (with other nuances that differentiate them) in psychopaths, narcissists, and patients with borderline personality disorder.

What determines where each of us falls on the empathy spectrum? Various regions of the brain and pathways may be involved. The disorder may be genetically determined (not through an "empathy gene"), but environmental factors (attachment styles) are also thought to have a significant influence. And this brings us to the crux of the matter. If a person with "zero empathy" suffers from some form of neurobiological disability, should they be held accountable if they commit a crime? If this disability prevents them from seeing the impact of their actions on the feelings of others do they deserve punishment? Baron-Cohen himself clarifies that punishment will be necessary to protect society—that the "disabled" person will repeat the crime—to make clear society's disapproval of such actions, and to convey a sense of justice to the victim and their loved ones. He also asks whether this disability is treatable and whether these serious deficits in empathy can be recovered.

Gazzaniga has also reflected extensively on this topic: "If traffic arises from cars and ultimately limits them, does the mind not limit the brain that generated it?" Remember that there is no absolute hierarchy in the brain's organization, no "general in command" of all brain systems (and we are not the "bosses" of our brains, as we tend to think): there are countless centers, "modules" that make important decisions.

Consciousness dynamically integrates a multitude of processes and systems that shape our conscious experience "on the fly." But if we are made up of an infinite number of modules, why do we have a sense of uniqueness? That psychological unity we experience arises from what he calls the "interpreter module," which generates explanations about perceptions, memories, and actions, and the links between them all. This allows for a personal narrative. This interpreter module is exclusively human and is the responsibility of the left hemisphere. Our subjective consciousness arises from the left hemisphere's relentless effort to bring order and explain fragments of information. But consciousness is a slow process; what has reached it … has already happened. This means that we construct our theories about ourselves after the events have taken place. The brain acts before we are aware of it. Even when the subject does not know the reasons for their actions, they are capable of inventing an explanation that seems appropriate for their behavior. Through brain neuroimaging, it is possible to predict what our behavior will be.

"Our interpreter module is cheating us," he says. It has created the illusion of the self, the feeling that we are the "commanding general" of all systems and make "free" decisions (a feeling that stems from the fact that we experience our brain as our own, which is otherwise a healthy experience). Perhaps we should abandon the concept of "free will," Gazzaniga reminds us. But radical determinism, according to which our behavior is the inevitable consequence of the laws of nature, physical forces, etc., is also invalid. Why strive for self-control if our behavior is predetermined? In other words, "not only do we believe that we control our actions through free will, but it is good for everyone to maintain that belief."

The solution proposed by Gazzaniga is to consider conscious thought as an **emergent property**, independent of all brain systems; it is on a higher plane than them, although ultimately dependent on them. This emergent property is not "mystical" in nature (he warns us), but rather involves the transition from one level of organization to another. Recalling his analogy with the circulation of vehicles, "you cannot analyze traffic at the level of the parts of a car." In the same way, responsibility is a dimension that arises from social exchange, that is, from the interaction of more than one brain. Responsibility and freedom are not found in the brain, but in the space between several brains. Control (and, by extension, self-control) does not appear at the level of neural mechanisms. It is an emergent property that arises from the brain and in turn limits it. Developing the cooperation necessary for the survival of large social groups caused humans to become less aggressive (Hare and Tomasello's process of "self-domestication"). This would have been incorporated into our genes, preferentially selecting systems that inhibit aggression: the social group limits behavior and influences the genome.

> And this is where the dilemma arises: **Who is responsible for the crime? The person or their brain?** Our knowledge of the brain is constantly growing, and yet forensic medicine continues to operate with concepts as old as volition, free will, and the "M'Naghten rule".

Based on current knowledge of neuroscience in a deterministic way, guilt would not exist, and without guilt, there should be no punishment or penalties. Case law dictates that past decisions by high courts set the path for future rulings in similar cases. But those rulings that created case law were handed down at a time when current scientific knowledge about the brain was not available.

How can this knowledge be explained to judges and juries? Defense attorneys are increasingly basing their arguments on neurobiological findings. Some studies suggest that judges and juries are more receptive to expert testimony when it is accompanied by brain images (CT, MRI, etc.) that "illustrate" the case. A more "scientific" explanation runs the risk of being disregarded in the absence of neuroimaging. There has been a tendency to impose lighter punishments after receiving explanations about determinism (if we convey that the offender is not ultimately responsible for their actions, but that these were caused by some alteration in their brain, it is judged that, after all, they do not deserve such a severe punishment). Nevertheless, it should be remembered that abnormal neuroimaging does not justify aggressive behavior or a lack of responsibility. If the judicial system considers that frontal lobe injuries exonerate an individual from their violent acts, this may provide an excuse for people with such injuries to commit crimes that they would not otherwise commit—or justify prophylactic measures being imposed on them.

It should be remembered that technical tests are admissible in courts of law only when they are widely accepted by the scientific community (Daubert Standard of Validity). However, the connectivity of our brains varies greatly from one person to another. When faced with an injury to a specific area of the brain in a particular patient, determining which circuits or functions may be affected is purely probabilistic. Therefore, these techniques are not particularly useful on their own. same ones used to explain whether a patient is criminally responsible or not. In the words of J. Fins and N. D. Schiff, "we should not place too much faith" in these techniques.

At the 2002 meeting of experts in San Francisco, considered the "founding document" of neuroethics, it was noted that in light of new findings "in fields ranging from genetics and brain imaging to the diagnosis and prevention of disease ... Neuroethics should examine how doctors, judges and lawyers, insurance company executives and politicians, as well as society in general, deal with all these findings."

Experts must be the "transmission belt" for the prudent application of scientific knowledge in court, responsible for reducing the wide gap between science and law in terms of language, objectives, and methodology.

We mentioned above how various studies show that the brain drives us to behave in a certain way even before we consciously make a decision. But **Brass** and **Haggard** have located a region in the dorsomedial frontal cortex related to "the capacity for self-control through the modulation of brain areas involved in motor preparation." The connections between this region and the premotor areas can inhibit actions, a predisposition that is greater in some individuals than in others. Free will would be demonstrated in our ability to "veto" a behavior whose potential for movement preparation has already been initiated by the brain. Or, as **Ramachandran** suggests, conscious minds may not have free will but rather "free non-will." There are people who do not inhibit their impulses, even though they can (irresistible impulse versus unresisted impulse). What magnitude of prefrontal injury is required to overcome the inhibitory function and attenuate responsibility? Neuroscience will never find the brain correlate of responsibility because it is a faculty of the person, not the brain. Most of us obey the law. Criminals do not. But they do not commit their crimes in front of the police. They are able to inhibit their impulses in the presence of law enforcement officers, based on their prior experience. In any case, science currently has no reliable evidence regarding the mental state of a defendant at the time they committed the crime. And if there were such evidence, various ethical and legal questions would arise: Is it lawful for judicial investigators and/or experts to be commissioned by the court to "read" an individual's mind? Would it be considered an invasion of privacy? What value would a court put on a person's refusal to undergo this type of test?

Perhaps the old debate between free will and determinism is nothing more than a (new) philosophical debate about what freedom is. The definition of freedom is very difficult for philosophers, let alone neuroscientists. It should also be remembered that "neuro-reductionism" often does not come from neuroscience, but is the result of excessive simplification by popularizers and the media.

We can simplify (greatly) the issue by assuming that we first make conscious decisions, even though when we carry out our actions, they are the result of millisecond discharges of action potentials in complex neural networks (and are therefore unconscious). Free will would be nothing more than "the planning of meaningful actions in the context of our goals."

Rapid advances in neuroscience tend to shift psychiatry away from the mind and toward the brain. Conveying to patients the idea that their illness is caused by a brain dysfunction that can only be treated with medication is a serious mistake. Not only is it false, it is also iatrogenic. In this way, the diagnosis becomes a label that the patient can adopt as part of their identity, justifying a lack of proactive attitude. Patient autonomy (a concept that has no place in the deterministic model) is essential to the therapeutic process.

Returning to the issue of accountability, Gazzaniga reminds us that our society lives in a fragile balance. If a deterministic explanation is accepted and the the offender as ultimately responsible for their behavior, Can a society function without punishment for those who break the rules? Let us remember that collaborative behavior was successful from an evolutionary perspective because it made sense at the group level (though not at the individual level). But without punishment, collaboration cannot be sustained. Recall Tomasello's theory of self-domestication: punishment allowed for the selection of the most collaborative temperaments.

We can analyze what a conviction should look like. There are three approaches:

- In *retributive justice*, each specific crime corresponds to an "objective" punishment (the offender gets "what they deserve").
- *Restorative justice* requires the offender to compensate for the damage caused.
- *Utilitarian justice* aims to deter the offender or others so that they learn from the example and the crime is not repeated. Prison sentences, fines, restraining orders, and professional disqualification may all be imposed; but utilitarian justice also contemplates rehabilitation through treatment or education.

This is where neuroscience might come into play. If we accept deterministic theories ("It wasn't the defendant's fault, it was his brain's fault"), punishment is not justified from the perspective of retributive justice, but it is justified from the perspective of utilitarian justice. And since it is considered that there are evolutionary reasons for punishing those who have caused harm, we can justify the sentences handed down by the legal system even if they do not represent a guide to moral truth (recall the ruling in the *Boixos nois* case cited a few pages above). Furthermore, although studies suggest that there are alterations in the brain function of psychopaths that predispose them to criminal behavior, these are currently only more or less possible hypotheses, and have not yet acquired the status of unquestionable scientific truth.

Meanwhile, we continue to consider the pragmatic criterion regarding the accountability of psychopaths because, as William Faulkner said, "You can trust bad people: they don't change."

The debate on the legal aspects of dual pathology often raises questions about the criminal activity of patients, their accountability, etc. However, there are more everyday issues with psychiatric-legal implications that often go unnoticed. One example is the (in)voluntariness of treatment, especially hospital admissions.

INVOLUNTARY ADMISSION OF PATIENTS WITH DUAL PATHOLOGY

Obviously, only medical reasons should justify the admission of patients to psychiatric hospitalization units. In practice, admission is determined by the patient's instability and difficulties in containing them at other levels of care (suicidal thoughts or attempts, hetero-aggressiveness, and psychotic symptoms). However, it is not uncommon for other reasons to be added or even to prevail: judicial authorizations processed due to family or social alarm generated by the patient's behavior and even judicial security measures as an alternative to the sentence that would result from criminal behavior.

In What Cases Should Admission Be Considered Involuntary?

It is not right to persuade a patient to sign a voluntary admission form when they are clearly not in a fit state to do so. If, shortly after admission, the patient requests voluntary discharge, would we grant it? Another widespread mistake is to follow the old idea that patients with certain conditions should not be admitted (drug use or personality disorders are common examples, especially if they are associated). Some clinicians cite the debatable effectiveness of admitting patients with dual pathology to reject these admissions (but this has more to do with their own nihilism than with clinical reality). They even add that if there are extraordinary circumstances that force us to admit them, this should be very brief. But scientific evidence is far from confirming this. It is true that making hospitalization too easy for some patients can reinforce attitudes of seeking care or dependence on others to cope with problems (external locus of control). However, Tyrer and Simmonds found that when outpatient treatment puts too much emphasis on avoiding hospitalization, the results are worse. The opposite tendency is also not uncommon: admitting patients uncritically for fear of the legal consequences of not doing so (defensive medicine), citing the risk of self- or other-directed aggression, despite the conviction that the risk is remote.

It is true that involuntary admission is more common in psychotic disorders than in affective disorders and personality disorders (in the latter, it is becoming less and less uncommon) and rare in other pathologies. But the law does not refer to diagnoses. Nor does it mention terms such as "reality testing" or "self- or hetero-aggressive risk." In other words, the criterion for involuntary admission in our legislation is the patient's lack of competence. "Safety" criteria do not apply.

Involuntary Admission from a Bioethical Perspective

The patient's **informed consent** is required prior to any diagnostic or therapeutic procedure. Admission to a psychiatric unit cannot be the exception. The three elements that constitute informed consent are (1) the patient's **voluntary** decision after having received (2) sufficient quantitative and qualitative **information** and (3) the patient's **competence** to give consent.

The Civil Procedure Act (LEC) 1/2000, in the chapter on "Processes concerning the capacity of individuals" are dealt with in Article 763 on *"Commitment due to mental disorder of a person who is not in a position to decide for themselves … ."* This refers to the patient's lack of competence to decide whether or not to be admitted to a psychiatric hospitalization unit (PHU). Remember that **competence** is "the patient's mental state that allows them to understand the situation they are facing, the values at stake, the alternatives, and the foreseeable consequences of each of them, in order to then make, express, and defend a decision that is consistent with their own scale of values," which will then be an autonomous decision. The term *autonomy* quickly brings us back to the **principles of bioethics**: non-maleficence, justice, beneficence, and autonomy. These are *prima facie* principles, i.e., they are mandatory as long as they do not conflict with each other. Ethical dilemmas arise when two or more of them conflict. If, in a given clinical situation, there is an indication for admission according to *lex artis* (beneficence) and the patient voluntarily accepts (autonomy), there is no ethical dilemma; the two principles operate in the same direction. If the professional believes admission is indicated and the patient refuses, the patient's autonomy must prevail as long as the patient is competent. And a patient is competent until proven otherwise; hence the need to argue in the medical record the reasons why we decided that admission should be involuntary. In cases where it is the patient who requests admission, and the professional does not consider it appropriate, there is no reason to admit them: autonomy does not take precedence over non-maleficence. A competent patient has the right to reject the alternative proposed to them (beneficence), but their preferences (autonomy) do not oblige us to perform an act that goes against *lex artis* (non-maleficence).

Competence must be assessed in relation to specific decisions at specific times: we assess whether a patient is competent at this precise moment to make this specific decision (the more complex the decision to be made, the more functionally preserved they must be to be considered competent).

Sometimes, patients with dual pathology have real difficulty in appreciating the risk of relapse in their consumption and show unusual optimism about their ability to maintain abstinence even in unfavorable circumstances. However, it is highly debatable whether this is sufficient to justify involuntary hospitalization. For a patient with dual pathology to have difficulty either understanding their clinical situation or processing information rationally (two of the criteria for competence), they must be in a state of acute intoxication. In this case, priority should be given to attention to possible physical complications and, therefore, to emergency care (or even care in an internal medicine ward) rather than possible (involuntary) admission to a psychiatric hospital unit. Nor should most detoxification and withdrawal treatments be subject to judicial authorization, as admission should be expressly accepted by the patient. Therefore, in dual pathology, involuntary admission should only be considered in situations where, if the patient is consuming psychoactive substances, they suffer a decompensation of other pathologies they may have (e.g., a psychotic episode) that makes them incompetent to make the decision about the admission they need.

Sometimes the judge understands that the patient-is not criminally responsible because at the time of committing the crime you had mental disorders that prevented you from knowing the illegality of your conduct or behaving differently. It is possible that alternative **security measures** may be imposed in lieu of the sentence, which may be outpatient measures or include psychiatric hospitalization (for a maximum period not exceeding the sentence that would have been imposed if he had been considered criminally responsible). A commonly associated problem is that hospitalization is prolonged even after the medical condition that led to criminal responsibility has subsided. After all, under the influence of psychoactive substances, many conditions are temporary. What should be done in these cases? Something similar occurs with the adoption of restraining orders in certain cases, for example when drug use has caused a psychotic breakdown and violent behavior has occurred in the family environment as a result. In these cases, doesn't a restraining order leave the patient helpless?

OTHER MEDICAL-LEGAL ASPECTS OF DUAL PATHOLOGY

Just a brief note on other common problems. Professionals' obligations regarding confidentiality (professional secrecy) may be waived in certain circumstances: to protect a greater good, in defense of the general interests of society. This includes epidemiological risks to the population (e.g., in cases of HIV infection) or the need to cooperate with the justice system: in criminal jurisdiction, assistance to the justice system takes precedence over professional secrecy, although the limits of the information that judges need to perform their duties must be very strictly defined. We must be very restrictive in the data we provide, limiting ourselves to those that are strictly relevant to the legal proceedings in progress. Along similar lines is the requirement of medical records by court order for criminal proceedings. It should be remembered that the obligation of professional secrecy for doctors is recognized in the Spanish Constitution and that breaching it is severely punished. However, there is a lack of specific regulation, which can lead to professionals being defenseless and finding themselves immersed in ethical conflicts when faced with the dilemma of disclosing information in court.

Another noteworthy topic, although not analyzed in depth in this chapter, is the prescription of off-label medications. This practice, which is rare in other fields, is the rule rather than the exception in patients with dual diagnosis. Most of these patients are prescribed medications that are only authorized for use in other conditions. It should be noted that although there is literature supporting such use in these cases, it must be justified in the medical record and the patient's informed consent must be obtained in accordance with the Patient Autonomy Law.

IMPLICATIONS OF LEGISLATION ON THE TREATMENT OF PATIENTS WITH DUAL DISORDERS

Although it may seem obvious, experience shows us that we must always remember that dual pathology (let us emphasize the term *pathology*) is the coexistence in the same person of an addictive disorder and another mental disorder—even though scientific evidence shows that these are not two diseases but different clinical manifestations with a common basis. Underlying neurobiological and environmental processes condition behavior. It is not a "vice"—a problem of "willpower" or "weakness of character"—as ignorance continues to claim. Rather, "No one chooses to have an addiction."

It is estimated that one-third of people diagnosed with a mental disorder will at some point in their development present a disorder associated with the use of psychoactive substances. Conversely, more than half of people who use psychoactive substances will meet the criteria for an additional diagnosis of a mental disorder. In the case of SUD and personality disorders, comorbidity is even more significant. The frequent legal implications of these diagnoses have already been mentioned above, and their coexistence is not additive but multiplicative in nature.

The very concept of dual disorder implies the need for a multidisciplinary model that integrates the two problems, rather than an ineffective model of parallel networks (one for mental health and another for addiction), as has unfortunately been the norm. To the extent that society and the politicians who represent it understand this, effective preventive and therapeutic measures can be implemented, rather than reducing the approach to the problem to a punitive one. But perhaps politicians need to take into account that voters' decisions have the same neurophysiological mechanisms as their own. Among other things, the brain has an enormous tendency to ignore all information that challenges our beliefs and could cause us to change our minds. That is why politicians appeal more to the emotional than to the rational.

In this regard, it is not surprising that terms such as "drug legalization" have always generated controversy, polarizing society around opinions on whether such a strategy would increase the use of psychoactive substances, its impact on their control and black market, on the possibilities of preventing their use, or the stigmatization of users.

However, methadone maintenance programs (MMPs), needle exchange programs (NEPs), the establishment of supervised drug consumption rooms ("narcosalas"), and other, similar harm reduction strategies have managed to focus attention on tertiary prevention. Although they are often criticized by some sectors of society, their results are undeniable, not only in terms of user health but also at the social level: the possibilities for social reintegration, the reduction of stigma, and, it must be said, the reduction of conflict perceived by the most reluctant have contributed to their gradual acceptance. Today, many governments have implemented harm reduction laws, policies, and programs. But we must remember that it is the needs of the consumer and not the demands of the most critical voices that are the most important criterion to take into account.

An example of how a decisive health policy health policy in this field can completely change the landscape is provided by Portugal. In 2001, our neighboring country changed the law that established prison sentences for the purchase and possession of drugs for personal use. It was concluded that drugs will never cease to exist in society and that the best way to reduce the harm they cause is not to ban them, but to decriminalize their possession and consumption. Portugal thus became a global benchmark in the fight against this problem. João Goulão is considered the mastermind behind this model, which he himself defined as "humanistic and pragmatic."

The new law converted what was previously a crime into an administrative offense. But more importantly, this legal measure meant treating the issue as a public health matter rather than a criminal problem. The law was accompanied by major changes in care. The peculiarity of the so-called Portuguese approach is not only the decriminalization of consumption, but also the introduction of harm reduction and social reintegration policies. In this way, users leave the judicial system and enter the health system, where they are guaranteed access to harm reduction tools, such as medical and psychological care, opioid substitution therapies (with methadone and naloxone), the provision of sterile syringes or condoms, access to all necessary information, and so on.

Contrary to the predictions of the most critical voices, there was no surge in consumption, nor did mafias proliferate around the black market for psychoactive substances. Drug use in Portugal remains illegal, but anyone caught with drugs for personal use is not sent to prison, but offered treatment programs or a fine. It is still a crime to possess these substances in quantities exceeding what is necessary for ten days' personal consumption (which would be equivalent to about 15 grams of cocaine or heroin and 20 grams of cannabis, as established by the Supreme Court). It is also still a crime to grow marijuana. The consumption of some substances has not decreased significantly. However, heroin consumption has declined, as have deaths from overdose and other side effects, such as HIV, tuberculosis, and hepatitis infections. In addition, prevention policies have succeeded in delaying the onset of consumption. The measures also greatly alleviated the saturation of the prison system. The "Portuguese Way" works, as these data show—and as evidenced by the fact that it has endured despite the alternation between progressive and conservative governments in the country.

REFERENCES

1. American Psychiatric Association. DSM-IV-TR. Breviario. Criterios diagnósticos. Barcelona: Masson, 2003.
2. American Psychiatric Association. DSM-5. Manual Diagnóstico y Estadístico de los Trastornos Mentales (5ª edición) (Tomos 1 y 2). Madrid: Editorial Médica Panamericana, 2014.
3. Appelbaum P, Roth LH. Clinical Issues in the Assessment of Competency. Am J Psychiatry. 1981;138(11):462–1467.
4. Appelbaum P, Mirkin S, Bateman A. Empirical assessment of competency to consent to psychiatric hospitalization. Am J Psychiatry. 1981;138 (9):1170–6.
5. Baron-Cohen S. Empatía cero. Nueva teoría de la crueldad. Madrid: Alianza Editorial, 2012.
6. Bello LA. Epidemiología, Factores Etiológicos y Modelos Asistenciales en Patología Dual. Miguel Hernández University, 2016.
7. Bobes J, Casas M, Gutiérrez M. Manual de Trastornos Adictivos (Addictive Disorders Manual). Enfoque Editorial S. C. Clayton R, 2011. Retrieved from https://bibliosjd.org/wp-content/uploads/2017/03/Manual.de_.Trastornos.Adictivos.pdf.
8. Carrasco JJ, Maza JM. Manual de Psiquiatría Legal y Forense (3ª edición). Las Rozas (Madrid): La Ley Actualidad, 2005.
9. Churchland PS. El cerebro moral. Lo que la neurociencia nos cuenta sobre la moralidad. Barcelona: Paidós Transiciones-Planeta, 2012.
10. De Wall F. Primates y Filósofos. La evolución de la moral del simio al hombre. Barcelona: Planeta, 2007.

11. Domoslawski A, Marcano A. Política sobre drogas en Portugal. Beneficios de la Descriminalización del Consumo de Drogas. New York: Open Society Foundations, 2011.
12. Drane JF. Competency to give an Informed Consent. A model for Making Clinical Assessment. JAMA. 1984;252:925–7.
13. Drane JF. The many faces of competency. Hasting Cent Rep. 1985;15(2):17–21.
14. Dutton K. La sabiduría de los psicópatas. Barcelona: Ariel, 2013.
15. Fernández-Hierro J, Muñoz K, Martínez Vico P. Los trastornos de personalidad en las UHP. En: Aparicio V, Angosto T (editores). El componente de Salud Mental en el Hospital General. Madrid: Spanish Association of Neuropsychiatry, 2015.
16. Garzón Díaz FA. La Neuroética, una nueva línea de investigación para la Bioética. Rev Latinoam Bioet. 2011;11(1):6–9.
17. Gazzaniga MS. ¿Quién manda aquí? El libre albedrío y la ciencia del cerebro. Barcelona: Paidós Transiciones-Plane-ta, 2012.
18. Gazzaniga MS. ¿Quién manda aquí? El libre albedrío y la ciencia del cerebro. Barcelona: Paidós Transiciones-Plane-ta, 2015.
19. Germán-Urdiola MJ. Tratamientos involuntarios y Enfermedad Mental. Pamplona: Thomson Reuters-Aranzadi, 2012.
20. Gorga M. Implicaciones éticas del conocimiento acerca del cerebro. Una aproximación a la Neuroética. Rev Colomb de Bioética. 2012;7(1):123–9. Bogotá: El Bosque, 2012.
21. Gracia D. Fundamentos de Bioética. Madrid: EUDEMA S.A, 1989.
22. Herreros B, Bandrés F. Bioética: de la globalización a la toma de decisiones. Paracuellos del Jarama (Madrid): Ademas Comunicación Gráfica S. L., 2012.
23. Johnson SC, Elbogen EB. Personality disorders at the interface of psychiatry and the law: Legal use and clinical classification. Dial Clin Neurosci. 2013;15:203–11.
24. Keysers C, Kaas JH, Gazzola V. Somatosensation in social perception. Nat Rev Neurosci. 2010;11(6):417–28.
25. Keysers C. The Empathic Brain. How the Discovery of mirror neurons changes our understanding of human nature. Social Brain Press, 2011.
26. López Frías FJ, Morales Aguilera P, Sebastian Solanes RF (editors). Bioética, Neuroética, Libertad y Justicia. Granada: Comares, 2013.
27. Lykken DT (2006). Psychopathy personality: The scope of the problem. In: C. J. Patrick (editor). Handbook of Psychopathy. New York, Guilford Press, 2006: 3–13.
28. Lynam DR, Widiger TA. Using a general model of personality to identify the basic elements of psychopathy. J Pers Disord. 2007;21(2):160–78.
29. Meffert H, Gazzola V, Den Boer J, Bartels AAJ, Keysers. Reduced spontaneous but relatively normal deliberate vicarious representations in psychopathy. Brain. 2013;136(8):2550–62. http://dx.doi.org/10.1093/brain/awt190.
30. Millon T. rastornos de la Personalidad. Más allá del DSM-IV. Barcelona: Masson, 1998.
31. Millon T. Trastornos de la Personalidad en la vida moderna (2ª edición). Barcelona: Masson, 2006.
32. Monahan J, Steadman HJ, Appelbaum P, Clark Robbins P, Mulvey EP, Roth LH *et al.* Rethinking Risk Assessment: The MacArthur Study of Mental Disorder and Violence. New York: Oxford University Press, 2001
33. Oldham JM, Skodol AE, Bender DS. Tratado de los Trastornos de la Personalidad. Barcelona: Masson, 2007.
34. World Health Organization. CIE-10. Décima Revisión de la Clasificación Internacional de las Enfermedades. Trastornos Mentales y del Comportamiento. Descripciones Clínicas y Pautas para el Diagnóstico. Madrid: Meditor, 1992.
35. Otero FJ (coordinator). Psiquiatría y Ley. Guía para la práctica clínica. Madrid: Edimsa, 2008.

36. Pueyo AA, Redondo S. Predicción de la violencia: Entre la peligrosidad y la valoración del riesgo de violencia. Papeles del Psicólogo. 2007;28(3):157–73.
37. Remmel RJ, Glenn AL, Cox J. Biological evidence regarding psychopathy does not affect mock jury sentencing. J Pers Disorders. 2019;33:164–84.
38. Sánchez-Caro J, Sánchez-Caro J. El consentimiento informado en Psiquiatría. Madrid: Díaz de Santos, 2002.
39. Santander F. Ethics and psychiatric practice. Madrid: AEN Estudios, 2000.
40. Schneider K. Las personalidades psicopáticas (1ª edición). Madrid: Morata, 1943.
41. Shedler J, Beck A, Fonagy P, Gabbard GO, Gunderson, Kernberg O, Michels R, Westen D. Refining Personality Disorder Diagnosis: Integrating Science and Practice. Am J Psychiatry 2004;161:1350–65.
42. Tomasello M, Carpenter M, Call J, Behne T, Moll, H. Understanding and sharing intentions: The origins of cultural cognition. Behav Brain Sci. 2005;28:675–735.
43. Tomasello M. A Natural History of Human Morality. Cambridge, MA: Harvard University Press, 2016.
44. Volkow N, Koob G, McLellan T. Neurobiologic Advances from the Brain Disease Model of Addiction. N Engl J Med. 2016;374:363–71.
45. Zimbardo, Ph. El efecto Lucifer. El porqué de la maldad. Barcelona: Paidós Ibérica, 2008.

8.2 PROPOSALS FOR A QUALITY APPROACH FOR DUAL PATHOLOGY PATIENTS IN THE CONTEXT OF CORRECTIONAL INSTITUTIONS

G. Flórez Menéndez and M. Pérez Rivas

SITUATION OF DUAL PATHOLOGY IN PRISONS

This chapter is marked by an epidemiological rule found in the general population: there is a high comorbidity between mental disorders and addictions. In the prison population, this dual pathology is even more dramatic, as both pathologies are more prevalent in this population. However, despite this epidemiological fact, the relationship between the two, and especially their treatment, has not been widely studied in this type of patient.

The following examples from the research serve as proof:

- In 2011, Fazel and Baillargeon published a review in *The Lancet* on the prevalence of health problems among prisoners worldwide. With regard to mental disorders, they reported a prevalence of 4% for psychosis, 10–12% for depression, and 40–70% for personality disorders (especially antisocial personality disorder). With regard to addictions, they reported a prevalence of 17–30% in men for problems related to alcohol consumption, with a prevalence of 10–24% in women; and with regard to illegal substances, the prevalence figures were 10–48% for men and 30–60% for women. However, as previously indicated, the authors do not analyze the relationship between the two types of disorders. Two aspects are clear: the prevalence rates of the different disorders are highly variable and depend on the methodology used in each study, and even so, it is clear that even for the lowest prevalence rates, the inmates who participated in the studies had a significantly higher prevalence of all disorders than the general population. The authors associated this generalized increase with the following factors: association with violent crime, scarcity of psychiatric care and forensic resources, and high prevalence of mental disorders related to the social drift that generates criminal behavior.[1]
- In 2012, MacDonald, Williams, and Kane analyzed the problem of addiction among the European prison population. Overall drug use was estimated to be between 1% and 51%. Once again, the disparity in the figures is striking, with intravenous drug use, which affected 2% to 22% of the population, being of particular concern. Cannabis was the most commonly used substance, followed by cocaine and heroin. This study does provide very broad figures on comorbidity: 74.5% of illegal drug addicts and 85.5% of alcohol addicts had a dual diagnosis. Finally, the authors indicate the need for a rehabilitative approach for these inmates, requiring more health resources both inside and outside prisons.[2]
- In 2019, Tyler *et al.* published the results of an epidemiological study conducted in a prison in the United Kingdom. They assessed 469 inmates (338 men and 131 women) and observed the following lifetime prevalences: 26.5% for personality disorders,

27.1% for anxiety disorders, 58.8% for mood disorders, 9.9% for psychotic disorders, 55.8% for problematic alcohol use, and 34.8% for drug dependence. Once again, these prevalences are higher than those of the general population. Without going into detail, the authors indicate that there is a high comorbidity among all disorders, affecting 47.5% of the sample.[3]

- In our country, Vicens *et al.* published an epidemiological study in 2011 conducted in a Spanish prison. They evaluated 707 male inmates. They obtained the following lifetime prevalences: alcohol addiction (46.4%), cannabis addiction (50.4%), cocaine and other stimulant addiction (57.6%), morphine derivative addiction (48.8%), mood disorders (41%), anxiety disorders (45.3%), personality disorders (80%) (66% met the criteria for more than one personality disorder), and psychotic disorders (10.7%). Dual pathology was not analyzed in this study.[4]

- López *et al.* published in 2016 in *Spanish Journal of Prison Health* an epidemiological study in two Andalusian prisons. The sample consisted of 472 males. The lifetime prevalence rates obtained were as follows: psychotic disorders (11.9%), affective disorders (31.4%), anxiety disorders (30.9%), personality disorders (79.9%), and drug abuse/dependence (65.9%). This study analyzes, albeit superficially, dual pathology, obtaining lifetime prevalence figures of 38.6% for axis I disorders and 84.9% for personality disorders.[5]

- In 2019, our research team at the Pereiro de Aguiar Penitentiary Center published a study in the *Spanish Journal of Prison Health* exclusively on personality disorders. The sample consisted of 204 inmates, 176 men and 28 women. The most prevalent for addiction were as follows: alcohol (20.8%), heroin (19.5%), cocaine (18.6%), and cannabis (15.8%). With regard to personality disorders, the following results were obtained: paranoid (14.2%), antisocial (18.6%), borderline (7.3%), histrionic (6.3%), narcissistic (21%), avoidant (8.3%), and more than one personality disorder (11.7%). Dual pathology was analyzed in this study, yielding the following results: having a personality disorder was associated with a higher prevalence of use of all the substances mentioned. Narcissistic disorder was associated with higher heroin use. Antisocial disorder was associated with higher heroin/cocaine/cannabis use. Paranoid and histrionic disorders were not associated with increased use of any of the substances. Avoidant personality disorder was associated with increased alcohol consumption, and borderline personality disorder was associated with increased heroin consumption. The results of this study allow us to indicate that the increase in the prevalence of addiction among inmates diagnosed with personality disorder is mainly dependent on antisocial personality disorder.[6]

In summary, national and international epidemiological studies confirm the high prevalence of mental disorders and addictions among prison inmates. There are clear indications, which need to be confirmed, that this high prevalence of both types of disorders translates into a high prevalence of dual pathology.

Unfortunately, as is often the case with this issue of comorbidity, research has not advanced much further in this field. There is no solid scientific evidence, even in the non-prison population, to enable specific recommendations to be made for assessment and, above all, treatment for each comorbidity scenario. Obviously, clinicians treating these inmates should be advised of the need to explore the presence of dual pathology and to draw up simultaneous treatment plans for each disorder they suffer from. These general guidelines are included in the Comprehensive Care Program for the Mentally Ill (PAIEM), which is applied in Spanish prisons and directly mentions dual pathology as a criterion for inclusion in the program. Curiously, mental disorders induced by the use of psychoactive substances are a criterion for exclusion from the program. However, the study of the program's results published in 2014 indicated that only 28% of the centers had a psychiatrist who collaborated more actively in the program.[7] These low figures indirectly reflect how little dual diagnosis has penetrated treatment plans.

PROPOSAL FOR PROTOCOLIZATION OF INTERVENTION IN THE PRISON ENVIRONMENT TO IMPROVE THE QUALITY OF CARE FOR DUAL PATHOLOGY PATIENTS ADMITTED TO PRISONS

The first step would be to conduct a multicenter epidemiological study representative of the Spanish prison population to confirm the extent of the clinical problem to be addressed.

The second step would be to include this type of patient in detail in the PAIEM and guarantee their specialized psychiatric and psychological care.

Once these first two steps have been completed, an individualized assessment of each case in each prison could be carried out in order to develop a therapeutic and rehabilitation plan for each patient based on their specific condition, as described in other chapters of this consensus document.

REFERENCES

1. Fazel S, Baillargeon J. The health of prisoners. Lancet. 2011;377(9769):956–65. doi:10.1016/s0140-6736(10)61053-7.
2. MacDonald M, Williams J, Kane D. Barriers to implementing through care for problematic drug users in European prisons. Int J Prison Health. 2012;8(2):68–84.
3. Tyler N, Miles HL, Karadag B, Rogers G. An updated picture of the mental health needs of male and female prisoners in the UK: prevalence, comorbidity, and gender differences. Soc Psychiatry Psychiatr Epidemiol. 2019;54(9):1143–52. doi:10.1007/s00127-019-01690-1.
4. Vicens E, Tort V, Dueñas RM, Muro Á, Pérez-Arnau F, Arroyo JM, Acín E, *et al.* The prevalence of mental disorders in Spanish prisons. Crim Behav Ment Health. 2011;21(5):321–2. doi:10.1002/cbm.815.
5. López M, Saavedra FJ, López A, Laviana, M. Prevalence of Mental Health problems in sentenced men in prisons from Andalucía (Spain). Rev Esp Sanid Penit. 2016;18(3):76–84.
6. Flórez G, Ferrer V, García LS, Crespo MR, Pérez M, Saiz PA. Personality disorders, addictions, and psychopathy as predictors of criminal behavior in a prison sample. Rev Esp Sanid Penit. 2019;21(2):62–79.
7. Sanz J, Gómez-Pintado P, Ruiz A, Pozuelo F, Arroyo JM. Programa de Atención Integral al Enfermo Mental en las prisiones españolas (PAIEM): valoración tras cuatro años de funcionamiento. Rev Esp Sanid Penit. 2014;16:91–102.

8.3 "THE PORTUGUESE MODEL": FROM THE DECRIMINALIZATION OF DRUG USE TO INTEGRATED RESPONSES TO ADDICTION

A. F. Vale Ferreira, A. J. Da Silva Barbosa, A. I. Da Silva Tavares, and J. A. Castel-Branco Goulão

CONTEXT

The problem of drug use in Portugal began to draw attention in the late 1970s and was linked to a number of factors, namely the fall of the dictatorial regime, the end of the colonial war in Africa, and the return of people from the colonies (including Portuguese soldiers), where cannabis use was already common, the opening of the country to the outside world with the implementation of democracy, and the emergence of LSD, heroin, and cocaine users, which led the government of the time to create three treatment centers (Lisbon, Coimbra, and Porto) under the Ministry of Justice, outside the scope of public health.

In the 1980s, above all, due to the widespread use of heroin, health services and professionals began to encounter the need to provide specific treatment responses for the dependent population (those existing at the time, both generalist and mental health services, were unable to respond) and, by the end of the decade, it had become a public health concern, leading the Ministry of Health to create the first drug treatment centers, first in Lisbon, then in Porto and the Algarve, and later spreading progressively to all districts of the country.

Throughout the 1990s, health professionals and society realized that the country had a serious drug use problem, due to the high rate of consumption, which became the main concern of the Portuguese people. Despite efforts, drug use continued to increase and the data on heroin users among those infected with HIV (60%) were particularly alarming. At the same time, criminalization, by generating fear of being treated as criminals, discouraged many users from seeking treatment and hindered the implementation of programs, such as needle exchange, despite being recommended by health professionals. These limitations affected both access to and continuity of medical care as full citizens and also hindered the implementation of effective and efficient public health measures in the areas of prevention, treatment, and rehabilitation for drug use and HIV infection, epidemics that proliferated simultaneously in the 1990s.

We can see how the problem of drug abuse drug use caused widespread social alarm, and political concern about this social issue became the subject of public debate. Called the "social scourge," it became the number one enemy of the 13th Constitutional Government, which, in its political program approved in November 1995, considered the situation of illegal drug use in Portugal to be very serious. Estimates pointed to around 100,000 socially vulnerable heroin users, most of whom injected the drug. In a 1997 Eurobarometer study, the Portuguese identified drug-related issues as the country's main social problem (Domostawski, 2011).

The problem of drug addiction was indeed prevalent, given the destructive effects of drug abuse on users' health, crime and the threat to security related to drug trafficking, the feelings of insecurity they cause due to petty crime associated with drug addiction, the risks to public health arising from certain patterns of behavior among users, the corrosive effects on the quality of life of affected families, the common social trajectory among users, and the type of opportunities they are unable to take advantage of due to their drug addiction. All of this has required an unprecedented effort of public debate, reflection, and proposals regarding alternative policies to address the problem of drugs and drug addiction as a society.

In the search for solutions to minimize the nature of the problems caused by the complexity of this issue, the state and civil society promoted an intense and rich public debate on the legal framework for illicit drug use. This discussion gained widespread attention in public opinion through media coverage and the participation of various public figures. It was a complex debate and, perhaps a disproportionate one, albeit appropriately so, in the context of the political strategy to be adopted in Portugal to address the drug problem. In any case, it allowed for the analysis of more tolerant legal regulatory models and other experiences practiced internationally. Issues such as decriminalization, legalization, and depenalization were widely discussed during this period.

Faced with the clear failure of repressive measures to combat the drug epidemic, a movement in favor of liberalization has emerged in Portugal. In this context, we highlight the proposals presented by youth associations from various parties and political leaders, who denounced the perverse effects of prohibitionist policies. But in a society such as Portugal's, which favors a mixture of prohibition and liberalization, the drug law continued to prohibit the market and tolerate consumption, just as the market allowed the sale and purchase of drugs in a context of total absence of rules.

THE PROCESS OF DECRIMINALIZATION

It was therefore during the 1990s that public and political discussions among professionals from various European countries began to take shape on the advantages and disadvantages of criminalizing drug use for users and for society in general. Based on cooperation and the exchange of concerns among health professionals involved in addiction treatment in several European countries, the first documents of ethical commitment appeared, treating the user as a full citizen and not as a criminal, with the right to medical care and social reintegration, and understanding drug addiction as an expression of their physical, psychological, and social suffering.

The first document, the *Declaration of Lisbon*, was prepared in 1992, within the framework of the 5th International Congress Meeting of Nations in Lisbon, by the Congress Delegates and was endorsed by them. Later, in 1994, the European Platform of Associations of Professionals Involved in Drug Addiction (ERIT) was established in Paris, with strong Portuguese participation and with the aim of reflecting, exchanging ideas, and cooperating with the governments of various countries so that policies in this area consider drug addicts as citizens with full rights and duties and facilitate access to treatment and respect for human rights, with coordinated policies adapted to needs and legislation, giving priority to prevention, treatment, and integration. All this, together with the imperatives of public health and the fight against exclusion, and a Europe based on exchange and collaboration, culminated in the 1996 Paris Proclamation, based on European citizenship, the minimization of harm, and quality healthcare (Patrício, 1997).

The increase in the number of drug users, the associated risks and harms, in particular of AIDS, viral hepatitis, and social disintegration, exacerbate the problems of a drug policy focused on outbreaks of social tension, insecurity, and poverty in the suburbs, on the streets, and in prisons, led at the end of the decade (1998) to the Constitutional Government of Portugal appointing a Group of Experts in health care and research, with the aim of drawing up recommendations for a more effective policy. After eight months, in 1999, the Group presented the results of its work in the form of a "National Strategy for the Fight Against Drugs," recommending the decriminalization of possession of drugs for personal use, both "hard" and "soft," as the most effective way to limit drug use and reduce the number of drug addicts.

The Committee also recommended that, in addition to legislative changes, the government should develop programs in the areas of prevention, reintegration, and harm reduction, in addition to expanding and improving the availability of drug treatment programs, thereby promoting universality, accessibility, and humanization in a practical and specific manner. Behind this new philosophy was the recognition of the concerns that professionals had been warning about for some years, as well as the concerns of families and society, the recognition of the need to respect human dignity, an understanding of the life choices and social circumstances of others, and constitutional support for the right to health. All of these served as the basis for changing the approach to the problem of drug use.

Thus, in a brief assessment ("Situation and Assessment of the Drug Problem in Portugal"), prepared by the Ad Hoc Commission for Monitoring and Assessing the Situation of Drug Addiction, Consumption, and Trafficking (1998), it was considered that the fight against trafficking was ineffective, there was no coordinated and articulated prevention, and it was difficult to find places for both outpatient consultation and hospitalization in public services. In addition, social reintegration was still in its infancy. Also, for this reason, the Government, through the initiative of the Deputy Minister of the Prime Minister, José Sócrates appointed a study committee—the Commission for the National Strategy to Combat Drugs—which brought together professionals and scientists to develop a proposal for a national strategy to combat drugs. In this way, the government sought to provide society with a national strategy to combat drugs and drug addiction, developed in dialogue with experts, institutions working in this area, and citizens themselves, having appointed a committee of renowned experts.

As already mentioned, the final report prepared by the Commission for the National Strategy for the Fight Against Drugs contained completely innovative proposals in the field of drug policy, namely the decriminalization of private drug use. The report presented to the government in October 1998 explicitly reflects the concern to decriminalize private consumption, as well as possession or acquisition for such consumption (CENCD, 1998), also suggesting the modification of legislation that punished drug use with prison sentences of up to three months.

This conceptual change introduced in Portugal reflects the exhaustion of the repressive model. In fact, prisons became "depositories for drug addicts" and the AIDS epidemic caused great social alarm ("the outbreak of drug use was a shock to the whole of society" [Poiares, 2001]), mobilizing political powers to implement more tolerant public policies in the field of drugs and drug addiction.

With the National Strategy for the Fight Against Drugs ("fight against the epidemic"), the political powers that be have opted to prohibit drug use solely as a social illicit act. This is not a measure of legalization or decriminalization; it only seeks to replace prohibition through criminal offense with prohibition through a more appropriate social offense. Based on this assumption, drug users are seen as individuals who require support rather than punishment.

Political discourse, based on medical and psychological concepts aimed at preventing risky behavior, moves away from the image of the criminal consumer, bringing to the fore the image of citizens in need of social and medical support, with a view to treatment and promoting abstinence. And when this is not possible, measures are put in place to minimize social and health damage. It should be noted, however, that drug use continues to be punished. Criminal penalties are imposed only for the use, possession, and illicit acquisition of all drugs for personal use. With this philosophy, the essential aim is to promote the treatment of the offending consumer, based on the motto "It is better to treat than to punish."

This National Strategy for the Fight Against Drugs (ENLCD) from 1999 also arose in a context marked by the emergence of new drugs, increased polydrug use, new patterns of alcohol and substance use such as cocaine, and the aging and increasing physical and mental deterioration of heroin users. The guiding principles of the ENLCD, defined in 1999, are (1) principles of international cooperation, prevention, humanism, pragmatism, security, coordination, and participation and rationalization of resources; (2) reinforcing the centrality of the human person; (3) active association with civil society; (4) proactive and proximity policies; and (5) prevention in the school and family environment. Recognition of the effectiveness of treatment, the need for national and sectoral action plans, integrated plans and responses, the fight against trafficking, the effectiveness of deterrence policies, the creation of knowledge, new responses to new addictions, and shared responsibility are guidelines that emerge from this evaluation process and lead to the decision to decriminalize drug use.

Contrary to what was customary, the government took into account all the recommendations of the Group of Experts, and in 2000 (Law No. 30/2000) the law decriminalizing the possession (amount considered for personal use) and consumption of drugs was published, removing it from the criminal sphere and orienting it toward the spheres of treatment and rehabilitation, in addition to making a significant investment in policies to deter consumption, either through increased budgets for prevention or through the creation of Drug Abuse Deterrence Commissions in all districts (joint commissions with experts from the justice and health sectors). The Commissions' mission was to inform people and deter them from using drugs, and had the power to impose administrative sanctions and, with their consent, refer people for treatment. This power ensured compliance with the international conventions by which Portugal was bound and also prevented the risk that such decisions, when applied to a single country, might turn it into a "drug paradise."

This new philosophy allows us to approach addiction as a disease that must be prevented, on the premise that addicts, being considered sick people, need help and treatment and are not criminals who should be imprisoned. This legislation, which has decriminalized possession by users, and this new strategy have consolidated the idea of "combating the disease and not the sick," including necessary measures for prevention and education, harm reduction, improved access to treatment programs (funded by the state), and the introduction of social reintegration programs.

THE IMPLEMENTATION PROCESS

In the 1990s, efforts and concerns increased to organize policies to address addiction in a coherent and comprehensive manner, along with the production of knowledge and the development of intervention strategies, conceived as a responsibility of society as a whole in the field of drug addiction and materialized in the need for coordinated networking. Important measures were taken, but some were lacking. It no longer makes sense to organize partial, scattered, or fragmented responses, because the complexity of the problem forces us to take comprehensive measures to increase the effectiveness of interventions and make the most of available resources. There were many institutions, both governmental and non-governmental, working in the social sphere, developing actions to improve the living conditions of the population; but these actions often ended up being fragmented, repetitive in some respects, focused on the same segment of the population and neglecting others, without the necessary methodological rigor, thus wasting human and material resources, despite the effort and commitment they provided (Ferreira, 1999). ENLCD 1999/2004, in addition to being a political framework of great importance, provided conceptual support for an articulated and integrated response, which in turn gave birth to the Institute of Drugs and Drug Addiction (IDT).

The IDT resulted from the merger of two services:

- The Drug Abuse Prevention and Treatment Service, which focuses on treatment and reports to the Ministry of Health
- The Portuguese Institute on Drugs and Drug Addiction, which is interministerial and focuses on social intervention policies

Excessive bureaucracy and some initial stagnation delayed the IDT's implementation and development, but even so, two crucial objectives were achieved: a 50% reduction in drug-related deaths and a reversal in the trend of HIV, HBV/HCV, and tuberculosis infections.

It is ENLCD 2005/2009 that definitively implements the conceptual model of integrated responses (comprehensive and integrated approaches), defining strategies for the various areas of intervention and reorganization of services, with the aim of significantly reducing the prevalence of drug use among the population and the social and health damage caused by the use and trade of illegal drugs, and ensuring a high degree of safety for the general public, while taking into account the achievements in the area of fundamental rights and freedoms.

A present, the IDT develops an integrated strategy to combat drugs and drug addiction, based on prevention of consumption, treatment and risk reduction, harm minimization, and social reintegration, ensuring the cross-cutting functioning of the national information system on drugs and drug addiction, promoting and stimulating research on the phenomenon, supporting the training of professionals involved in this field, supporting the functioning of the Drug Addiction Deterrence Commissions in all districts, ensuring cooperation with external entities, and studying and proposing legislative and administrative measures in this field and accompanying their implementation.

The intervention is now organized and unified by axes, covering Cross-Cutting Areas:

1. Coordination (internal, intra- and interministerial; and external, civil society and international cooperation), information, research, training, evaluation, and legal reorganization)
2. Demand reduction (prevention, deterrence, risk reduction and harm minimization, treatment and reintegration)
3. Supply reduction

It was also defined that all vectors of the demand reduction axis would be developed by strategic areas: universal, selective, and indicated; for vectors: prevention and deterrence (non-addicts).

THE INTEGRATED RESPONSE MODEL

Demand reduction is undoubtedly the core of the intervention, the essential support for ENLCD and the main pillar for the success of the decriminalization of drug use. This strategic axis, enshrined in the European Strategy (EUELCD 2005–2012), was subdivided into vectors that together constituted the technical intervention of the Ministry of Health in the field of drug addiction.

These vectors, whose strategic importance is unquestionable, were directly attributable to the adoption of the guiding principles enshrined in the ENLCD, their operational effectiveness in the field, and the strong cohesion between them (prevention, deterrence, risk reduction and damage minimization, treatment, and social reintegration). In this regard, a strategic reorientation of interventions was chosen, an integrated response model capable of ensuring the consistency and coherence of actions and optimizing results from the perspective of health benefits, based on the following principles:

- **Focus on citizens**: Intervention in drug addiction is not an end in itself, and should focus not on substances, but rather on citizens and their objective and subjective needs. The excessive bureaucracy sometimes observed in service providers and healthcare authorities must be rationalized and organized in accordance with the overall satisfaction of these needs, taking into account that individuals have an active voice and a shared responsibility in defining their life project, in terms of equal rights and duties of citizenship. Therefore, services should be constituted as managers of citizens' own health capital, with citizens themselves responsible for deciding whether to use these services. This perspective does not invalidate a proactive attitude in intervening in situations of greater risk to the individual and the community. This perspective is present in all vectors of intervention and embodies the notion of integrated responses aimed at strengthening and self-managing each individual's possible state of health, approaching them as an indivisible whole, regardless of the services they use.

- **Territoriality**: To improve knowledge, intervention, and evaluation, the focus should be on localized and territorial management and planning. Proximity interventions can be carried out and adapted, avoiding the dispersion of responses and devices, and defining the role and function of each entity and/or actor in the territory shared with others. In the field of IDT, its internal organization must be restructured, decentralizing powers and promoting the emergence of regional potential and decentralized management. The perception of realities and phenomena is felt more strongly and perceived better at the local level, so it must start from an analysis of local needs/proposals in order to build intervention plans that respond to territorial diagnoses, identifying priorities for the initiation or continuation of interventions. Externally, it is important to define with local actors the degrees of co-responsibility and, in technical and financial terms, the type of management that best suits the needs of a given territory.
- **Integrated approaches and responses—integrated intervention at the internal and external levels**: Approaches and responses must be developed in an integrated manner, without separating individual and social realities. Services must organize their operational intervention by creating comprehensive response mechanisms that constitute a coherent network of action capable of addressing the complexity and cross-cutting nature of the drug problem and related issues. Partial and reductive views have led to scattered, fragmented interventions with no measurable results that would allow us to understand the real scope, characteristics, and trends of this problem:
    - **Internal level**: The integrated response model is developed **internally** by the integrated response centers (IRCs), which are public health and local intervention centers of an operational and administrative nature, composed of multidisciplinary technical teams that work in the community on their own and in collaboration with other public and private entities, promoting integrated and territorially defined responses for prevention, treatment, social reintegration, and harm reduction for people with addictive behaviors/dependencies.
    - **External level**: This is developed following a community intervention approach, which is reflected in the Integrated Response Operational Plan (IROP), a structural measure at the integrated intervention level, which aims to reduce the demand for psychoactive substances, seeking to enhance the synergies available in the territory. The IROP is based on the principles of:
        - *Territoriality* (the territory as the center of intervention)
        - *Integration* (coordinated and concerted work at the local level)
        - *Partnership* (based on a culture of sharing)
        - *Participation* (raising awareness among all stakeholders to improve understanding of the problems)

These principles build a global network of integrated and complementary responses, with the aim of increasing the scope, accessibility, effectiveness, and efficiency of interventions, targeting specific groups that do not generally use public health services. The implementation and execution of the IROP is achieved through the implementation of Integrated Response Programs (IRP).

IRPs can be projects or interventions with or without direct financial support from the state, which integrate interdisciplinary and multisectoral approaches and responses, in accordance with some or all areas of intervention, such as prevention, treatment, risk reduction, harm minimization, and social reintegration. IRPs allow for the reorganization of available resources in areas where there are no ongoing interventions or where resources are not sufficiently utilized, strengthening actions based on identified needs (Silva *et al.* 2008).

Deterrence: The current legal and regulatory framework applicable to illicit drug use (Law No. 30/2000 and complementary regulations) incorporates a set of principles and strategies arising from the deterrence paradigm, which is based on an integrative and complementary philosophy and approach in the field of demand reduction that transcends the perspective of mere decriminalization. This integrative perspective includes a network of complementary local responses that work in the same direction and correspond to the real needs of the consuming population.

The drug abuse deterrence committees, with territorial jurisdiction in law enforcement matters, work closely with the community to mediate between situations of drug use and the application of punitive measures. Without discrediting the accused for engaging in illegal behavior, it seeks to intervene and tailor decisions to the specific situation of the accused, taking into account their personal circumstances and context. Punitive measures may include referral of the accused to support structures (depending on their psychosocial diagnosis and the support available to them) or more punitive measures.

In terms of the results to be achieved, the aim is to that the implementation of this law will contribute to reducing illicit drug use in a fair and equitable manner, in accordance with the needs of the accused, whether preventive, health-related, therapeutic, or punitive, and will further several objectives:

- *Ensure efficiency in law enforcement*, guaranteeing adequate and fair monitoring, with technical quality and satisfying the actual needs of accused consumers. Until now, those responsible have invested heavily in deterrence, which has led to uncertainty and instability among internal stakeholders, partners, and consumers. This situation has an effective impact on law enforcement, on the legitimacy of the current legislative framework itself, and on the credibility, respect, and dignity of the responsible entities.

- *Establish and maintain coordination between partners working in the field of drug addiction*, so as to ensure that the specific interventions of each service at the local level are complementary and that there is in-depth knowledge of the available responses. In this way, it is possible to develop mediation work with structures that offer responses that meet the actual needs of the accused, facilitating the referral of addicted users for treatment in order to provide them with the necessary social and health care and to act in situations of drug addiction where there is a lack of specialized support.

- *Building a comprehensive network of integrated and complementary responses*, in the context of risk reduction and damage minimization, with public and private partners. It must be based on a logic of proximity and citizen-centeredness, promoting values such as citizenship, participation, and accessibility, and creating the necessary conditions to ensure the sustainability of the responses implemented.
- *Provide a wide range of programs* for prevention, treatment, social reintegration, risk reduction, harm minimization, and deterrence, covering a broad spectrum of approaches, from legal, psychological, social, and/or pharmacological perspectives, always guided by ethical principles and in line with currently available scientific evidence, ensuring timely access to existing programs (integrated and complementary) for all those who need and want them.

CONCLUSIONS

The trajectory of drug policies in Portugal has been marked by different cycles that have followed international trends. In this matter, Portugal has shown a dual position and, at times, even an ambivalent attitude.

First, due to the commercial interests of opium from Macao, Portugal followed the political guidelines advocated by England and France, opting to apply political models for regulating the distribution of opium and legally controlling its consumption.

Subsequently, influenced by the strategic power established by the United States in various international forums (namely, through the International Conventions on Psychotropic Substances of 1961, 1971, and 1988), it followed the prohibitionist trend, which essentially manifested in repressive action against illicit drug use.

Currently, the positions adopted are influenced by the European Union Guidelines, through the European Strategy on Drugs, which assigns responsibilities to Member States for strengthening health policies (Barbosa, 2006).

In this context, the processes of globalization and Europeanization of drug policy have given rise to different periods of regulation of illicit drug use:

- In the first period, policy measures were derived from a fiscalization perspective, which only covered the regulation of the opium trade (the period of basic drug products).
- In the second period, through the imposition of international conventions, the political discourse advocated a repressive approach, which resulted in the application of punitive measures and the launch of prophylactic and health campaigns (the "drug-crime" period).
- The third period expresses aims of clinical, psychosocial, and social reintegration in relation to illicit drug use (the "drug-disease" period).

- Currently, due to social and political concerns arising from the epidemic spread of AIDS among injecting drug users, we are witnessing the emergence of a fourth period, with the appearance and legitimization of policies to deter and reduce harm in order to mitigate risks to individual and collective health (period of "drug epidemic").

The recognition of the failure of prohibitionist measures, together with the epidemic outbreak of AIDS among drug users, has changed the political approach to the drug problem. Consequently, and in accordance with the European Union's recommendations on drugs and drug addiction, the Portuguese state has been investing in humanistic and public health measures as alternatives to repressive models aimed at preventing individual and collective health, which have been enshrined in the National Strategy for the Fight Against Drugs (ENLCD).

We believe that ENLCD has contributed decisively to the implementation of innovative public policies and that its design and structuring principles remain relevant, regardless of social developments in the field of drugs and addiction, both nationally and internationally.

By proposing the decriminalization of private consumption, rather than insisting on purely repressive and ineffective measures, the ENLCD also contributed to a paradigm shift in international drug policy, complementing measures that promote respect for human dignity and the right to health and social reintegration of people with addictive behaviors and dependencies.

Decriminalization was adopted and introduced in the context of a comprehensive, integrated, and inclusive drug policy that includes a set of other complementary and coordinated measures to help people with addictive behaviors reduce risks and harm, begin treatment, and return to society in better health and with prospects for greater social autonomy.

Twenty years after its implementation, the Portuguese experience of decriminalizing drug use, free from prejudice and moralism, has shown that through tolerant, pragmatic, and humanistic strategies, it is possible to reduce drug use, reduce the percentage of drug users infected with HIV, decrease crime rates related to drug use, and increase public safety.

The integrated response model has been adopted as a strategic instrument of Portuguese policy, promoting proximity to citizens and social contexts, thus improving patients' access to social and health care in terms of addictive behaviors and dependencies.

Investment in integrated intervention, based on two pillars (citizen-centeredness and territoriality), has led to a paradigm shift in the field of responses to address the problems caused by addictive behaviors.

The adoption of the principle of territoriality allowed for the geographical delimitation of interventions, mobilizing public, private, and social solidarity entities for the design and development of coordinated and concerted projects in the field.

Recognition of the principle of participation, through community intervention methodologies that involve different social agents in the construction of territorial diagnoses (identification of needs, open areas, and definition of intervention priorities) has promoted shared responsibility in the management of problems related to addictive behaviors and dependencies.

Through joint and coordinated work, embodied in a culture of sharing and based on network intervention strategies, it has been possible to strengthen existing interventions, optimize community resources, and promote the complementarity of actions, thereby improving the efficiency and effectiveness of various public policies to address issues related to addictive behaviors and dependencies.

REFERENCES

Barbosa J. Entre a regulação dos riscos psicoativos e a defesa dos direitos de cidadania: o Serviço Social no seio das Capítulo 8 El abordaje de la vertiente legal y ética de la patología dual 111 políticas de redução de danos. Tese de Mestrado. Lisbon: FCH - UCP, 2006.

Domostawski A. Política da droga em Portugal: os benefícios da descriminalização do consumo de drogas. Open Society Foundations, 2011.

Ferreira A. Saúde e Prevenção Primária das Toxicodependências. O contributo do CIAC-Norte. Drug Addiction Magazine. 1999;5(3): 41–7.

Patrício Luís. Face à Droga - como (re)agir?. Serviço de Prevenção e Tratamento da Toxicodependência (SPTT). Lisbon: Ministry of Health, 1997.

Poiares CA. Droga, lei & saber, abordagem psicocriminal". Em: Torres N, Ribeiro JP (Org.). A pedra e o charco, sobre o conhecimento e intervenção nas drogas. Almada: Ímanedições, 2001: 89–105.

Presidency of the Council of Ministers (1999). Aprova a Estratégia Nacional de Luta Contra a Droga (1999-2004). Diário da República, 1ª Série-B, nº 122 de 26-05-1999.

Presidency of the Council of Ministers (2006). Plano Nacional de Luta Contra a Droga e a Toxicodependência (2005-2012). Diário da República 1st Series, no. 180 of 09-18-2006.

Silva M, Cruchinho M, Carvalho S. Aspetos metodológicos do diagnóstico social do Plano Operacional de Respostas Integradas - PORI. Revista Toxicodependências. 2008;14(1):73–84.

8.4 TOXICOLOGICAL ASPECTS IN THE APPROACH TO DUAL-PATHOLOGY PATIENTS

A. M. Bermejo Barrera, P. Cabarcos Fernández, I. Álvarez Freire, and M. J. Tabernero Duque

The use of drugs of abuse and psychoactive substances is a global public health problem. In addition to significant clinical repercussions, it has numerous medico-legal implications.

Chronic and acute intoxication currently has a high incidence in all hospitals, mainly in emergency departments, at the expense of acute drug intoxication.

There has also been a considerable increase in mental health problems resulting from the use of these types of substances, as well as other types of diverse pathologies.

Many people with addictive behaviors are also diagnosed with mental illnesses, and vice versa. In daily clinical practice, it is important to be able to distinguish between psychiatric symptoms and symptoms induced by substances, as this makes a significant difference in terms of treatment. To do this, in the case of addictions, it is essential to confirm the diagnosis using analytical techniques that determine the degree of addiction and the type of substances consumed. Today, it can be stated categorically that there is a high correlation between mental health problems and addictions. When these two disorders coexist in the same patient, it is called dual pathology. While it is true that addictions can be very varied, ranging from addictions to legal substances (such as tobacco or alcohol) to illegal substances such as drugs or certain behaviors such as shopping or sex addictions, here we will focus on those addictions caused by the use of drugs of abuse and psychoactive substances.

For decades, pediatricians have been concerned about drug use during pregnancy, due to the perinatal repercussions it entails. Although urine tests on newborns and opioid withdrawal syndrome have often shown this type of consumption, in recent years, with the increase in drug use in the population, including women of childbearing age, there has been great concern about the effects on the fetus. In some cases these appear later and cannot be diagnosed in the first days of life. That is why, in recent years, toxicology has also advanced in this field, developing analytical methods that allow the analysis of biological samples for this purpose. From a medical-legal point of view, the repercussions of drug use are, on the one hand, deaths caused by adverse reactions to the consumption of these types of substances, mainly cocaine, heroin, ecstasy, and alcohol, and, on the other hand, deaths caused indirectly, such as traffic accidents, workplace accidents, and even, currently, a large number of suicides. In the case of deaths due to adverse reactions, acute non-cardiogenic pulmonary edema is usually the mechanism of death in the case of opiates, and cardiovascular complications in the case of cocaine and stimulants. Legal problems arising from drug use are also very important, either because of the antisocial behavior they can generate or because of the large number of crimes that can occur under their influence, such as illicit trafficking and distribution; crimes against public health, property, and road safety; assault, and abuse. All of this has significant legal implications, which is why there is extensive legislation in place for this type of crime.

In general, crimes might be classified according to the type of substances consumed. For example, crimes against property are more frequently committed by opiate users due to the urgent need for consumption caused by their dependence. In contrast, crimes of assault and abuse are more common among chronic users of ethyl alcohol and stimulants such as cocaine or amphetamines. Finally, in the case of cannabis, the crimes committed are generally related to illicit trafficking or crimes against public health.

Special mention should be made of sexual assaults, the incidence of which has increased dramatically in recent years and where, despite the headlines in the press, alcohol and commonly used psychoactive substances are behind many cases.

In short, the problems arising from drug use from a criminal law perspective range from the modification of criminal responsibility in the case of crimes committed as a result of addiction to psychoactive substances (Articles 20.2 and 21.2 of the Criminal Code) to the special legal treatment of drug addiction with the application of security measures (Article 102.1) or the application of conditional suspension of the sentence (Articles 80 and 87).

Even today, there are articles in the Criminal Code that refer to road safety offenses, such as Articles 340 and 343.

ROLE OF TOXICOLOGY IN DRUG ADDICTION

For all the above reasons, it is essential to have a toxicology laboratory in order to confirm the presence or absence of drugs in all possible cases.

To this end, a **toxicological investigation** must be carried out, which is divided into a pre-analytical phase, which includes sample collection, shipment, reception, and storage, and an analytical phase proper. In this latter phase, the possible presence of drugs in the samples submitted will be investigated, using *screening* methods and confirmation methods.

In the case of drugs of abuse, screening methods are of the immunoassay type, which provide rapid results, are easy to perform, and do not require prior sample preparation. However, these analytical methods can produce false positive results due to cross-reactions between compounds with similar chemical structures. For this reason, it is essential to confirm the results using other analytical techniques, such as chromatography with different types of detection, especially mass spectrometry, which is widely used today.

Once the result has been confirmed, it is necessary to quantify the toxin to determine whether that concentration can justify a clinical picture or medical-legal repercussions.

To carry out the toxicological investigation, the laboratory may use different biological matrices, depending on each specific case and the purpose of the analysis.

Thus, in drug addicts who are brought before the courts, hair and urine samples are usually analyzed; for drug testing in road traffic, saliva or exhaled air; in acute intoxications received in hospital emergency departments, blood, urine, and gastric contents; and in cases of sexual assault, blood, urine, and hair.

For diagnosing drug exposure during pregnancy, meconium, umbilical cord blood, and hair are the samples used are the biological samples to be used for this purpose.

In any case, a very important part of toxicological analysis is its correct interpretation, for which, in addition to knowing the advantages of each biological sample, it is essential to understand the metabolic processes of these substances, and the pharmacological activity of each of their metabolites.

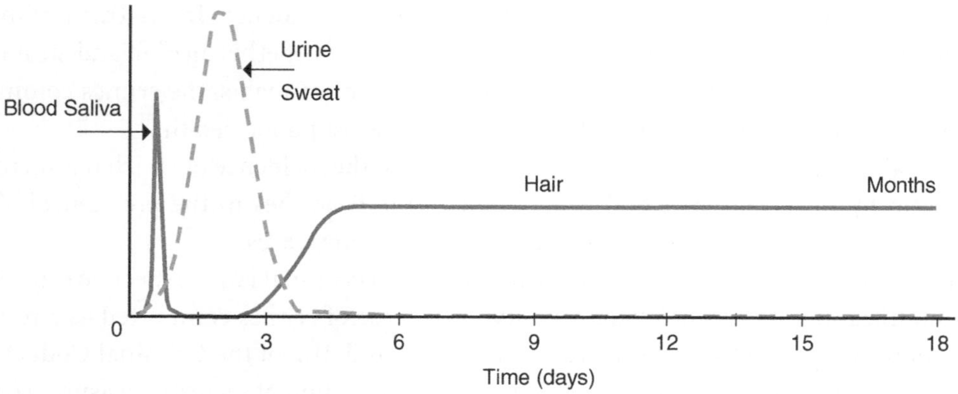

FIGURE 8.1 Biological sample detection windows.

Blood and urine have traditionally been the most commonly used biological samples for toxicological analysis, as the mechanism by which drugs are incorporated into them is well known, thus facilitating the interpretation of the analysis results. The significant developments that have taken place in the field of toxicology in recent years have enabled the use of other types of matrices that can be useful in the field of drug addiction, such as hair and saliva, which offer multiple advantages over conventional matrices, although this has required the use of highly sensitive analytical techniques due to the low concentration of toxins found in them.

The choice of sample type is determined by multiple factors, but obviously the purpose of the analysis is the fundamental factor. Therefore, it is necessary to know the detection windows for each, and the appearance and disappearance of drugs in them (Figure 8.1, Table 8.1).

Thus:

- To demonstrate recent consumption or the possibility of being under the influence of drugs, the only biological samples that can be used are blood and saliva.
- To demonstrate habitual use or use in the preceding hours, urine and keratin matrices are the samples of choice.
- To demonstrate previous consumption, hair is undoubtedly the ideal biological sample to use.

TABLE 8.1 Time of Appearance and Disappearance of Drugs in Biological Samples

Matrix	Appearance	Disappearance
Blood	1–2 hours	<24 hours
Saliva	1–2 hours	24–36 hours
Urine	2–4 hours	3–6 days
Sweat	2–4 hours	3–6 days
Hair	1 week	

Another highly relevant aspect to consider is **sample collection**, so it is important to assess the possibility of finding the least invasive, fastest method that requires the least specialized personnel and minimizes the possibility of adulteration or contamination.

With a good selection of the biological sample to be analyzed and using the appropriate analytical technique, accurate results can be obtained, the correct interpretation of which is essential in this field.

The biological samples most commonly analyzed in the case of drug testing from a medico-legal point of view are urine and blood as standard samples, and hair and saliva, as alternative samples. However, other biological samples can also be used, such as gastric contents, bile, meconium, and others in the field of clinical and *postmortem* toxicology.

Blood is the only biological sample that allows us to prove that an individual is under the influence of a drug, and furthermore, the concentrations found in the blood correlate with the clinical condition and degree of intoxication. It is therefore highly relevant in the case of crimes against road safety, or any type of criminal offense, in which the presence of drugs at the time the offense was committed may justify a change in the individual's behavior and, therefore, modify their criminal responsibility.

However, it does have some drawbacks. Collection is invasive and requires specialized personnel. It is also a complex sample that requires preparation prior to analysis, and in which drug and metabolite concentrations are lower than in other types of samples, such as urine, so analytical techniques with sufficient sensitivity and specificity to detect and quantify them must be used. In addition, when dealing with cadaveric blood, there is a risk of hemolysis, which greatly complicates the analysis. Furthermore, most toxins disappear from the blood within the first 24 hours, or even sooner, as is the case with ethyl alcohol or substances with short elimination half-lives, so late collection can lead to false negatives.

A sufficient quantity must be collected and stored under appropriate conditions, with particular emphasis on refrigeration, as the concentrations of toxic substances such as cocaine or ethyl alcohol can be altered if they are not stored in the right conditions.

Another conventional sample widely used in toxicology is **urine**. This sample has great advantages over blood. The first of these is that, even though the concentration of drugs in urine is influenced by urinary volume, which in turn depends on multiple factors, such as volume of fluid ingested, physical activity, and even weather conditions, it is undoubtedly a sample where the toxin is concentrated, as the kidney is the natural route of elimination for such substances, facilitating their detection even when highly sensitive analytical techniques are not available. It is also a sample that, due to its simple composition, allows for rapid screening tests (immunoassays) that do not require sample preparation or specialized personnel to perform and that also provide results in a short period of time. Its collection is non-invasive, a large amount of sample is obtained, and no trained personnel are required. However, the process must be supervised to prevent substitution or adulteration.

Despite these advantages, urine sampling also has some limitations. The first and most important of these is that the toxic concentrations found do not correlate with clinical status, as this is a cumulative sample, so the results must be interpreted correctly. Thus, a positive urine test only indicates previous exposure in the preceding days, and can never be used to justify a clinical picture, let alone a change in behavior at a specific moment. It should also be noted that there are no commercially available immunoassays for all drugs of abuse, and even fewer for new psychoactive substances.

In general, a sufficient amount is collected to allow for preliminary screening and subsequent confirmation, and storage at 4°C is sufficient, without the need to add any preservatives.

Gastric contents are only of interest in cases where it is suspected that the drug was consumed via the digestive tract, as might be the case with amphetamines and other psychoactive substances. This sample can be very useful in an emergency department or in cases of fatal poisoning.

The main advantage of this sample is the extremely high concentration of drugs that can be detected without having undergone metabolic processes, which greatly simplifies detection.

However, unlike urine, it is not possible to use immunoassays for preliminary screening, nor can such samples be analyzed without a laborious prior process of extracting the toxin, which prevents analytical results from being obtained in a few minutes.

It is a biological sample in which only qualitative analyses are normally performed, since the concentration of toxins in it only provides information on the amount of toxin ingested, but without any clinical relevance except for confirmation of toxin ingestion.

The three biological samples mentioned above are now referred to as "conventional samples," as they have been routinely used in all toxicology laboratories and offer the main advantages of knowledge of drug incorporation mechanisms, analysis methods, and interpretation.

In contrast to these, so-called alternative samples are currently used, so named because they can replace conventional samples. Thus, as shown in Figure 8.1, saliva can be an alternative sample to blood, since the detection windows for the toxin are similar; sweat can be an alternative to urine; and hair, unlike all the others, has the largest detection window and is completely different from the other samples.

The main advantages of these samples are that they are difficult to tamper with and can be collected non-invasively. Furthermore, with current knowledge, it is possible to interpret the results obtained from a toxicological point of view. On the other hand, the concentration of drugs in these samples is lower, so they require the use of highly sensitive analytical techniques.

It is also important to mention the possibility of using meconium or umbilical cord blood to assess drug exposure during pregnancy, a procedure that is currently used routinely in some hospitals for this purpose.

Saliva or oral fluid is a biological sample that has been used for several decades to analyze certain drugs, offering the possibility of conducting pharmacokinetic studies without the need for blood draws. Today, its main use in this field is the analytical control of drugs of abuse in road traffic.

Saliva is a biological fluid produced constantly by the salivary glands, reaching a volume ranging from 0.5 to 1.5 liters per day, depending on various factors, and even higher when subjected to stimulation processes.

Most drugs reach saliva from the blood through a simple process of diffusion through the lipid membrane that separates them, with saliva thus representing a mirror image of the blood, although there are small variations in concentration between them, due to the physicochemical properties of each drug. For this reason, a saliva test can replace a blood test to demonstrate the presence of any drug at a given moment and, due to the large number of screening devices on the market, its use is now a reality in the control of drug abuse in driving.

Its simpler biological composition relative to blood has allowed the development of rapid analysis kits for preliminary screening. In addition, it is easy and quick to collect, non-invasive, and difficult to tamper with.

However, it has its limitations, such as the difficulty, mainly from a medical-legal point of view, of interpreting the results. This is partly due to the multiple factors that can vary the concentrations found: salivary pH, the collection method, etc.

The volume of sample collected can also be a limitation, since even though it is possible to perform a rapid test that requires only a small sample, this must be confirmed using more specific analytical techniques, as there is always the possibility of cross-reactions that might lead to false positives. The volume obtained is influenced by many factors that can affect saliva production, such as hydration, exposure to olfactory stimuli, or even certain types of pathologies. Although saliva production can be stimulated to obtain a larger sample volume, this is not recommended, as it is now known that this can lead to dilution of the sample and, therefore, to obtaining a false negative.

Sweat, as a means of eliminating toxins from the body, is an alternative sample to urine for drug testing, with the main advantage of a longer detection window due to the way it is collected.

It is produced by the sweat glands in quantities that can reach up to more than 1 liter per day, depending on multiple factors, such as ambient temperature and humidity, physical exercise, hormonal factors, etc.

As with saliva, most drugs easily reach sweat through passive diffusion processes, a process conditioned by the chemical structure of each drug.

It is an easy and unique biological sample, collected through patches that can cover 7 to 14 days of drug exposure, without the need for more frequent testing, which is a great advantage over urine, whose detection window is much smaller. For example, some substances, such as cocaine, reach sweat within 2 hours of exposure and can be detected up to four days later. These are breathable patches, in which sweat is collected through an absorbent pad and the drug accumulates for the desired period of time. Those currently in use are easy to apply and remove and impossible to falsify, as each one has an identification number, making it impossible to replace them.

One disadvantage worth mentioning is that, unlike with urine or saliva, there are no rapid screening tests available, due to the mechanism of drug elimination, which requires a minimum amount of time for a detectable amount to be present. Therefore, the patch must be worn for at least 24 hours before it can be analyzed, and more sensitive analytical techniques, such as chromatographic techniques, must be used. In addition, there is no possibility of pharmacokinetic interpretation of the results, as there are many factors that can influence them, such as sweat pH, uneven distribution of glands, etc. Nevertheless, it is a biological sample of great interest that allows periods of abstinence of 7 to 14 days to be monitored without the need for more frequent analysis, as is the case with urine, which would require analysis at least every two or three days.

Hair is undoubtedly the most widely used alternative biological sample in the field of drug addiction, especially in the medico-legal sphere, without detracting from its clinical applications, which have become increasingly well known in recent years.

Although the initial application of hair analysis was for the detection of metals, since the 1970s it has been extended to the analysis of organic compounds, including drugs of abuse. Thus, in 1979, Baumgartner began to determine heroin in hair using immunological methods, and since then, analytical methods have been developed for the determination of all types of toxins, including pharmaceuticals, drugs, environmental contaminants, etc. To this end, analytical methods have been developed using different analytical techniques that currently allow for all types of determinations, even when the concentrations found are low. Today, hair is the only biological sample that allows for the detection of consumption prior to collection, which is why it is widely used in the field of drug addiction, replacing conventional periodic urine tests.

It is now well known how toxins are incorporated into hair, including drugs of abuse. This incorporation occurs in several ways: the blood that irrigates the hair follicles, the secretions of sweat and sebaceous glands at that level, and, not least, incorporation through external contamination, which must be taken into account when performing the analyses to avoid giving a false positive result.

There is considerable individual variability in the concentration of toxins in hair, due to multiple factors, such as the structure of the hair itself (cuticle, medulla, and cortex), and factors that depend on the drug itself, such as its lipophilicity, chemical structure, and affinity for melanin. All these factors must be taken into account when interpreting the analytical results, not considering the quantitative value as an absolute result, as is the case with analyses in other biological matrices. However, it is a biological sample that allows the severity of consumption to be assessed, and even the individual pattern of drug dependence to be identified. It is therefore a very useful biological sample that complements those mentioned above.

Hair offers many advantages as a biological sample. The first of these is the possibility of detecting previous consumption, since drugs are incorporated into the hair 7–10 days after consumption and remain there indefinitely without undergoing further metabolic processes. It is also important to note that it is easy to collect without using invasive methods or invading privacy, coupled with the fact that it does not require the addition of any preservatives. All of this has facilitated a large number of large-scale epidemiological studies, which are generally spread out over time.

Its applications, as mentioned above, are increasingly extensive. Hair analysis is used to evaluate adherence to detoxification treatments, the influence of drug use on certain psychiatric and cardiovascular pathologies, and to monitor drug use during pregnancy.

Another important advantage is the possibility of analyzing hair from any part of the body (armpit, pubic hair, beard, etc.) when scalp hair is not available or is unsuitable due to its length. In this case, the biology of each type of hair must be taken into account when interpreting the analytical results, which is obviously more difficult than in the case of hair, as its growth rate is not known with certainty.

However, certain limitations must be taken into account. The first is the possibility of a false positive due to external contamination if the pre-analytical phase, which includes decontamination procedures, is not performed correctly. Another limitation is that, due to the high variability between individuals, there is no exact correlation between the dose consumed and the concentration detected.

Furthermore, it has not yet been possible to establish the minimum detectable dose, so a negative result does not always rule out drug exposure, a fact that must be taken into account when using it as a sample for the diagnosis of chemical submission.

Finally, it is important to highlight the slowness of the disappearance of drugs from the hair after cessation of use, making it possible to detect them several months after the start of the abstinence period, particularly for drugs such as cocaine, which, due to their chemical structure, are easily incorporated into the hair.

All these limitations have been noted in studies evaluating the difficulty of interpreting analytical results in some cases.

The most relevant characteristics of all the samples mentioned are listed in Table 8.2.

Meconium is the first fecal matter eliminated by newborns during the first days of life. Its formation begins approximately in the twelfth week of gestation, and all the toxins to which the fetus was exposed are deposited in it. As is well known, these toxins reach the fetus through the placenta, which metabolizes them and eliminates them into the amniotic fluid, subsequently producing their reabsorption. In this way, they will accumulate in the

TABLE 8.2 Comparison Between Different Biological Samples

	Saliva	**Blood**	**Urine**	**Hair**
Sample collection	Non-invasive	Highly invasive	Intrusion into privacy	Non-invasive
Primary analyte	Toxic	Toxic and metabolites	Metabolites	Toxic
Analyte concentration	Low	Very low	Very high	Medium
Interpretation	• Pharmacokinetic studies • Potential correlation with impairment • Determines the free fraction in blood	• Pharmacokinetic studies • Potential correlation with impairment	• Limited use • No correlation with clinical status • Does not estimate blood concentration	• Limited if not hair
Potential problems	• Contamination • Changes in pH during collection affect S/P • Small sample size • No reference material	• Limited collection • Complex composition	• Adulteration • pH changes during storage • Excretion varies with pH	• External contamination • Complex sample

meconium, and therefore their analysis will allow us to evaluate the possible exposure of the fetus to toxins during the last six months of gestation. In addition to having this large detection window, this sample is simple to collect—directly from the diaper—and collection remains possible for at least 3 or 4 days.

The main disadvantage of meconium samples is their complex composition, which has prevented the development of rapid tests that can be implemented in neonatal services, and the laborious extraction procedure, even in the toxicology laboratory itself.

Furthermore, it is recommended that collection be done as soon as possible, as meconium is eliminated over several days, so its composition is variable, leading to different analytical results depending on the day of collection.

Even so, its current use for monitoring drug use during pregnancy is, together with the possibility of analyzing analysis of maternal pubic hair shaved at the time of delivery, the best tool available for this purpose.

REFERENCES

1. Bermejo AM, Tabernero MJ. Determination of drugs of abuse in hair. Bioanalysis. 2012;4(17):2091–4.
2. Bermejo M, Tabernero MJ, Strano-Rossi S, Álvarez I, Cabarcos P. Muestras Biológicas en Toxicología. Manual de Adiciones para Médicos Especialistas en Formación.. Socidrogalcohol, 2010: 285–309.
3. Musshoff F, Madea B. Analytical pitfalls in hair testing. Analytical and Bioanalytical Chemistry. 2007;388(7): 1475–94.
4. Suarez Garcia A, Álvarez Freire I, Bermejo AM, Cabarcos Fernández P, Tabernero Duque MJ. Duration of detection of cocaine and metabolites in hair after discontinuation of abuse. Microchemical Journal. 2020;153:104335.
5. Torales J, Castaldelli-Maia JM, da Silva AG, Campos MW, González-Urbieta I, Barrios I. Even More Complex…. When Mental Disorder Meets Addiction in Youth: Dual Pathology. Curr Drug Res Rev. 2019;11(1):40–43.
6. Wada M, Ikeda R, Kuroda N, Nakashima K. Analytical methods for abused drugs in hair and their applications. Analytical and Bioanalytical Chemistry. 2010;397(3):1039–67.

8.5 ETHICAL ASPECTS IN THE APPROACH TO DUAL-PATHOLOGY PATIENTS

M. J. Tabernero Duque, P. Cabarcos Fernández, I. Álvarez Freire, C. C. Cossío Uribe, and A. M. Bermejo Barrera

INTRODUCTION

Drug Use and Dual Pathology

Drug use is a problem with significant repercussions, not only for the individual but also for their environment and society as a whole.

According to the World Health Organization (WHO), *addiction* is a disease caused by repeated consumption of one or more psychoactive substances, to the point that the user becomes intoxicated periodically or continuously, shows a compulsive desire to consume the preferred substance (or substances), has enormous difficulty voluntarily stopping or modifying consumption of the substance, has enormous difficulty voluntarily interrupting or modifying consumption of the substance, and is determined to obtain psychoactive substances by any means (WHO, 1994).

Addiction is characterized by a set of signs and symptoms involving biological, genetic, psychological, and social factors. It is a progressive and serious disease, characterized by continual episodes of lack of control, distorted thinking, and denial. It is thus understood to be a chronic and recurrent condition that affects the brain's structure and functioning, altering the reward system.

When an addictive disorder is combined with a mental disorder, this is referred to as *dual pathology*. These patients require specialized care focused on their specific needs.

Currently, in addition to drug addictions, there are also behavioral addictions, which refer to those that are not due to a dependence on substances such as alcohol, cocaine, or other drugs, but rather to types of behavior dependent on certain daily activities that are beyond the person's control and limit their life (gambling, shopping, online activities, etc.). Among all behavioral addictions, gambling is the one most frequently described as associated with other mental disorders.

Among the essential characteristics of patients with dual pathology are: lack of awareness of the disorder (with difficulties in accepting and/or communicating that they have an addiction), identification with only one of the disorders (mental or addictive), greater use of emergency services and psychiatric hospitalization, maladjustment and difficulty in adhering to treatment (high relapse rate), great vulnerability and difficulty coping with stressful life events, and a consequent higher likelihood of unemployment and social exclusion (more pronounced in women with dual diagnosis).

Depending on the order of appearance of these diseases and the relationship of influence established between them, three mechanisms have been proposed to explain the development of dual pathology (Confederación Salud Mental España, 2020):

1. The primary disorder is addiction, which induces the development of a mental disorder. This usually occurs in patients with preexisting vulnerability.

2. Addiction is caused by the use of substances used to treat or alleviate symptoms due to a psychiatric disorder.
3. The two processes share the same risk factors (stress, personality or genetic traits, environmental circumstances) that induce their onset.

Patients with dual pathology are characterized by (Confederación Salud Mental España, 2020):

- Lack of awareness or denial of illness or addiction
- Usually admitting to only one of the two disorders (addiction or mental illness)
- Frequent use of emergency services and higher frequency of hospital admissions
- Social/family/work maladjustment
- Difficulty adhering to treatment, and high frequency of therapeutic failures, relapses, and treatment refusals
- High vulnerability, with low stress tolerance
- Gender differences in relation to the substance causing addiction (in women, the most common addictions associated with mental disorders are related to alcohol and tranquilizer use; in men, cocaine, heroin, and cannabis are most prevalent)
- Greater risk of women with dual pathology of gender-based violence and social and labor exclusion
- Seeking health care less frequently

Treatment and Prevention: Drug Addiction

Drug addiction treatment consists not only of caring for people affected by addiction, but also of early intervention for drug users who are not yet affected by it, and preventive measures aimed at delaying the age of onset of use and preventing it from becoming a problem for the individual or their environment.

This care also includes strategies and advice for patients' families and communities to alleviate the stress they generally suffer and improve the support they can provide to the patient in the process of withdrawal.

With regard to prevention, the fundamental approach is based on a balance between reducing risk factors and promoting protective factors.

Today, prevention faces new challenges: new forms of addiction (pathological gambling, social media, online shopping), the perception of normality in alcohol and cannabis use by minors, the debate on the legalization of cannabis, and the continuous emergence of new psychoactive substances on the market. In addition, it is necessary to adapt to new social contexts and the different forms of relationships in which consumption occurs (especially social media).

Programs for the prevention of drug addiction and other addictive disorders are developed in different areas: education, family, community, and leisure and free time.

The human and social cost of drug addiction is undeniable, not only in terms of the economic cost of care provided by the public health system (prevention and health promotion measures, medical care, and treatment), but also in terms of the risks associated with public safety and social impact (risks to driving and public health, intimate partner and sexual violence, the environment, and the impact on family, work, and society).

Purposes of Medicine

In the current conception of medicine, it is undeniable that healthcare professionals must not only recognize the disease, but also the patient's reaction to that disease. Health is not only the absence of disease, but a state of physical, psychological, social, and spiritual balance that provides the person with harmony with themselves and their environment. Illness involves a loss of this balance, leading to a state of discomfort, physical pain, and psychological suffering, compounded by fear of the unknown. Each patient's reaction to a disorder depends not only on the illness itself, but also on their personality and their personal, family, and social circumstances.

In 1996, the Hastings Center indicated that there are four purposes of medicine: to prevent illness, to cure, to care, and to help to die in peace (Fundació Grifols, 2004). To achieve these objectives, it is essential to establish an appropriate clinical relationship, based on a social contract founded on the trust that the patient places in the knowledge and commitment of the physician. This relationship is based on three fundamental pillars: trust, mutual respect, and truthfulness. Healthcare personnel are responsible for ensuring that the dignity of the patient is respected in this relationship.

To this end, it is essential to respect confidentiality, privacy, the right to information and participation in decision-making, and the right not to be discriminated against on the basis of origin, beliefs, situation, or economic, cultural, or social capacity. The trust established between the therapist and the patient is essential in order to reach an accurate diagnosis and thus address the treatment of any illness in the most appropriate manner.

ETHICAL ASPECTS IN THE TREATMENT OF DUAL-PATHOLOGY PATIENTS

General Considerations

In human relationships (and therefore in healthcare relationships), there are no ethically neutral acts. Bioethics aims to assist in decision-making by incorporating values into facts.

In the healthcare field, bioethics, now fully established, is beginning to advance in the study of ethical conflicts generated in different specialties, pathologies, and areas of treatment, identifying problems and establishing frameworks of agreement to propose courses of action (rather than seeking indisputable consensus or definitive solutions).

At the healthcare level, this means addressing the conflicts of values arising from the clinical relationship. The ethics of clinical care (clinical or healthcare bioethics) involves all professionals who care for patients with addictive and mental disorders (doctors, psychologists, nurses, social workers, etc.).

Drug addiction raises conflicts of values at many different levels, constituting a complex problem in which very diverse interests interact (not only health-related, but also political, economic, social, and cultural) and which, in many scenarios, health professionals end up addressing through their moral intuitions.

Bioethical reflection aims to assist in the decision-making process in situations of ethical and clinical uncertainty, addressing some of the problems that arise (such as the criteria for choosing between different programs: drug-free, maintenance, or harm reduction).

The treatment of addictive disorders, as part of clinical intervention, has undergone conceptual modifications and changes. From attempts to explain all aspects of addictive behavior and its therapeutic intervention, to the tendency to justify non-quantitative assessment methodologies due to the diversity of nuances in the therapeutic process. Currently, the trend is toward standardization of care, although there are still significant differences in how it is implemented and in existing opinions regarding intervention methodologies.

Beauchamp and Childress's *principlism* has been the best-known practical theoretical system of medical ethics principles in the healthcare field, although it is not the only one. It proposes four general principles as axiological poles of medical ethics that can guide the resolution of conflicts, dilemmas, or situations of ethical-clinical uncertainty (Escobar López, 2012). Patients with an addictive disorder and a psychiatric disorder have defining and specific characteristics. The implication and use of these four basic principles of bioethics in health care for patients with dual pathology involves integrating and understanding these specificities in order to adapt to their demands. Below are some considerations based on the four principles aimed at this patient population:

- **Non-maleficence**: Confidentiality, use of validated and proven therapeutic techniques, accredited and trained therapists, accurate diagnosis (important to avoid the risk of stigmatization), a range of therapeutic options, and the existence of concomitant disorders.

- **Justice**: Equal opportunities for all; non-discrimination and non-marginalization, which are obvious for any patient, take on special importance here. It is essential to bear in mind the concept of equity in relation to the high demands of some of these patients and, therefore, adaptation to their specific needs.

- **Respect for autonomy**: A multitude of issues that take on special relevance in relation to the capacity/competence to decide, voluntariness, lack of legal capacity, substitution of criminal sanctions for treatment, complications and risk to third parties, pregnancy, dual diagnosis, etc.

- **Beneficence**: The well-being of the patient, the therapist's main objective, must take into account their wishes and free choice, since a benefit imposed or achieved through coercion or compulsion does not respond to the bioethical values pursued in clinical practice.

Healthcare ethics must always take into account the consequences (real or foreseeable) of clinical activity. When it comes to behavioral disorders or disturbances, the interpretation of the principles of beneficence and autonomy can sometimes be conflicting or even contradictory in relation to the consideration of values and opinions about appropriate treatment.

Several models of the clinician–patient relationship have been described that outline how the relationship with the patient as a moral subject is established and how decision-making is guided based on one principle or another. The oldest and most prevalent has been the paternalistic model, which, although it gave rise to medicine, has been enriched over time by various philosophical theories, such as utilitarianism (the obligation to seek the greatest possible happiness for the greatest possible number of people, regardless of the right to information, truthfulness, or confidentiality). In this model, it is the physician who, based on the principle of beneficence, makes all decisions with the conviction of knowing what is best for the patient. The autonomist model recognizes the prevalence of patient autonomy as the basis for decision-making and implies a moral obligation between the therapist and the patient, assuming that the patient has the capacity to understand and the right to make decisions about their life. This model also seeks the greatest possible happiness for the patient, but always focusing on their wishes and needs, and their full understanding of the situation (Emanuel and Emanuel, 1992).

However, autonomy (and freedom in the decision-making that this implies) is not the only value that must be taken into account in all cases (Morera Pérez, 2022). As Diego Gracia says, "Any value, taken to its ultimate consequences, becomes tyrannical because it damages many other values" (Gracia, 2013). It is necessary to consider the therapeutic possibilities, seeking what the professional considers best and most appropriate for a specific patient (beneficence) and respecting each patient's individual choice (autonomy), avoiding any harm or contraindication (non-maleficence) and always respecting equity and protection of third parties (justice), which today can be considered shared decision-making.

Drug addiction carries a heavy emotional and ideological burden that gives rise to extreme positions and often confrontational stances (legalization vs. criminalization, drug-free programs vs. substitution programs, marginalization versus integration or normalization, etc.).

When addiction and mental disorder coexist, a conflict arises between the patient and society (life–freedom dilemma) in relation to the establishment of limits (law–individual autonomy, society's actions to prevent harm to third parties, society's obligations to individuals who are irresponsible by their own choice, social, health, and economic costs assumed by society due to free and autonomous, etc.), which transcends the clinical relationship. While the latter requires personal and individualized care, society demands a comprehensive approach to the disease, including issues unrelated to clinical care (in relation to legal, social, political, economic, and even criminal aspects).

Thus, the care of these patients raises specific ethical issues and problems that we must consider:

- Assessment of the costs and benefits of actions in a health system that promotes universal coverage
- Confidentiality (conflict situations arise in relation to diagnosis and follow-up)

- Patient autonomy: The need to obtain informed consent for preventive and/or therapeutic procedures. Difficult balance between autonomy and paternalism, taking into account the need for support and the difficulties of the process
- Choice of therapeutic interventions that are minimally restrictive of patient freedom.
- Consideration and acceptance of the patient, and their rights and needs
- Professional competence, training, and updating of knowledge
- Definition of the limits of professional work
- Satisfaction of the interests of patients, families, and the community, especially when there is conflict between them
- Justice: In addition to the aforementioned need for fairness and non-discrimination, and the significant risk of stigmatization of these patients, consideration of the special protection required by the most vulnerable and the defense of incapacitated or marginalized patients
- The need to establish a clinical relationship based on mutual trust and respect, allowing the patient to make decisions after considering the information and voluntarily, avoiding prejudices or preconceived opinions that may influence the therapist's attitude

Clinical Relationship

The therapeutic relationship is the basis of healthcare work, and mutual trust and respect are essential to it. Only through an appropriate clinical relationship is it possible to establish a therapeutic plan in which the patient feels involved and jointly responsible.

Many patients with mental disorders take years to seek professional help due to the social stigma associated with it and social, economic, or other obstacles that hinder their access to health care.

Drug-dependent patients suffer from an illness, since drug addiction is an illness, but it is a marginalized illness that carries a very high social stigma, and this conditions how it is approached and treated, especially considering that patients often do not recognize the existence of a pathology.

Dual pathology adds a diagnosis of mental illness to drug addiction. This represents a different situation, something more than the sum of two illnesses. The coexistence of both pathologies in the same patient makes diagnosis difficult, increasing the possibility that one of the two processes will remain hidden. For example, the effects of drug use may be attributed to symptoms of mental illness. There are clinical indicators and analytical markers that help one make a correct diagnosis.

The professional must establish a therapeutic bond with the patient that helps them become aware of the existence of both pathologies and build a relationship of trust that facilitates adequate and prolonged follow-up over time. Only by establishing a definitive diagnosis can we move forward in addressing the disease, as it is necessary for the patient to be adequately involved in the treatment and recovery process. It is a fact that patients with dual pathology have a high rate of treatment dropouts, lack of motivation, changes and alternations between care teams, and relapses.

In order to establish stable therapeutic relationships that motivate the patient and provide the relationship with the therapist with the necessary trust, constant support and a therapeutic process that is continuously reviewed and adapted to the individual needs of each patient is required, with individualized interventions and the establishment of achievable short-term goals. Given that treatment is a long and ongoing process, it is necessary to understand and readjust the patient's expectations, maintaining constant motivation to prevent relapse or abandonment and promote adherence to treatment and the well-being derived from achieving personal goals.

Comprehensive, coordinated care provided by a team of trained professionals equipped with the necessary resources helps to develop long-term strategies and resolve conflicts that arise over time.

In these patients, it is particularly important to consider advance healthcare planning, which helps to promote their autonomy by providing them with tools for decision-making and confidence to resolve any conflicts that may arise, thereby strengthening their bond with therapists. In this way, patients are aware of their situation and its evolution, enabling them to develop a fuller life and set goals that help them develop their own life project.

Autonomy

A patient-centered care model considers autonomy to be the cornerstone of the clinical relationship, encouraging decision-making that reflects the patient's own life plan. However, this autonomy requires one essential condition: the patient's ability and competence to deliberate and make their own decisions, to take into account realistic expectations, and to achieve clear and realistic goals. Autonomy is a concept with philosophical roots that refers to self-governance, while capacity, understood as the operational function of autonomy, is a concept with psychological roots that refers to the subject's ability to perform.

In the healthcare setting, the task at hand is health decision-making (Cossio, 2020). Patients with decision-making difficulties, with diminished capacity or competence, may have problems fully exercising this right to autonomy. Leaving aside the criteria used to determine the degree of capacity, it is clear that patients with dual pathology may need support in making decisions. The therapeutic relationship can provide this support by understanding their wishes and preferences, establishing adequate communication that allows for knowledge of their needs and expectations, and helping with advance care planning that is progressive throughout the evolution of the process and care.

In order for patients to fully exercise their autonomy, it is necessary to promote the knowledge and social skills that are essential for decision-making. A correct self-perception of one's own identity and possible vulnerabilities, through the review and knowledge of the reality that surrounds them, facilitates the exercise of their autonomy.

According to the Convention on the Rights of Persons with Disabilities (Spain, *Law 8/2021*), equal recognition before the law of persons with disabilities should be a universal achievement, and people's biological characteristics should not determine whether or not they can exercise their rights. In cases where they are unable to decide for themselves, support should be provided to enable them to make responsible choices. The problem arises when undue influences affect or harm the dignity of the patient. The aim is to offer the necessary support and assistance without interfering with their wishes and life plans or making value judgments based on prejudices or unfounded assumptions.

Confidentiality

The fundamental ethical basis for confidentiality is the professional's respect for the autonomy of their patient, which obliges them to protect their personal information and preserve their privacy. Professional secrecy is the basis of a relationship of trust between therapist and patient.

Legally speaking, professional secrecy is considered a means of protecting fundamental rights, but not a fundamental right in itself. Professionals also have other duties, and fulfilling these duties may conflict with their duty of confidentiality. That is why there are well-known exceptions to this duty.

Patients have the right to privacy and confidentiality of information relating to their health processes, and it is the professional's obligation to safeguard this right.

They also have the right to access the information contained in their medical records. However, in the case of psychiatric patients, some authors differentiate between two types of information in medical records: on the one hand, objective facts and data, and on the other, the therapist's personal judgments or reflections. The latter constitute subjective information, interpretations, or hypotheses that do not necessarily have to be shared (Ramos Montes, 2012).

Confidentiality is particularly important in psychiatry due to the intimate nature of the information involved and the prejudices and stigmas associated with mental illness, meaning that the disclosure of information can seriously damage the patient's dignity.

Most potential conflicts relating to the confidentiality of information concern three aspects: the need for teamwork (multidisciplinarity and relations between different agencies or institutions), third-party access to information (e.g., in the case of intervention by judicial bodies), and the patient's inability to consent and therefore decide on the handling of their health information. These cases must be addressed in accordance with legal regulations and criteria of good professional practice. Thus, the information disclosed must be strictly necessary for the required purpose and, whenever possible, the patient should be included in the process, explaining the reasons for the exceptional nature of the situation.

Psychiatric reports are another potential source of conflict. It is necessary to prepare the report with a clear understanding of its purpose and to include only the information that is required and necessary for that purpose, avoiding subjective or unconfirmed data.

In competent patients, the patient's authorization is required to disclose the information (except in cases provided for by law). Consulting the patient about whether they consent to its use, as well as communicating the type and extent of the information required and its purposes, helps to strengthen the doctor–patient relationship by involving them in decision-making. Extreme caution is necessary in the case of particularly vulnerable patients (minors, incompetent patients), always informing them, taking into account their ability to understand.

Each specific case must be analyzed from an ethical standpoint, seeking a solution that is tailored to the patient's preferences as far as possible in order to avoid conflicts and strengthen the trust that the patient has put in their therapist, but also considering other possible implications (potential for homicidal behavior, gender violence, child abuse, or risk of suicide: substance use is a major risk factor for suicide, and it is estimated that 40% of people with dual pathology have suicidal thoughts (Confederación Salud Mental España, 2020).

Decision-Making

Traditionally, mental disorders have been understood as a situation of incapacity or incompetence on the part of the patient, assuming the existence of an abnormal perception of reality and internal conflicts that prevent self-control. This stigma associated with mental illness greatly conditions the development of a self-managed life project (Kong, 2017).

When patients refuse the care or treatment proposed by their doctor, or choose the least appropriate option for their situation, professionals are faced with a problematic situation, a conflict of values, or even the dilemma of carrying out what they consider to be the most appropriate course of action as opposed to recognizing autonomy through respect for the patient's freedom to make decisions.

Here it is essential to assess the patient's capacity and competence, which forms part of the qualification of consent to the proposed intervention. The criteria for decision-making capacity are sometimes changeable, as the patient's situation may vary over time. Patients go through different phases and psychological reactions after a diagnosis of mental illness, and this can limit their ability to decide. In many cases, their family members and loved ones may also experience similar reactions and phases. Therefore, it is sometimes important for this consideration to vary, depending on the clinical situation and the patient's decision at any given moment.

It is necessary to recognize patients' capacity to choose and therapeutic needs, their clinical situation at the time of treatment, and their right to refuse therapy; this is complicated when it is necessary to take into account other opinions (from relatives or family members) in patients who are legally incapable of making decisions (whether permanently or temporarily). The new Law 8/2021, reforming civil and procedural legislation to support persons with disabilities in the exercise of their legal capacity (Spain, *Law 8/2021*), provides for a reconsideration of these situations by revising the concept of capacity/incapacity with a new perspective that takes into account the need for support in exercising capacity and developing one's own decision-making process.

In some cases, it will still be necessary to turn to the patients' legal representatives and take their choice into consideration (decisions by proxy). The basic objective is that this representative should be someone who truly knows the patient's values and wishes and is capable of adapting to the demands of the specific situation in which they find themselves. In some cases, the patient does not have suitable representatives who can perform this role because there are no individuals who are familiar with their values and wishes. In these situations, the support of a professional (not directly involved in the care work) who can assist in decision-making to achieve the most appropriate outcome in the patient's best interests is particularly valuable.

In order to preserve the autonomy of patients when they are no longer competent to make decisions for themselves, a type of advance decision-making has been proposed that allows their wishes, preferences, and needs to be taken into account. The decision can be set out in an *advance directive* (AD) or *advance care directive* (ACD), which is an expression of the principle of autonomy, in anticipation of a hypothetical future situation, with the limitations that this anticipation entails. *Advance care planning* (ACP) refers to preparing for future medical decisions in a hypothetical situation in which individuals are no longer able to express their wishes or make decisions for themselves. It is a more useful and realistic concept than an AD, as it evolves with the situation, adapting as circumstances change. It arises as a result of a new way of understanding the clinical relationship. It is also referred to as *advance statement*, in reference to different types of measures depending on their objectives, the involvement of professionals, the presence or absence of a third party, and prior assessment of the competence or nature of the content.

The aim is for professionals to plan medical care with the patient, anticipating future situations and making decisions on how to proceed in the event of events that may occur in the near or distant future. This involves knowledge and understanding of the patient's personal values and preferences and may include a trusted person who will be responsible for making care decisions if the patient is unable to do so.

Medical care is thus understood as a continuous process that is not occasional, sporadic, or fortuitous, but rather carefully devised.

Psychiatric patients may require this planning due to the possibility that their illness might affect their ability to understand and perceive themselves or the reality around them, meaning that the decisions they make within the context of their illness might not reflect their preferences and values, or their own life plan.

Its purpose is to promote patient autonomy and self-determination, improving intra-family and care relationships, as it facilitates communication and promotes alliances and support for conflict resolution. In addition, it involves the patient in the care process, thereby reducing situations of refusal, abandonment, or rejection of treatment, as well as relapses, avoiding or limiting as much as possible the use of legal action and involuntary measures.

This advance planning for psychiatric patients must address the issue of the patient's capacity for autonomous decision-making and, therefore, whether other elements should be considered (e.g., indications, appropriate use of resources, or family or third-party interests). It is also necessary to be aware of the possibility of limits to what can be anticipated or planned in advance.

The content that should be reflected in the PAAS (Morera, 2022), in a very general way, has to do with:

- Preventive measures (to detect relapse early and limit damage: symptoms or signs that should trigger intervention, key people to involve, intervention strategies)
- Therapeutic decisions (preferences for pharmacological treatment, dose limits based on personal experience, specific routes of administration or forms of pharmacological presentation, preferences for place of treatment and alternatives to hospitalization,

situations in which voluntary admission would be acceptable or the need for involuntary admission, preferences for emergency care)

- Other decisions (information to third parties, permitted visits, support during hospitalization and access to communications, dietary preferences, and persons who should take over the patient's personal responsibilities during a period of incapacity)
- Appointment of a representative for healthcare decision-making (their participation in the discussion and decision-making process, and any limits that may be established).

To promote patient protection, taking into account their particular needs and circumstances, community support and the application of flexible care models that adapt to specific circumstances and demands are essential, as these vary greatly even in each patient at certain points in the progression of their illness and the combined effects of their addiction (Confederación Salud Mental España, 2020). It is necessary to change the perception that people with dual pathology are difficult cases and therefore require exceptional measures that prevent respect for their free decision.

Other Considerations

Dual pathology requires a comprehensive healthcare approach, including the individual, their family and social environment, and the community as a whole. When we talk about public health, we are referring to care for the community and the sick individual, understanding that every individual action also has an impact on society as a whole (public safety, economy, health, etc.). The objective must be patient care and its effects on collective health. In the case of addiction, it is particularly evident that drug use affects not only the user, but also the addict's environment and society as a whole, which could be affected. in some way at some point due to this consumption.

The Royal Decree on the Basic Portfolio of Services of the National Health System and other state and regional regulations related to addiction care establish universal and free healthcare coverage and establish a principle of equity (which requires actions proportional to needs) and solidarity (prioritizing the protection of the most vulnerable groups).

The aim is to provide a response tailored to the needs of each patient and to promote their full social integration.

Drug addiction care consists of care for people affected by addiction and also early care for drug users not yet affected by it.

Given the characteristics of drug dependence disorders, strategies and advice are also needed for families with the aim of alleviating the stress they generally suffer and improving the support they provide to their family member in the process of withdrawal. It is also necessary to provide information and support to people in the family environment who are at particular risk or in a situation of drug abuse.

As with any psychiatric illness, the family plays an essential role in understanding and diagnosing dual pathology; and their active involvement in the therapeutic process and in monitoring progress contributes to recovery and social inclusion. The family can be an important source of support and is considered an essential protective factor, but it is necessary to collaborate with them, support them, and provide them with all the tools they need to bear the burden of caring for these patients. Conflicts in family relationships are common, and it is necessary to try to reduce the burden that families bear, which can lead to abandonment or confrontation due to an inability to cope with the consequences of a long-term process. It is also important to avoid overprotection and encourage autonomy, so that the patient is able to take on greater responsibilities and, in doing so, partially relieve the family of the total burden of the situation, promoting shared responsibility. Accurate information and training on mental health and addiction are also necessary to get everyone involved in resolving potential conflicts and problems that arise in everyday relationships. Families must play an active and positive role and be aware of their role in the patient's treatment and care process.

It is essential to highlight the importance of self-determination and the participation of patients and their families in the therapeutic process, as well as knowledge of the effects of treatments that help in choosing the one best suited to personal needs or rejecting those that fall short of their expectations or specific context. Patients with dual pathology are vulnerable and require special adaptability that protects their environment and specific values and avoids the feeling of helplessness that they often experience and that leads to rejection or constant relapse.

Coordination between professionals and family members involved must be improved, as must the availability of different resources, and criteria for access to care must be made more flexible, since patients who use drugs are often not accepted into specific care programs from which they might benefit. Intervention is necessary, adapting to the needs of the individual and the existing resources.

In order to deal with these types of pathologies correctly, with skill and knowledge, a change in attitudes is necessary. The shift from a paternalistic medical tradition to a model that respects the patient's decision-making involves respecting values such as good practice, autonomy, and beneficence, which in the case of psychiatric illnesses too often clash with less clear-cut values such as security, social peace, and public tranquility. Some of the general risk factors for mental disorders, such as social exclusion or economic inequality, cannot be addressed directly by psychiatrists.

Universal interventions in the general population require a public mental health approach and the involvement of other professionals or sectors such as education.

The conflict that arises between beneficence and autonomy is difficult to manage and requires a continuous process of dialogue (deliberation), striking a balance between respecting patients' wishes and the difficulty of exercising their freedom and autonomy in certain circumstances and moments, due to the effects of their own illness. Despite the obvious need to respect the right to free decision-making and choice, based on each person's personal life plan, support and guidance are needed to promote these values, while understanding the particular needs of each case and the specific context in which they arise. Professionals must bear in mind the importance of deliberation in this process.

In summary, more in-depth knowledge is required, specific training that includes communication skills and abilities, professional development, assessment of abilities, and techniques for handling difficult situations and decisions. Resources and strategies are also needed to help with the proper approach and planning of care. Guidelines or protocols for action are an important tool to help and support professionals in the correct management of different situations: establishing specific objectives, planning content, anticipating possible difficulties and knowing resolution strategies, and trying to understand and disseminate the values at stake so that they are accepted by professionals, patients, and their families. This requires an attitude of constant dialogue with a willingness to modify whatever is necessary to adapt to each specific situation.

It is also necessary to ensure continuity of care, together with the accessibility and availability of the necessary resources to provide the best possible care. This requires professionals to act responsibly, especially with patients who have greater difficulty accessing the healthcare system or who lack a social and/or family support network, and who require more time, effort, and commitment so that they feel involved in their own recovery process and valued in their particular circumstances.

REFERENCES

Spanish Mental Health Confederation. Apuntes sobre patología dual. Propuestas de la Red Salud Mental España. Madrid: Spanish Mental Health Confederation, 2020.

Cossio UC. Pacientes sin capacidad de decisión. Medical Ethics, 2020: 327–335 (CIB Publishing Fund, CES Publishing).

Emanuel EJ, Emanuel LL. Four Models of the Physician-Patient Relationship. JAMA. 1992;267(16):2221–6.

Escobar López MT. Bioética más allá del principialismo. Latin American Journal of Bioethics. 2012;12(2):6–9. Retrieved November 09, 2022, from http://www.scielo.org.co/pdf/rlb/v12n2/v12n2a01.pdf

Spain. Ley 8/2021, de 2 de junio, por la que se reforma la legislación civil y procesal para el apoyo a las personas con discapacidad en el ejercicio de su capacidad jurídica. BOE-A-2021-9233.

Gracia D. Construyendo valores. Madrid: Editorial Tria-castela, 2013: 66.

Hastings Center. Los fines de la medicina: el establecimiento de unas prioridades nuevas. Translation by the Victor Grifols Foundation. Notebooks of the Victor Grifols and Lucas Foundation. The aims of medicine. 2004:11.

Kong C. Mental Capacity in Relationship. Decision-Making, Dialogue, and Autonomy. Cambridge: University Press, 2017.

Morera Pérez B. Planificación anticipada de la asistencia en psiquiatría: criterios y marco de aplicación. EIDON. 2022;57:3–28.

WHO. Lexicon of Alcohol and Drug Terms. Madrid: Spanish Ministry of Health and Consumer Affairs, 1994.

Ramos Montes J, Gabaldón Fraile S. La confidencialidad en el ámbito de la discapacidad intelectual y la enfermedad mental. Bioètica & Debat. 2012;18(67):8–13.

CHAPTER 9

Is Prevention Possible in Dual Pathology?

F. Otero Lamas, A. F. Vale Ferreira, A. I. Da Silva Tavares, and A. Piñón Blanco

Prevention in dual pathology, in the strict sense, refers to specific strategies to reduce the incidence, prevalence, and recurrence of addictive disorders that occur simultaneously or sequentially with another mental disorder throughout the life cycle. From this perspective, a review of the literature would lead us to infer that the prevention of dual pathology, as such, is nonexistent and it could be said that we do not have specific preventive strategies for this clinical condition, which is characterized by high prevalence, complexity of care, and poor prognosis, among other features. However, this assessment may not be entirely accurate.

It should be borne in mind that, in the field of mental health, the availability of effective and standardized preventive strategies is still in its infancy. The systematic development of science-based prevention programs and studies to test their effectiveness spans only a few decades, during which most of the contemporary scientific, technical, and policy contributions that summarize knowledge in this field have been made, such as the World Health Organization (WHO) publications on mental health promotion,[152] mental health promotion,[153] and mental disorder prevention[154] and the series of reports by the US National Academy of Sciences on mental disorder risk reduction,[1] prevention of mental, emotional, and behavioral disorders among children and youth,[2] and promotion of healthy mental, emotional, and behavioral development in children and young people.[3] In Europe, the European Commission's Green Paper on Mental Health[4] and the contributions of projects such as MINDFUL (Mental Health Information and Determinants for the European Level),[5] IMHPA (Implementing Mental Health Promotion Action),[6] CAMHEE (Child and Adolescent Mental Health in Enlarged European Union),[7] ROAMER (Roadmap for Mental Health Research in Europe)[8,9] and, more recently, the European College of Neuropsychopharmacology Network on the prevention of mental disorders and the promotion of mental health.[10,157]

The WHO 2013–2030[156] comprehensive mental health action plan still proposes, as a global goal, that 80% of countries have at least two national and multisectoral mental health promotion and prevention programs in place by 2030 and includes general

DOI: 10.4324/9781003786153-9

strategies for promoting mental health and preventing mental disorders throughout life, focusing on: (1) laws and information campaigns against discrimination and human rights violations; (2) promoting the rights, opportunities, and care of people with mental disorders; (3) fostering basic individual attributes in the formative stages of life (such as early childhood programs, life skills and sex education, programs to support the development of secure, stable, and enriching relationships between children, their parents, and caregivers); (4) early intervention through the identification, prevention, and treatment of emotional or behavioral problems, especially in childhood and adolescence; (5) provision of healthy living and working conditions (including improvements in work organization and evidence-based stress management schemes in both the public and private sectors); and (6) protection programs or community protection networks that address child abuse and other forms of violence at the domestic and community levels, and social protection for the poor. To this end, states are invited to take the lead and coordinate multisectoral strategies that combine universal and specific interventions to promote mental health and prevent mental disorders, and to integrate these actions into national mental health and health promotion strategies. There is also a continued emphasis on the need to raise awareness of the magnitude of the disease burden associated with mental disorders and the availability of effective intervention strategies for mental health promotion and mental disorder prevention.

Mental disorders and substance use disorders are the main contributors to the global burden of disease, and their role is increasing, especially in developing countries.[11] According to data from the 2010 global burden of disease study, mental disorders and addictive disorders already accounted for almost 23% of the total global indicator of years lived with disability and almost 30% when referring specifically to the group of noncommunicable diseases.[11,12] In the European Union, it is estimated that 164.7 million people (more than 38% of the population) suffer from at least one mental disorder each year[12] and that the economic costs of mental illness may exceed 4% of GDP in several European countries.[13] On the other hand, half of all cases of mental disorders develop before the age of 14, although most are not detected or treated until later;[14,15,155] furthermoree, substance use disorders are common among children and young people with mental disorders. Children with emotional or behavioral disorders start using substances earlier and are at greater risk of developing problematic substance use disorders or substance use disorders,[16,17] and the prevalence rates of comorbid psychiatric disorders in young people treated for substance use disorders are consistently high in all studies, with total psychiatric comorbidity ranging from 61% to 88%.[18] Furthermore, mental and substance use disorders are the leading causes of health-related disability in children and young people,[15,19,20] who, between the ages of 0 and 24, constitute no less than 49% of the world's population.[21]

In turn, the prevalence of disorders due to use of substances concurrent with other psychiatric disorders is also very high, varying between 15% and 80% depending on the population samples analyzed and the methodology used.[22] People with dual pathology tend to be underdiagnosed and undertreated, while experiencing a high burden of morbidity and mortality, including premature drug-related death and increased risk of suicide. It has also been shown that people with dual pathology are significantly more likely to attend emergency departments, be hospitalized, and receive primary care than those with substance use disorders or mental disorders not related to concurrent substance use.[23]

Considering the enormous impact that mental disorders have on the health of the population, it is paradoxical to note the still insufficient funding dedicated to mental health research.[24] A study in the United Kingdom[25] reported that only approximately 5% of total health research resources had been allocated to mental health research and that, in turn, less than 4% of this funding had been applied to prevention research between 2014 and 2017. On the other hand, only 26% of the money spent on mental health research is allocated to projects on children and young people, despite the fact that 75% of mental illnesses begin before the age of 24.[26]

In this general context, the prevention of dual pathology has also been historically conditioned by other issues, such as conceptual controversies, the intrinsic complexity of the phenomenon, and the development of a specific body of knowledge on the genetic, epigenetic, neurobiological, and environmental factors that contribute to the development of this type of disorder. Despite advances in understanding the underlying mechanisms, further research is still needed on the common risk factors that may contribute to both addictive disorders and other mental illnesses, how mental illnesses may contribute to the development of addictive disorders, and how addictive disorders may contribute to the development of other mental illnesses.[158] It is precisely these etiopathogenic considerations that would point us to different mechanisms for approaching the effective prevention of dual pathology. Thus, programs developed to promote mental health and prevent mental disorders (such as those specifically aimed at preventing substance use disorders and other addictions) could also be considered useful in the prevention of dual pathology. In addition, improved identification of common and specific risk and protective factors would allow for more effective development of preventive strategies for both dual pathology and specific mental disorders.[27,28] However, research in this field is very complex, due, among other reasons, to the enormous variability of interactions between biology and environment,[29–32] which gives rise to dynamic and heterogeneous interindividual responses, even in the presence of the same risk and protective factors. Advances in knowledge about epigenetic mechanisms should contribute not only to the development of personalized therapeutic strategies but also to the availability of preventive resources that improve individual biological resilience to environmental risk factors.[32,33]

On the other hand, the promotion of mental health and the prevention of mental disorders should be approached from the perspective of the life course or life cycle,[34,35] since the interaction of certain risk and protective factors can be particularly relevant depending on the stage of development in which they occur.[36,37] This implies that it is necessary to consider the prenatal, perinatal, early childhood, childhood, adolescence and youth, adulthood, and old age periods differentially, as they represent specific intervals of vulnerability that must be taken into account when establishing the objectives of interventions and the time frame for the strategies to be developed, which, in turn, may encompass one or more of these periods. In a recent meta-analysis on the age of onset of mental disorders worldwide,[38] the authors report peaks at 14.5 and 30.5 years for the age of onset of any mental disorder. In the category of substance use or addictive behavior disorders, the peaks in age of onset are at 19.5 and 44.5 years. Although these data reinforce the importance of prioritizing prevention interventions in the earliest periods of development, they also point to the need to focus on older ages. On the other hand, the evolution of the population pyramid in our environment, with a progressive reduction in the population under 20 years of age and a continued increase in the population over 65 years of age, urges us to pay adequate attention to the prevention of dual pathology in older people.

> Another element that contributes to the complexity of research and implementation of prevention strategies is their typological diversity, which, historically, has been categorized according to the most classic taxonomies of primary, secondary, and tertiary prevention[39]; universal, selective, and indicated prevention[40]; integrative models based on the above that incorporate other concepts such as mental health promotion or personalized medicine, in which, for example, risk is identified based on genomic analysis[3]; up to the most recent classifications focused on the function or purpose of the intervention, which differentiate between environmental, developmental, or informational preventive measures.[41]

Furthermore, the multidimensional nature of mental health means that strategies for promoting it and preventing mental disorders go beyond the health sector itself and involve all levels of social organization. In this regard, we have a multitude of publications on experiences and programs of all kinds and types in each of the different areas of action and, to a lesser extent, studies that provide us with information on their quality, effectiveness, risk-benefit ratio, applicability, and efficiency. Although it is not the purpose of this chapter to review all the evidence, we can agree that a considerable number of specific prevention programs for mental disorders and substance use disorders have proven to be effective and cost-effective, that the implementation of these programs remains limited, and that there is still a need to converge towards a holistic and structural model in which each actor contributes specific interventions in their field but with synergistic effects within a global framework of comprehensive action.[42] Thus, despite the advances in theoretical and applied knowledge that have taken place in recent decades, we are still far from satisfactorily resolving some issues, which, for example, were already raised in a 1978 report produced in the US, which concluded that efforts to prevent mental illness and promote mental health were not structured, focused, or coordinated and received insufficient attention at the federal, state, and local levels.[43]

For practical reasons, we will restrict this chapter to the health sector and how it can contribute to this holistic and structural approach by incorporating a preventive approach based on consideration, detection, and treatment into routine healthcare practice, and early intervention and action on the main known risk factors affecting mental health. Although we will focus primarily on issues related to promotion and primary prevention, it is worth mentioning that secondary or tertiary prevention measures in adults with addictions or other mental disorders can also be considered, from a transgenerational perspective, as primary prevention measures. For example, effective treatment of dual pathology, reduction of its complications, or prevention of relapse would, in turn, represent forms of primary prevention for the offspring of affected individuals.

PREVENTION SITUATION IN THE CONTEXT OF DUAL PATHOLOGY

Reviewing the state of prevention in dual pathology necessarily involves doing so from a dichotomous perspective, since the effective segregation between mental health structures and those that treat addictive disorders is still a widespread reality. On the one hand, the situation of mental disorder prevention, which has been addressed marginally by national health systems, and, on the other, the prevention of drug addiction and other addictive disorders, which has received greater attention from specific sectoral structures, such as the National Plan on Drugs in Spain or the Intervention Service for Addictive Behaviors and Dependencies (SICAD) in Portugal.

A recent publication on preventive strategies for mental health,[44] provides a comprehensive review of the current situation regarding mental health prevention, the evidence supporting primary prevention in psychiatry, the cost-effectiveness of mental health prevention, the role of mental health professionals in mental health prevention, and a compilation of the main risk factors, risk markers, proposals for early detection, and preventive interventions categorized according to sensitive periods of intervention. It also provides timely reflections on the factors that hinder progress in prevention in psychiatry, examples of primary preventive interventions in mental health, and a set of key messages for the prevention of mental health disorders, which highlights the need to: (1) translate scientific evidence on cost-effective preventive interventions into public health initiatives, clinical practice, and service delivery systems; (2) increase social, professional, and political awareness of the advances and importance of mental health prevention and promotion; (3) shift clinical practice toward risk-oriented detection and intervention; (4) provide interventions designed for each stage of development to minimize the impact of risk factors; (5) promote multidisciplinary and multilevel interventions (psychological, social, family, and legal); take a multidisciplinary and multilevel approach (psychological, social, family, and legal); (6) promote healthy lifestyles that include nutrition and exercise; and (7) encourage school-based interventions (aimed at children, parents, and education professionals).

In a recent systematic review on cost-effectiveness,[45] most studies showed that interventions for prevention and mental health promotion were cost-effective, and targeted prevention was found to be more so than universal prevention. In children and adolescents, screening plus psychological interventions in schools were the most cost-effective interventions for the prevention of mental disorders, while interventions for parents had good evidence for promoting mental health. In adults, strong evidence supported screening plus psychological interventions for the prevention of mental disorders, and workplace interventions targeting employees in general were also cost-effective. There is no conclusive evidence for preventive interventions for mental disorders or mental health promotion in older adults.

We know that the etiology of mental disorders is multifactorial and an expression of a complex interaction between genetic vulnerability and environmental variables. In the absence of genetic biomarkers for clinical use, family history of mental disorders remains the main indicator of the risk of developing a mental disorder throughout life and, therefore, a risk factor that must be taken into account at all stages of the life cycle. Similarly, social adversity and stigma are risk factors that can have an impact throughout life.

With regard to the prenatal period, known risk factors include exposure to tobacco, alcohol, illicit drugs, medications, and toxins; nutritional problems; immune activation secondary to maternal infections; exposure to stress; and maternal psychopathology. In the perinatal period, risk factors include obstetric complications, premature birth, perinatal trauma, postpartum depression, severe social deprivation due to institutionalization, malnutrition, and attachment disorders.

Adverse experiences during childhood and adolescence play an important role in the development of physical and mental health problems in adulthood. Childhood exposure to chronic stress causes changes in the development of the nervous, endocrine, and immune systems, leading to impaired cognitive, social, and emotional functioning, increased allostatic load, and the adoption and persistence of behaviors that are harmful to health.[46–48] A large number of adverse childhood experiences have been identified, including problems at home such as domestic violence, substance abuse, mental illness, divorce, and incarceration; problems of emotional and physical neglect; problems of physical, emotional, and sexual abuse; and other problems such as bullying, isolation, socioeconomic status, separation or death of parents, and others.[49] The impact of adverse childhood experiences on neurobiology, mental health, and somatic health in later adulthood has been extensively studied[50,51] and evidence indicates that the risk is dependent on the number of adverse experiences suffered, and is higher for depression, post-traumatic stress disorder, borderline personality disorder, and substance abuse. Adverse childhood experiences were attributed to approximately 30% of anxiety cases and 40% of depression cases in North America and more than a quarter of both conditions in Europe.[52] Up to 24 adverse childhood experiences were associated with an increased risk of common mental disorders or suicidal tendencies in a recent comprehensive review of systematic reviews and meta-analyses,[53] which also emphasizes the need to further develop, evaluate, and implement interventions to prevent adverse childhood experiences or reduce their impact.

From adolescence onwards, the consumption of alcohol and other drugs play a particularly significant role as risk factors for the development of mental disorders. For example, the high potency of marijuana sold today is associated with an increased risk of dependence, cognitive impairment, and psychiatric problems.[54–56] THC administration can induce transient psychotic experiences in healthy individuals, and cannabis use is a risk factor for the development of psychosis or schizophrenia. Early age at onset of use and the use of more potent cannabis strains further increase the risk of psychosis. Cannabis use is also associated with a decrease in the age of onset of psychosis and, in people at high clinical risk, can exacerbate psychotic symptoms and advance the onset of psychosis.[57] On the other hand, cannabis use in adolescence is associated with an increased risk of developing major depression and suicidal tendencies in young adulthood, especially suicidal ideation.[58]

In adulthood and older adulthood, important risk factors include stress, social and economic adversity, health problems, chronic diseases and functional limitations, drug abuse, alcoholism and other addictions, and abuse.[59]

However, despite the multitude of studies on risk and protective factors for mental disorders conducted in recent decades, we must be aware that the knowledge generated is still limited, due, among other issues, to multiple methodological problems and the intrinsic complexity of the task, which must take into account phenomena of equifinality (multiple factors can lead to the same disorder) and multifinality (the same etiological factor can cause different mental disorders). A recent general review[60] analyzed 1,180 associations between putative risk or protective factors and mental disorders. Among these, 497 were non-significant, 507 were weak associations, and 176 were more robust associations, although only 21 met the criteria for the strongest associations.

Regarding addiction disorders, there are a large number of studies on risk and protective factors related to the use of legal or illegal substances,[61] but there is less evidence available on factors specifically related to the development of addictive disorders themselves. It is obvious that substance use is the main factor in the genesis of a substance use disorder, but fortunately, only a portion of all users develop a clinical entity requiring treatment. For example, the US Substance Abuse and Mental Health Services Administration reported that in 2018, approximately 164.8 million people aged 12 and older (60.2% of the population) used substances (tobacco, alcohol, or illicit drugs) during the past month, 139.8 million drank alcohol, and 31.9 million used an illicit drug. In the same year, approximately 20.3 million people aged 12 or older suffered from a substance use disorder related to alcohol or illicit drug use, 14.8 million suffered from an alcohol use disorder, and 8.1 million had an illicit drug use disorder.[62] Although there are variations depending on the substance studied and patterns of polydrug use, in general, we could consider that around 1 in 7 drug users develop a substance use disorder, as reported in a transnational study with more than 90,000 respondents,[63] which found that an individual's personal risk of transitioning to more severe drug use is associated with the substance use history of their age cohort, as well as their own history of involvement with drugs and alcohol.

In 2013, the first edition of the International Standards on Drug Use Prevention was published, summarizing the evidence on drug use prevention worldwide with the aim of identifying effective strategies. In 2018, the updated second edition[64] provided an overview of recent systematic reviews and describes the interventions and policies found to improve drug use prevention outcomes. In addition, it identifies the main components and characteristics of an effective national prevention system. This work builds on, acknowledges, and complements the work of many other organizations, such as the European Monitoring Center for Drugs and Drug Addiction, the Canadian Center on Substance Abuse and Addiction, the Inter-American Drug Abuse Control Commission (CICAD), the Colombo Plan for Cooperative Economic and Social Development in Asia and the Pacific, and the National Institute on Drug Abuse (NIDA), which have developed other standards and guidelines on various aspects of drug use prevention.

Various publications and tools from the European Monitoring Centre for Drugs and Drug Addiction (EMCDDA), such as the *Resource Kit for Prevention and Evaluation*,[65] the *European Quality Standards for Drug Prevention*,[66] the *Guidelines for the Evaluation of Drug Prevention*,[67] the *European Prevention Curriculum: A Handbook for Decision-Makers, Opinion-Makers and Policy-Makers in Science-Based Prevention of Substance Use*[68]; and the

Database of Programs to Reduce Drug Use (https://www.emcdda.europa.eu/best-practice_en), among others, have also contributed to the advancement and quality of drug dependence prevention in Europe.

Although, from a public health perspective, reducing substance use in the general population is a highly desirable goal, from a clinical standpoint it might be more beneficial to have interventions that target the risk and protective factors more specifically related to the development of addictive disorders and the possibility of identifying vulnerable individuals in advance through psychological, health, environmental, and social behavior characteristics that can predict the pathological evolution and its degree of severity. We know that both individual phenotypic characteristics and environmental factors can help us predict the development of addictive disorders, but most research separates these factors according to the individual or the environment, and given the large number of variables proposed and their complex etiopathogenic relationships,[69] it is difficult to translate this knowledge into clinical practice. Currently, artificial intelligence provides us with *machine learning* tools that have potential utility for healthcare practice, as they would allow us to combine both etiological dimensions and quantify their prominence to help, for example, detect young people who are at high risk of developing substance use disorder before and after the onset of use,[70,71] predict comorbid substance use disorders in people with ADHD,[72] or predict which children will develop mental health symptoms in adolescence.[73] A systematic review of risk and protective factors for drug abuse among adolescents[74] classified them into three main domains: individual, family, and community factors. The individual risk factors identified were high-impulsivity traits; rebelliousness; impaired emotional regulation; low religious involvement; catastrophic pain; school task compliance; total screen time and alexithymia; experience of abuse or negative upbringing; psychiatric disorders such as behavioral problems and major depressive disorder; previous exposure to e-cigarettes; behavioral addiction; low perceived risk; high perceived accessibility of drugs; and high attitude toward using synthetic drugs. Family risk factors included prenatal maternal smoking; poor maternal psychological control; low parental education; neglect; poor supervision; uncontrolled pocket money; and the presence of substance-using family members. A community risk factor was having peers who abuse drugs. Protective factors found were individual traits of optimism; high level of mindfulness; having social phobia; having strong beliefs against substance abuse; desire to maintain health; high parental awareness of drug abuse; school integration; structured activity; and strong religious beliefs.

Another recent publication[75] reviewed the literature between 1989 and 2019 to identify risk factors for developing substance use disorders and found that for each age group (children, young adults, adults, and older adults) there are certain developmental and life stressors, and that common risk factors across all age groups included adverse childhood experiences, trauma, chronic health problems, environmental factors, family history, social determinants, grief, and loss. Despite the similarities, the contextual factors and life challenges associated with these risks varied across different stages of life.

Although we have extensive knowledge on the long-term negative effects of adverse childhood experiences and their impact on physical and mental health,[50] research on their relationship to the diagnosis of substance use disorder is still scarce. Available studies suggest that there is a higher prevalence of adverse childhood experiences in the population with substance use disorders than in the general population, and a positive association with the development and severity of these disorders in adolescence and adulthood.[76] In a recent study on the lifelong health consequences and associated annual costs of adverse childhood experiences, they were reported to account for approximately 34.1% of illicit drug use in Europe and 41.1% in North America.[52]

A systematic review and meta-analysis of longitudinal studies on early risk and protective factors for gambling problems[77] identified typically small-to-medium effects for a variety of early factors that predict the development of gambling problems. Overall, this review identified 13 individual thematic risk factors (frequency of alcohol use, antisocial behaviors, depression, male gender, cannabis use, illicit drug use, impulsivity, number of gambling activities, severity of gambling problem, sensation seeking, tobacco use, violence, temperament), one relational thematic risk factor (peer antisocial behaviors), one community thematic risk factor (low academic performance), one individual thematic protective factor (socioeconomic status), and two relational thematic protective factors (parental supervision, social problems) that were significantly associated with subsequent gambling problems.

Similarly to other mental disorders, when analyzing the degree of evidence from studies on risk and protective factors for addictive disorders, most associations obtain weak or insignificant evidence, and few risk factors identified groups at risk for the development of selective prevention strategies.[78]

The overlap between risk and protective factors identified for both mental disorders and addictive disorders should be studied in greater depth, as this could contribute to improving the effectiveness of preventive intervention from the perspective of dual pathology.

In an initiative organized by the Prevention and Early Intervention in Mental Illness and Substance Use Centre of Research Excellence (PREMISE) of the National Health and Medical Research Council of Australia,[42] a group of 80 prevention experts, bringing together research leaders, government representatives, advocacy and leadership groups, people with lived experience, funding partners, and others, agreed that the highest priority for prevention research is to better understand and focus on risk and protective factors, which means investing in prospective cohort studies to determine how certain factors affect rates of mental and substance use disorders, investing in long-term outcome studies to determine whether prevention programs actually prevent or simply delay the onset of disorders, investing in long-term outcome studies to determine whether prevention programs actually prevent or simply delay the onset of disorders, and examining the role and influence of a wide range of disorder-specific and transdiagnostic risk and protective factors across different developmental periods and life stages. The second priority was to strengthen links between research areas through better collaboration, with a holistic and interdisciplinary approach, and to share research methods and data on open access platforms. Other priorities included involving diverse stakeholders throughout the research process from conceptualization to implementation, evaluating and refining prevention programs in the real world, and improving data collection, management, sharing, and harmonization. To this end, they considered it essential to establish a national framework and strategy for the prevention of mental and substance use disorders and to invest in and improve the sustainability of prevention programs.

As things stand, the Mental Health Strategy of the Spanish National Health System (SNS) for the period 2022–2026[79] still considers prevention in an incipient and fragmented way, through the formulation of generic proposals for the specific approach to promoting mental health among the population and preventing mental health problems, preventing, early detection, and care for suicidal behavior, and promoting mental health and the prevention and early detection of mental health problems in childhood and adolescence, as set out in three of its ten strategic lines, Lines 2, 3, and 5:

Strategic Line 2. Promotion of the Mental Health of the Population and Prevention of Mental Health Problems

2.1 *Promote Mental Health in the Community and Among Specific Groups*

2.1.1. Have a comprehensive plan for promoting mental health and preventing mental disorders (either on its own or included in a general plan) within the framework of the Health Promotion and Prevention Strategy in the Spanish National Health System, with priority given to the program for promoting psychosocial development during the first five years of life through primary care services.

2.1.2. Promote and disseminate new models of equal and healthy relationships between women and men, based on respect for individual preferences, opinions, beliefs, and abilities, incorporating a gender perspective into all actions in the field of mental health.

2.1.3. Promote that all plans, programs, projects, and regulations subject to environmental impact studies and assessments incorporate health impact assessments (both physical and mental), thereby promoting people's mental health.

2.1.4. Promote interventions specifically aimed at raising awareness, advising, and informing those responsible for institutions in different fields (education, environment, labor, justice, health, etc.) about the relationship between their actions and mental health, highlighting the central role of mental health as a generator well-being and productivity, as well as the negative socioeconomic consequences of ignoring them.

2.1.5. Promote mechanisms for the early identification of abuse of vulnerable groups, especially children, adolescents, and the elderly, by strengthening community networking.

2.1.6. Carry out specific awareness-raising actions aimed at the media, incorporating them as active agents with the power to transform public opinion.

2.2 *Prevent the Emergence of Mental Health Problems, Substance Use Disorders, and Addictions in the Community*

2.2.1. Develop and evaluate community interventions in areas at high risk of social exclusion, discrimination, poverty, and marginalization, in order to act on the social determinants, including gender determinants, of mental health problems and substance use disorders and addictions.

2.2.2. Develop and evaluate interventions within the scope of the 2017–2024 National Strategy on Addiction and the action plans that implement it (and, where appropriate, with the plans developed in the different autonomous communities), with the aim of reducing substance and non-substance addictions.

2.2.3. Consider behavioral addictions, or non-substance addictions, such as those derived from problematic or pathological gambling behaviors, and promote measures for their early detection and direct intervention in the gambling capacity of this type of participant and in the young population under 18 years of age, cyber addiction, and its consequences.

2.2.4. Promote the development of what has been termed "social capital" by supporting activities that increase citizen participation, encouraging mutual support groups, first-person movements, and all kinds of community initiatives for the prevention of loneliness, the improvement of stress management in stressful life situations, and the promotion of resilience.

2.2.5. Establish and evaluate collaborative interventions between social services, primary care, and mental health services to prevent mental health problems, with a special focus on the most vulnerable populations (social exclusion, gender violence, history of mental health problems in the family, caregivers, people with chronic health problems, disabilities, etc.).

2.2.6. Promote actions to support prevention and occupational health services aimed at preventing work-related stress, harassment, and work-related mental disorders.

2.2.7. Include specific prevention and awareness programs in schools, incorporating them into educational programs, always with a cross-cutting perspective, and using materials, resources, and first-hand experiences.

2.2.8. Promote health promotion and mental health problem prevention campaigns among people in prisons, prison psychiatric hospitals, and other vulnerable groups.

Strategic Line 3. Prevention, Early Detection, and Care for Suicidal Behavior

3.1 *Early Detection and Prevention of Suicidal Behavior*

3.1.1. Raise awareness and improve information for the general public through awareness-raising, consciousness-building, and information campaigns promoted by public institutions, the media, and social organizations dedicated to the cause.

3.1.2. Detect early and prevent suicide risk.

3.2 *Improve Care for People at Risk of Suicide*

3.2.1. Promote the development of integrated care processes for people at risk of suicide.

3.2.2. Support and encourage forms of mutual aid among survivors of suicide attempts and people with suicidal ideation.

3.2.3. Support and encourage forms of mutual support among family members in the community for people grieving a suicide.

3.2.4. Establish counseling and support for professionals who have experienced suicide in their workplace.

3.2.5. Facilitate and promote direct access for adolescents with mental health problems by developing specific programs for those who express suicidal ideation.

3.2.6. Develop an efficient, coordinated, and integrated telephone helpline network to improve the approach to people at risk of suicide.

Strategic Line 5. Mental Health in Childhood and Adolescence

5.1 *Promotion of Mental Health in Childhood and Adolescence. Prevention and Early Detection of Mental Health Problems at These Ages*

5.1.1. Promote protective factors in education, such as resilience, self-esteem, social skills, decision-making and conflict resolution skills; ensure a positive and safe school environment; develop prosocial behaviors that help others and promote physical health.

5.1.2. Plan preventive and mental health promotion activities in coordination with other health and non-health resources.

5.1.3. Develop programs and protocols in the educational, health, and community spheres to promote positive parenting, including families in situations of social, developmental, and psycho-affective risk.

5.1.4. Establish training and awareness programs for the educational community on the symptoms and treatment of mental health problems and combat stigmatization.

5.1.5. Ensure accessibility to mental health support in the educational setting by establishing partnerships with community support networks and resources.

5.1.6. Incorporate screening procedures that allow for better identification of major depressive disorder in adolescents who attend primary healthcare services. Integrate these types of tools into the care process itself, ensuring access to early treatment and adequate follow-up.

5.1.7. Design specific actions to raise awareness and prevent ICT abuse in children and adolescents and non-substance addictive behaviors (cyber addiction and cyberbullying).

5.1.8. Include specific prevention programs in dysfunctional family environments that enable the identification of situations of abuse, violence, mistreatment, or vulnerability, both in terms of child abuse and gender violence, due to their particular impact on the mental health of those who suffer them.

5.1.9. Strengthen training in discrimination and monitoring of mental health problems in Educational Guidance Teams, school psychologists, school nurses, and social workers, establishing relationships and synergies with mental health services, offering the educational community behavioral support and promotion of mental well-being, identification and evaluation of early interventions, individual and group counseling, and referral to community services.

However, the implementation of this set of proposals in the corresponding Mental Health Action Plan 2022–2024,[80] with €100 million in funding from the Spanish government, is confined to a limited number of objectives more related to the early detection and treatment of suicidal behavior than to its prevention per se, and to the continuity of the prevention of addictive behaviors with and without substances, prioritizing the implementation of programs that have proven effective, the evaluation of the effectiveness of existing programs, and the adaptation of existing and recognized evaluated programs (in good practice portals or scientific publications) to local circumstances and their application by local corporations or NGOs.

On the other hand, also in Spain, prevention has been one of the top priorities of the National Plan on Drugs since its inception in 1985. For more than three decades, specific actions to prevent drug use and other addictive behaviors have been funded on an ongoing, albeit uneven, basis due to the idiosyncrasies of each of the 19 territorial entities that make up the country. Prevention activities, carried out mainly by local authorities and NGOs, have been supported by technical reference documents on their theoretical[81] and scientific[61] bases and have traditionally covered universal, selective, and targeted prevention strategies in different areas of action: school, family, youth, work, and community. Recently, environmental prevention strategies have also been incorporated.[82] In some cases, such as Galicia, specific publications were available on the preventive processes and the portfolio of services in the field of prevention of the Galician Plan on Drugs[83] and on the instruments for the evaluation of the programs included in the portfolio of services in the field of drug addiction prevention.[84] The evaluation of the 2009–2016 National Drug Strategy[85] describes that, depending on the programs implemented and their territorial coverage, prevention activity in Spain can be grouped into three categories: (1) programs that seem to form a basic portfolio common to all autonomous communities and with broad coverage, such as school, family, community, alternative leisure, and programs for minors at risk; (2) programs that are implemented in most territories but not all, such as programs in universities, the workplace, and early detection and intervention; and (3) programs that exist in some territories but not in most, such as programs for pregnant women and traffic accident prevention. Schools continue to be the focus of most programs, with activities aimed at students and their families. The priority strategy is skills education for schoolchildren and training in educational guidelines for families. The main targets of these prevention programs were students, young people participating in alternative leisure programs, parents, and vulnerable minors. In terms of quality, just over half of the territories have a portfolio of services and/or a catalogue of preventive programs, and the accreditation of programs based on quality criteria was still deficient in most of the autonomous communities. The overall assessment of the results obtained by the prevention activities carried out over the years is based on the three main objectives (delaying the age of onset of drug use, reducing the prevalence of drug use, and reducing the harm associated with drug use), but there are no studies that focus on the impact on the evolution of dual pathology.

The strategic objectives for prevention in the current National Strategy on Addiction (ENA) 2017–2024[86] are:

1. Reduce the presence and promotion of drugs and other behaviors that can lead to addiction
2. Limit minors' access to drugs and other behaviors that can lead to addiction
3. Promote social awareness of the risks and harms caused by drugs and addictions, increase the perception of the risks associated with consumption and certain addictive behaviors (gambling, ICT), and encourage citizen participation in this regard
4. Reduce the unjustified perception in society, and especially among minors, that drug use, primarily cannabis and alcohol, is "normal"
5. Develop personal skills and abilities that reduce vulnerability to drug use and other behaviors that can lead to addiction

6. Promote healthy behaviors and lifestyle habits, healthy use of new technologies, and healthy leisure alternatives that are incompatible with substance abuse and other addictive behaviors
7. Detect early and prevent high-risk consumption (consumption by minors, pregnant women, while driving, etc.)

For the development of the ENA, the 2018–2020 Action Plan on Addictions[87] proposed: (1) promoting the incorporation of environmental/structural prevention measures into prevention programs, especially those implemented at the local level; (2) contributing, through communication activities, to increasing awareness of the social risks associated with drug use and other addictions; (3) promoting the inclusion of non-substance addictions in prevention regulations, plans, and programs; (4) increasing the population coverage of the most effective family prevention programs; (5) early detection of risk cases in schools and social and health settings; (6) incorporating a practical approach to gender perspective in prevention programs; (7) promoting the expansion of safe and healthy leisure programs in collaboration with the hospitality and tourism sector; and (8) generalizing early detection and brief intervention programs for at-risk drinkers and including minors as target populations for these programs. The current Action Plan on Addictions 2021–2024[88] includes: (1) promoting the incorporation of environmental/structural prevention in addiction policies and specific measures in prevention programs; (2) improving the quality and scope of addiction prevention programs nationwide and in all areas of intervention; (3) improving the quality of addiction prevention programs in leisure contexts; (4) promoting the development of non-substance addiction prevention (pathological gambling, but explore other potential areas such as video games, screens, networks, pornography, etc.); (5) generalizing early detection and brief intervention programs for people with risky consumption in primary health care and extending their implementation to other resources; and (6) promoting addiction prevention actions in the workplace and in the field of road safety.

On a practical level, in Spain, prevention programs developed by local corporations and NGOs have funding mechanisms through competitive bidding at the national and regional levels. For example, in 2022, the granting of state financial aid to local authorities for the development of addiction prevention programs[89] has a budget of €4,200,000 and aims to develop addiction prevention programs, including behavioral addictions, as well as risk reduction in minors and young people, in one or more of the following areas of intervention: (1) family prevention, (2) environmental or structural prevention, (3) alternative leisure activities to the consumption of psychoactive substances with addictive potential, (4) risk reduction in nightlife contexts, (5) socio-educational prevention for vulnerable minors, and (6) community prevention. In the case of the call for applications for financial aid to private nonprofit entities at the state level for the implementation of supra-community programs on addiction in 2022,[9] the budget forecast is €4,296,490. In addition, another €500,000 is available for the consolidation of the most valuable addiction prevention programs, including their digitization, through competitive grants to private, nonprofit, state-level entities for the development of projects in the field of prevention and treatment of addictions for the year 2022 within the framework of the Recovery, Transformation, and Resilience Plan, financed by the European Union's–NextGenerationEU.[91] At the regional level, Galicia is contributing an additional €680,000 per year to co-finance projects for the prevention of addictive behaviors promoted by private nonprofit entities[92] and €837,821/year to co-finance projects promoted by city councils, associations of city councils, or groups of city councils.[93] Funding covers programs aimed at schools, families, young people, communities, and others, with a special focus on activities related to the prevention of cannabis use, pathological gambling, and problems related to the use of the internet and ICT.

PROPOSAL FOR INTERVENTION IN THE FIELD OF DUAL PATHOLOGY PREVENTION

If addictive disorders and other mental disorders share neurological pathways, overlapping genetic risk factors, and common environmental risk factors, forming a clinical reality of complex management and prognosis that requires a specific approach,[23] then the development of dual pathology prevention not only seems necessary but should also be a priority in the research and implementation of preventive strategies in mental health.[42]

In a statement by the UNODC/WHO Informal Scientific Network at the 63rd session of the Commission on Narcotic Drugs, recommendations were made for national health systems interested in developing coordinated, multi-system interventions to address the needs of people with dual diagnosis, reflecting the unanimous consensus reached by the members of the Network:[94]

1. Dual pathology should be addressed as an integral part of universal health coverage.
2. Policymakers should devise strategies to address the common biopsychosocial factors associated with the development of dual pathology.
3. The high prevalence and related disability of dual pathology require active intervention by policymakers at the systems level and active advocacy by health professionals.
4. Service providers must be trained in the management of dual pathology, and sufficient financial support must be provided for this purpose.
5. Systematic screening for other mental disorders, using validated instruments administered by trained healthcare providers, is an essential component of adequate care for people with substance use disorders.
6. Adequate treatment must be made available and accessible, regardless of the point of entry into the care systems, in accordance with the principle of "no wrong door."
7. Sex- and gender-based knowledge and a stigma-free approach are necessary for the effective management of dual disorders.
8. Age-specific interventions are required throughout life, especially for minors and the elderly.

9. Science-based prevention interventions that address common risk factors, such as early life adversity, should be available for children living with parents and/or caregivers with dual disorders.
10. Attention should also be paid to other vulnerable and at-risk populations, in accordance with local needs.
11. Access to services for dual pathology in the criminal justice system must be ensured, particularly in prison settings, juvenile detention, or correctional facilities.
12. Data collection and analysis should be encouraged to monitor the magnitude of the problem, the quality of care, and the results of policies and interventions.
13. The implementation and expansion of effective and efficient interventions, taking into account cultural and country-specific characteristics, is a priority.

In practical terms, national health systems could contribute more to the prevention of dual pathology by incorporating systematic consideration, early detection, and specific actions targeting the main known risk factors into healthcare practice, using a holistic, structural, multidisciplinary, and transdiagnostic approach[95] involving healthcare professionals from different specialties, such as obstetrics, pediatrics, child and adolescent mental health, and primary care, among others, and developing effective coordination mechanisms with the corresponding educational, social, and community resources.[96]

Gynecology consultations and family planning services may be ideal for developing preventive measures for dual pathology during the preconception stage.[97] The detection of risk factors and the implementation of interventions aimed at reducing or avoiding their subsequent influence on the gestational period can provide an excellent opportunity to effectively prevent prenatal exposure to tobacco, alcohol, illicit drugs, medications, and toxins, as well as problems related to nutritional issues, exposure to stress, and maternal psychopathology. It should be noted that delaying these tasks until the gestation period means acting too late, especially in unplanned pregnancies where interventions may occur late in the first trimester and, in the best-case scenario, only serve to reduce damage that is already occurring to fetal development.

Information on prevalence of substance use during pregnancy is limited and varies depending on the methodology used. In the US, it has been reported that between 4% and 7.4% of pregnant women use illegal drugs[98] and that more than 20% admitted to using one or more substances, including alcohol and/or tobacco, according to data from the 2020 National Survey on Drug Use and Health.[99] Studies conducted in Spain, using biological sample analysis, report figures between 8% and 16% for drug use during pregnancy.[100,101,102,103,104]

Obstetric care must have a decisive impact on the prevention of dual pathology by addressing known prenatal and perinatal risk factors from a biopsychosocial perspective.[105] This issue is so important that it has been suggested that, given all the scientific evidence available on the possibility of modifying gestational determinants that cause disease, failure to take the necessary preventive measures may mean that healthcare professionals are collectively and individually responsible for preventable diseases in children.[97]

During this period, in addition to addressing the problem of prenatal exposure to substances of abuse and toxins, it is also important to adequately address the mental health pathology of parents,[106,107] promote interventions that address unfavorable socioeconomic circumstances,[108,109] and provide knowledge and skills for future parenting, among other strategies.[110]

A recent systematic review on primary prenatal prevention of mental illness through micronutrient supplementation during pregnancy[111] identified studies with four types of prenatal maternal dietary interventions to promote fetal brain development and reduce the subsequent risk of mental illness. Higher serum concentrations of vitamins A and D appear to promote brain development and reduce the risk of schizophrenia, but their potential toxicity limits their use to the currently recommended amounts. Folic acid has benefits for fetal brain development and later child behavior and cognition, but it has not been shown to specifically prevent schizophrenia. Omega-3 fatty acids have been associated with a reduced risk of premature birth and wheezing in childhood, but they increase the risk of subsequent schizophrenia and ADHD symptoms in childhood. Phosphatidylcholine supplements appear to promote fetal brain development and subsequent infant behavior.

Although it has been shown that certain environmental influences, such as maternal diet during pregnancy or children's diet, cause epigenetic changes during critical periods of development and can affect our well-being and mental health throughout life, we are still far from sufficiently understanding how they work and their impact on different stages of development to be able to provide individualized dietary recommendations.[112] Therefore, further research is needed on which dietary components are truly important for mental health, including in psychiatric disorders, as well as for whom, under what circumstances, and in what specific doses these nutritional interventions have preventive effects and therapeutic efficacy.[113,114]

Complementary to interventionsdeveloped during the prenatal and perinatal stages, pediatric care is crucial for adequately addressing the prevention of dual pathology. Evidence indicates that some interventions in children aged 0 to 3 years can be effective in promoting healthy development, particularly in infants from high-risk environments. A recent review[115] emphasizes the importance of including mothers, partners, and children to make the intervention more effective and reviews the evidence on the effectiveness of programs based on cognitive-behavioral principles, training in practical skills on how to care for the baby, focusing on the development of attachment or bonding between parents and children, developing parents' reflective functioning skills, the co-parenting relationship between parents, and the importance of building broader support networks.

There is evidence to suggest that preventive interventions targeting parents with mental illness could reduce the risk of mental disorders in their children by 40%[116] and that preventive interventions targeting children of parents with mental disorders can achieve not only a significant reduction in the incidence of mental illness in children, but also a decrease in internalizing symptoms in the year following the intervention.[117]

Various general measures that form part of standard clinical practice, such as promoting adequate nutrition,[112] physical exercise[118,119] and preventing childhood obesity[120] are also useful for preventing dual pathology. However, given their enormous importance, it is necessary to improve the level of attention paid to adverse childhood experiences and trauma by implementing specific primary prevention strategies (such as programs that prevent child abuse and neglect, programs that increase family and community stability and resilience, and programs that teach positive and effective parenting skills); secondary prevention (programs that identify and intervene in families experiencing violence and abuse, trauma-informed care to identify and intervene immediately, psychological first aid that reduces the psychological impact of trauma); and tertiary prevention (trauma-informed care, programs that identify and reduce associated risk behaviors, social awareness campaigns).[121] A WHO study of 51,945 adults in 21 countries[122] found that eradicating childhood adversities, especially those associated with maladaptive family functioning (e.g., parental mental illness, child abuse, neglect), would reduce any lifetime mental disorder by 29.8%, and the reduction is even greater when considering only cases that begin in adolescence (32.3%) and childhood (38.2%). Although this is a complex task that involves legislative action, public administrations, the education system, community social resources, and families themselves, healthcare personnel play a leading role, which will depend on their specific training in identifying adverse childhood experiences and developing strategies for their prevention and for the care of patients who have experienced them.[49,123,124] In this area, pediatrics, primary care, and emergency services can also contribute to improving this population's access to selective and indicated prevention programs that should be available in their community.

Prevention of dual pathology must be present at all stages of pediatric care and continue throughout adolescence. Although there is ample evidence on effective intervention programs from an early age[42,125–128] and on how to improve children's and adolescents' access to mental health care,[129] further research is still needed so that this body of knowledge can be translated into standardized interventions that also take into account the differential effects of gender, age groups, socioeconomic status, geographic settings, and other contextual factors.

In the clinical setting, it would be of great interest to have tools capable of predicting individual risk for the development of mental disorders, but research in this field also faces multiple difficulties.[130,131] The SBIRT (Screening, Brief Intervention, and Referral to Treatment) model can be useful as a strategy for preventing addiction[132] and other mental disorders[133] through early detection and intervention with people who have a high probability of developing them. In the field of addiction, SAMHSA (Substance Abuse and Mental Health Services Administration)[133] recommends the use of SBIRT from pediatric age onward, in routine health checkups, as a tool for the periodic identification of risk behaviors, or during visits for acute processes.[134] Another example would be psychometric interviews used to detect individuals at high clinical risk of psychosis as clinical tools for indicated prevention.[10,135]

The role of primary health care in the prevention of dual pathology is also relevant,[136,137] especially from adolescence onward, but above all in older people.[138,139] Algorithms have been developed and validated to predict the onset of major depression, anxiety disorders, and alcohol abuse in primary care, with results similar to those used to predict cardiovascular risk, for example,[140] and there are a variety of tools for detecting mental health problems in adults that can be used in primary care settings.[141] A clinical trial conducted in Spain, using a prediction algorithm and individualized preventive actions, achieved a 21% and a 23% reduction, respectively, in the incidence of depression and anxiety in a population of 3,326 non-depressed patients registered with 140 family doctors in 70 health centers in seven Spanish provinces.[142] A meta-analysis on the effectiveness of psychological and educational interventions for the primary prevention of depression in primary health care found that such interventions were effective, although the effect size was small.[143]

The implementation of specific measures for the promotion of mental health and the prevention of dual pathology in older people are another urgent need that requires further development and is of particular concern to primary health care,[144] and also to the community[145] and other specialties involved in health care for this age group. These latter should incorporate into their procedures the detection of and intervention on known risk factors, such as stress, social and economic adversities, health problems, chronic diseases and functional limitations, medication abuse, alcoholism and other addictions, and abuse.[59] A recent comprehensive review of biopsychosocial factors predictive of mental health in older adults,[146] found that some biological factors, such as age, sex, physical function, health conditions, and chronic diseases; psychological factors, such as affect, personality traits, and subjective well-being; and social factors, such as smoking, physical activity, sleep quality, daily activities, social support, marital status, loneliness, religion and spirituality, and conditions in early life. Another example of research in this field is the MINDMAP project, funded by the European Union, which aims to identify opportunities in the urban environment for promoting the mental well-being and functioning of older people in Europe by bringing together European cities with longitudinal urban aging studies, focusing on mental health planning policies and programs dedicated to older adults, ranging from health promotion to the need for nursing care, and on the importance of early detection of the preclinical stages of frailty, including the mental components of functional competence.[147,148]

The importance of the prevention of dual pathology in older people is evident when we consider that the population is aging much faster than in the past; it is estimated that between 2020 and 2030 the percentage of the world's population over the age of 60 will increase by 34%. Currently, the number of people aged 60 and over exceeds that of children under 5, and by 2050 it will exceed that of adolescents and young people aged 15 to 24.[149] We can conclude that addressing mental health promotion and mental disorder prevention from a dual pathology perspective represents a pragmatic and coherent approach in terms of translational neuroscience. In the short term, it may be useful to promote the convergence of available resources, traditionally dissociated as they relate to addictions or other mental disorders, and avoid duplication of parallel actions on common risk and protective factors; but above all, it is urgent to adapt efforts to the real magnitude of the problem and its consequences for public health. This paradigm shift should be considered at all levels, from social organization to public policy and from research to the implementation of intervention programs. In this task, in order for the prevention of dual pathology to acquire structural characteristics, the healthcare system plays a central role and the different professions and specialties that it comprises must contribute decisively. In the medium and long term, it is necessary to develop a new conceptual framework based on neuroscience that is capable of integrating the underlying neurobiological mechanisms, the affected neurodevelopmental processes, individual differences, and contextual factors to guide the design of more personalized preventive interventions, in line with the principles of precision medicine.[150,151,152]

REFERENCES

1. Institute of Medicine (US) Committee on Prevention of Mental Disorders. Mrazek PJ, Haggerty RJ (eds.). Reducing Risks for Mental Disorders: Frontiers for Preventive Intervention Research. Washington (DC): National Academies Press (US), 1994. PMID: 25144015. National Academies Press (US), 1994. doi: 10.17226/2139. https://www.ncbi.nlm.nih.gov/books/NBK236319/
2. National Research Council (US) and Institute of Medicine (US) Committee on the Prevention of Mental Disorders and Substance Abuse Among Children, Youth, and Young Adults: Research Advances and Promising Interventions. O'Connell ME, Boat T, Warner KE (eds.). Preventing Mental, Emotional, and Behavioral Disorders Among Young People: Progress and Possibilities. National Academies Press (US), 2009. doi: 10.17226/12480 https://www.ncbi.nlm.nih.gov/books/NBK32775/
3. National Academies of Sciences, Engineering, and Medicine; Division of Behavioral and Social Sciences and Education; Board on Children, Youth, and Families; Committee on Fostering Healthy Mental, Emotional, and Behavioral Development Among Children and Youth. Fostering Healthy Mental, Emotional, and Behavioral Development in Children and Youth: A National Agenda. National Academies Press (US), 2019. doi: 10.17226/25201 https://www.ncbi.nlm.nih.gov/books/NBK551842/
4. European Commission. Green Paper: Improving the mental health of the population. Towards a strategy on mental health for the European Union. Brussels: Health and Consumer Protection Directorate General, 2005. https://ec.europa.eu/health/ph_determinants/life_style/mental/green_paper/mental_gp_en.pdf
5. Wahlbeck K. MINDFUL-Mental health information and determinants for the European level: Final technical implementation report. September 14, 2006. https://ec.europa.eu/health/ph_projects/2003/action1/docs/2003_1_11_frep_en.pdf
6. Jané-Llopis E. "Mental health promotion and mental disorder prevention in Europe". J Public Ment Health. 2006:5(1): 5–7. https://doi.org/10.1108/17465729200600002
7. Puras D, Gerasimos Kolaitis G, Tsiantis J. Child and adolescent mental health in the Enlarged European Union: Overview of the CAMHEE project. Int J Ment Health Promot. 2010;12(4): 3–9doi: 10.1080/14623730.2010.9721821
8. Haro JM, Ayuso-Mateos JL, Bitter I, Demotes-Mainard J, Leboyer M, Lewis SW, *et al.* ROAMER: Roadmap for mental health research in Europe. Int J Methods Psychiatr Res. 2014 Jan;23(Suppl 1):1–14. https://doi. org/10.1002/mpr.1406
9. Forsman AK, Wahlbeck K, Aarø LE, Alonso J, Barry MM, Brunn M, Cardoso G, Cattan M, de Girolamo G, Eberhard-Gran M, Evans-Lacko S, Fiorillo A, Hansson L, Haro JM, Hazo JB, Hegerl U, Katschnig H, Knappe S, Luciano M, Miret M, Nordentoft M, Obradors-Tarragó C, Pilgrim D, Ruud T, Salize HJ, Stewart-Brown SL, Tó-masson K, van der Feltz-Cornelis CM, Ventus DB, Vuori J, Värnik A; ROAMER Consortium. Research priorities for public mental health in Europe: Recommendations of the ROAMER project. Eur J Public Health. 2015;25(2):249–54. https://doi.org/10.1093/eurpub/cku232

10. Fusar-Poli P, Cappucciati M, Rutigliano G, Schult-ze-Lutter F, Bonoldi I, Borgwardt S, *et al.* At risk or not at risk? A meta-analysis of the prognostic accuracy of psychometric interviews for psychosis prediction. World Psychiatry. 2015;14(3):322–32. https://doi.org/10.1002/wps.20250
11. Whiteford HA, Degenhardt L, Rehm J, Baxter AJ, Ferrari AJ, Erskine HE, *et al.* Global burden of disease attributable to mental and substance use disorders: Findings from the Global Burden of Disease Study 2010. Lancet (London, England). 2013;382(9904):1575–86. https://doi.org/10.1016/S0140-6736(13)61611-6
12. Wittchen HU, Jacobi F, Rehm J, Gustavsson A, Svensson M, Jönsson B, *et al.* The size and burden of mental disorders and other disorders of the brain in Europe 2010. European Neuropsychopharmacol. 2011;21(9):655–79.
13. OECD/EU. Health at a Glance: Europe 2018: State of Health in the EU Cycle, OECD Publishing, Paris, 2018. https://doi.org/10.1787/health_glance_eur-2018-en
14. Patel V, Flisher AJ, Hetrick S, McGorry P. Mental health of young people: A global public-health challenge. Lancet (London, England). 2007;369(9569):1302–13. https://doi.org/10.1016/S0140-6736(07)60368-7
15. Erskine HE, Moffitt TE, Copeland WE, Costello EJ, Ferrari AJ, Patton G, *et al.* A heavy burden on young minds: The global burden of mental and substance use disorders in children and youth. Psychol Med. 2015;45(7):1551–63.
16. Armstrong TD, Costello EJ. Community studies on adolescent substance use, abuse, or dependence and psychiatric comorbidity. J Consult Clin Psychol. 2002;70(6):1224–39.
17. Harford TC, Yi HY, Chen CM, Grant BF. Psychiatric Symptom Clusters as Risk Factors for Alcohol Use Disorders in Adolescence: A National Study. Alcohol Clin Exp Res. 2015;39(7):1174–85. https://doi.org/10.1111/acer.12767
18. Couwenbergh C, van den Brink W, Zwart K, Vreugdenhil C, van Wijngaarden-Cremers P, van der Gaag RJ. Co-morbid psychopathology in adolescents and young adults treated for substance use disorders: A review. Eur Child Adolesc Psychiatry. 2006;15(6):319–28. https://doi.org/10.1007/s00787-006-0535-6
19. Gore FM, Bloem PJ, Patton GC, Ferguson J, Joseph V, Coffey C, *et al.* Global burden of disease in young people aged 10-24 years: A systematic analysis. Lancet (London, England). 2011;377(9783):2093–102. https://doi.org/10.1016/S0140-6736(11)60512-6
20. Sawyer SM, Afifi RA, Bearinger LH, Blakemore SJ, Dick B, Ezeh AC, *et al.* Adolescence: A foundation for future health. Lancet (London, England). 2012;379(9826):1630–40. https://doi.org/10.1016/S0140-6736(12)60072-5
21. United Nations Population Fund (2022). World Population Dashboard. https://www.unfpa.org/data/world-population-dashboard
22. Torrens Mèlich M. Patología dual: situación actual y retos de futuro. Addictions. 2008;20(4):315–20. http://dx.doi.org/10.20882/adicciones.255
23. Hakobyan S, Vazirian S, Lee-Cheong S, Krausz M, Honer WG, Schutz CG. Concurrent Disorder Management Guidelines. Systematic Review. J Clin Med. 2020;9(8):2406. doi: 10.3390/jcm9082406
24. Wykes T, Haro JM, Belli SR, Obradors-Tarragó C, Arango C, Ayuso-Mateos JL, Bitter I, Brunn M, Chevreul K, Demotes-Mainard J, Elfeddali I, Evans-Lacko S, Fiorillo A, Forsman AK, Hazo JB, Kuepper R, Knappe S, Leboyer M, Lewis SW, Linszen D, Luciano M, Maj M, McDaid D, Miret M, Papp S, Park AL, Schumann G, Thornicroft G, van der Feltz-Cornelis C, van Os J, Wahlbeck K, Walker-Tilley T, Wittchen HU; ROAMER consortium. Mental health research priorities for Europe. Lancet Psychiatry. 2015;2(11):1036–42. https://doi.org/10.1016/S2215-0366(15)00332-6
25. MQ Transforming Mental Health. 2021; UK Mental Health Research Funding 2014–2017. https://doi.org/10.21955/amrcopenres.1114943.1

26. Fusar-Poli P. Integrated Mental Health Services for the Developmental Period (0 to 25 Years): A Critical Review of the Evidence. Fusar-Poli P. Front Psychiatry. 2019;10:355. https://doi.org/10.3389/fpsyt.2019.00355
27. Kendler KS, Prescott CA, Myers J, Neale MC. The structure of genetic and environmental risk factors for com- psychiatric and substance use disorders in men and women. Archives of general psychiatry. 2003;60(9):929–37.
28. Cerdá M, Sagdeo A, Johnson J, Galea S. Genetic and environmental influences on psychiatric comorbidity: A systematic review. J Affect Disord. 2010;126(1–2):14–38. https://doi.org/10.1016/j.jad.2009.11.006
29. Tsuang MT, Bar JL, Stone WS, Faraone SV. Gene-environment interactions in mental disorders. World Psychiatry. 2004;3(2):73–83. https://www.ncbi.nlm.nih.gov/pmc/articles/PMC1414673/pdf/wpa020073.pdf
30. Jaffee SR, Price TS. Gene-environment correlations: A review of the evidence and implications for prevention of mental illness. Molecular Psychiatry. 2007;12(5):432–42. https://doi.org/10.1038/sj.mp.4001950
31. Assary E, Vincent JP, Keers R, Pluess M. Gene-environment interaction and psychiatric disorders: Review and future directions. Semin Cell Dev Biol. 2018;77:133–43. https://doi.org/10.1016/j.semcdb.2017.10.016
32. Kular L, Kular S. Epigenetics applied to psychiatry: Clinical opportunities and future challenges. Psychiatry Clin Neurosci. 2018;72(4):195–211. https://doi.org/10.1111/pcn.12634
33. Kaplan G, Xu H, Abreu K, Feng J. DNA Epigenetics in Addiction Susceptibility. Front Genet. 2022;13:806685. doi: 10.3389/fgene.2022.806685
34. Teicher MH, Samson JA, Anderson CM, Ohashi K. The effects of childhood maltreatment on brain structure, function and connectivity. Nature reviews. Neurosci. 2016;17(10):652–66. https://doi.org/10.1038/nrn.2016.111
35. Mikkelsen B, Williams J, Rakovac I, Wickramasinghe K, Hennis A, Shin HR, *et al.* Life course approach to prevention and control of non-communicable diseases. BMJ (Clinical research ed.). 2019;364:l257. https://doi.org/10.1136/bmj.l257
36. Stanis JJ, Andersen SL. Reducing substance use during adolescence: A translational framework for prevention. Psychopharmacology. 2014;231(8):1437–53. https://doi. org/10.1007/s00213-013-3393-1
37. Jordan C J, Andersen SL. Sensitive periods of substance abuse: Early risk for the transition to dependence. Dev Cogn Neurosci. 2017;25:29–44. https://doi.org/10.1016/j.dcn.2016.10.004
38. Solmi M, Civardi S, Corti R, Anil J, Demurtas J, Lange S, *et al.* Risk and protective factors for alcohol and tobacco related disorders: An umbrella review of observational studies. Neurosci Biobehav Rev. 2021;121:20–28. https://doi.org/10.1016/j.neubiorev.2020.11.010
39. Caplan G. Principles of Prevention Psychiatry. Basic Books, 1964.
40. Gordon RS Jr. An operational classification of disease prevention. Public Health Rep. 1983; 98(2):107–9. https://pubmed.ncbi.nlm.nih.gov/6856733/
41. Foxcroft DR. "Form ever follows function. This is the law." A prevention taxonomy based on a functional typology. Addictions. 2014;26(1):10–14. https://doi.org/10.20882/adicciones.123
42. Baker S, Deady M, Birrell L, Ross K, Fitzpatrick S, Newton N, *et al.* Prevention of mental and substance use disorders: Shaping priorities for research and implementation. Mental Health & Prevention. 2021;24:1–6. https://doi.org/10.1016/j.mhp.2021.200211
43. President's Commission on Mental Health (1978). Report to the President from the President's Comission on Mental Health. U.S. Government Printing Office, 1978.
44. Arango C, Díaz-Caneja CM, McGorry PD, Rapoport J, Sommer IE, Vorstman JA, McDaid D, Marín O, Serrano-Drozdowskyj E, Freedman R, Carpenter W. Preventive strategies for mental health. Lancet Psychiatry. 2018;5(7):591–604. https://doi.org/10.1016/S2215-0366(18)30057-9

45. Le LK, Esturas AC, Mihalopoulos C, Chiotelis O, Bu-cholc J, Chatterton ML, *et al.* Cost-effectiveness evidence of mental health prevention and promotion interventions: A systematic review of economic evaluations. PLoS Med. 2021;18(5):e1003606. https://doi.org/10.1371/journal.pmed.1003606
46. Danese A, McEwen BS. Adverse childhood experiences, allostasis, allostatic load, and age-related disease. Physiol Behav. 2012;106(1):29–39. https://doi.org/10.1016/j.physbeh.2011.08.019
47. Newman L, Judd F, Olsson CA, Castle D, Bousman C, Sheehan P, *et al.* Early origins of mental disorder - risk factors in the perinatal and infant period. BMC Psychiatry. 2016;16:270. https://doi.org/10.1186/s12888-016-0982-7
48. Agorastos A, Pervanidou P, Chrousos GP, Baker DG. Developmental Trajectories of Early Life Stress and Trauma: A Narrative Review on Neurobiological Aspects Beyond Stress System Dysregulation. Front Psychiatry. 2019;10:118. https://doi.org/10.3389/fpsyt.2019.00118
49. Jones CM, Merrick MT, Houry DE. Identifying and Preventing Adverse Childhood Experiences: Implications for Clinical Practice. JAMA. 2020;323(1):25–2. https://doi.org/10.1001/jama.2019.18499
50. Hughes K, Bellis MA, Hardcastle KA, Sethi D, Butchart A, Mikton C, *et al.* The effect of multiple adverse childhood experiences on health: A systematic review and meta-analysis. Lancet Public Health. 2017;2(8):e356–66. https://doi.org/10.1016/S2468-2667(17)30118-4
51. Herzog JI, Schmahl C. Adverse childhood experiences and the consequences on neurobiological, psycho-social, and somatic conditions across the lifespan. Front Psychiatry. 2018;9:420. https://doi.org/10.3389/fpsyt.2018.00420
52. Bellis MA, Hughes K, Ford K, Ramos Rodriguez G, Sethi D, Passmore J. Life course health consequences and associated annual costs of adverse childhood experiences across Europe and North America: A systematic review and meta-analysis. Lancet Public Health. 2019;4(10):e517–28. https://doi.org/10.1016/S2468-2667(19)30145-8
53. Sahle BW, Reavley NJ, Li W, Morgan AJ, Yap MBH, Reupert A, *et al.* The association between adverse childhood experiences and common mental disorders and suicidality: An umbrella review of systematic reviews and meta-analyses. Eur Child Adolesc Psychiatry. 2022;31(10):1489–99. https://doi.org/10.1007/s00787-021-01745-2
54. Murray RM, Quigley H, Quattrone D, Englund A, Di Forti M. Traditional marijuana, high-potency cannabis and synthetic cannabinoids: Increasing risk for psychosis. World Psychiatry. 2016;15(3):195–204. https://doi.org/10.1002/wps.20341
55. Wilson J, Freeman TP, Mackie CJ. Effects of increasing cannabis potency on adolescent health. Lancet Child Adolesc Health. 2019;3(2):121–8. https://doi.org/10.1016/S2352-4642(18)30342-0
56. Hindley G, Beck K, Borgan F, Ginestet CE, McCutcheon R, Kleinloog D, *et al.* Psychiatric symptoms caused by cannabis constituents: A systematic review and meta-analysis. Lancet Psychiatry. 2020;7(4):344–53. https://doi.org/10.1016/S2215-0366(20)30074-2
57. van der Steur SJ, Batalla A, Bossong MG. Factors moderating the association between cannabis use and psychosis risk: A systematic review. Brain Sci. 2020;10(2):97. https://doi.org/10.3390/brainsci10020097
58. Gobbi G, Atkin T, Zytynski T, Wang S, Askari S, Boruff J, *et al.* Association of cannabis use in adolescence and risk of depression, anxiety, and suicidality in young adulthood: A systematic review and meta-analysis. JAMA Psychiatry. 2019;76(4):426–34. https://doi.org/10.1001/jamapsychiatry.2018.4500
59. Jané-Llopis E, Gabilondo A (eds.). Mental Health in Older People. Consensus paper. Luxembourg: European Communities, 2008. https://ec.europa.eu/health/ph_determinants/life_style/mental/docs/consensus_older_en.pdf
60. Arango C, Dragioti E, Solmi M, Cortese S, Domschke K, Murray RM, *et al.* Risk and protective factors for mental disorders beyond genetics: An evidence-based atlas. World Psychiatry. 2021;20(3):417–36. https://doi.org/10.1002/wps.20894

61. Becoña E. Factores de riesgo y protección. In: Becoña E (eds.). Bases científicas de la prevención de las drogodependencias. Madrid: Government Delegation for the National Plan on Drugs, 2002. https://pnsd.sanidad.gob.es/profesionales/publicaciones/catalogo/catalogoPNSD/publicaciones/pdf/Bases_cientificas.pdf
62. Substance Abuse and Mental Health Services Administration. (2019). Key substance use and mental health indicators in the United States: Results from the 2018 National Survey on Drug Use and Health (HHS Publication No. PEP19-5068, NSDUH Series H-54). Rockville, MD: Center for Behavioral Health Statistics and Quality, Substance Abuse and Mental Health Services Administration.
63. Degenhardt L, Bharat C, Glantz MD, Sampson NA, Al-Hamzawi A, Alonso J, Andrade LH, Bunting B, Cia A, de Girolamo G, De Jonge P, Demyttenaere K, Gureje O, Haro JM, Harris MG, He Y, Hinkov H, Karam AN, Karam EG, Kiejna A, Kovess-Masfety V, Lasebikan V, Lee S, Levinson D, Medina-Mora ME, Mneimneh Z, Navarro-Mateu F, Piazza M, Posada-Villa J, Scott K, Stein DJ, Tachimori H, Tintle N, Torres Y, Kessler RC; WHO World Mental Health Survey Collaborators. Association of cohort and individual substance use with risk of transitioning to drug use, drug use disorder, and remission from disorder: Findings from the world mental health surveys. JAMA Psychiatry. July 1, 2019;76(7):708–20.
64. United Nations Office on Drugs and Crime and the World Health Organization 2018. International Standards on Drug Use Prevention, Second updated edition. Vienna. ISBN 978-92-4-151448-4. https://www.unodc.org/documents/prevention/UNODC-WHO_2018_prevention_standards_E.pdf
65. European Monitoring Centre for Drugs and Drug Addiction (2010). Prevention and Evaluation Resources Kit (PERK), Publications Office of the European Union, Luxembourg. https://www.emcdda.europa.eu/system/files/publications/617/Manual4PERK_214413.pdf
66. European Monitoring Centre for Drugs and Drug Addiction (2011). European drug prevention quality standards: A manual for prevention professionals, Publications Office of the European Union, Luxembourg. https://www.emcdda.europa.eu/system/files/publications/646/TD3111250ENC_318193.pdf
67. European Monitoring Centre for Drugs and Drug Addiction (2012). Guidelines for the evaluation of drug prevention. A manual for program planners and evaluators, Publications Office of the European Union, Luxembourg. https://www.emcdda.europa.eu/system/files/publications/678/188138_EMCDDA_Guidelines_382952.pdf
68. European Monitoring Centre for Drugs and Drug Addiction (2019). European Prevention Curriculum: A handbook for decision-makers, opinion-makers and policy-makers in science-based prevention of substance use, Publications Office of the European Union, Luxembourg. https://www.emcdda.europa.eu/system/files/publications/11733/20192546_TDMA19001ENN_PDF.pdf
69. Vanyukov MM, Tarter RE, Conway KP, Kirillova GP, Chandler RK, Daley DC. Risk and resistance perspectives in translation-oriented etiology research. Transl Behav Med. 2016;6(1):44–54. https://doi.org/10.1007/s13142-015-0355-7
70. Jing Y, Hu Z, Fan P, Xue Y, Wang L, Tarter RE, *et al.* Analysis of substance use and its outcomes by machine learning I. Childhood evaluation of liability to substance use disorder. Drug Alcohol Depend. 2020;206:107605. 10.1016/j.drugalcdep.2019.107605
71. Hu Z, Jing Y, Xue Y, Fan P, Wang L, Vanyukov M, *et al.* Analysis of substance use and its outcomes by machine learning: II. Derivation and prediction of the trajectory of substance use severity. Drug Alcohol Depend. 2020;206:107604. https://doi.org/10.1016/j.drugalcdep.2019.107604
72. Zhang-James Y, Chen Q, Kuja-Halkola R, Lichtenstein P, Larsson H, Faraone SV. Machine-Learning prediction of comorbid substance use disorders in ADHD youth using Swedish registry data. J Child Psychol Psychiatry Allied Discipline. 2020;61(12):1370–9. https://doi.org/10.1111/jcpp.13226

73. Tate AE, McCabe RC, Larsson H, Lundström S, Lich-tenstein P, Kuja-Halkola R. Predicting mental health problems in adolescence using machine learning techniques. PloS One. 2020; 15(4):e0230389. https://doi.org/10.1371/journal.pone.0230389
74. Nawi AM, Ismail R, Ibrahim F, Hassan MR, Manaf MRA, Amit N, *et al.* Risk and protective factors of drug abuse among adolescents: A systematic review. BMC Public Health. 2021;21(1):2088. https://doi.org/10.1186/s12889-021-11906-2
75. Afuseh E, Pike CA, Oruche UM. Individualized approach to primary prevention of substance use disorder: Age-related risks. Subst Abuse Treat Prev Policy. 2020;15(1):58. https://doi.org/10.1186/s13011-020-00300-7
76. Leza L, Siria S, López-Goñi JJ, Fernández-Montalvo J. Adverse childhood experiences (ACEs) and substance use disorder (SUD): A scoping review. Drug Alcohol Depend. 2021;221:108563. https://doi.org/10.1016/j.drugalcdep.2021.108563
77. Dowling NA, Merkouris SS, Greenwood CJ, Oldenhof E, Toumbourou JW, Youssef GJ. Early risk and protective factors for problem gambling: A systematic review and meta-analysis of longitudinal studies. Clin Psychol Rev. 2017;51:109–24. https://doi.org/10.1016/j.cpr.2016.10.008
78. Solmi M, Radua J, Olivola M, Croce E, Soardo L, Salazar de Pablo G, *et al.* Age at onset of mental disorders worldwide: Large-scale meta-analysis of 192 epidemiological studies. Mol Psychiatry. 2022;27(1):281–95. https://doi.org/10.1038/s41380-021-01161-7
79. Ministry of Health. (2022a). Estrategia de Salud Mental del Sistema Nacional de Salud. Madrid. https://www.sanidad.gob.es/areas/calidadAsistencial/estrategias/saludMental/docs/EstrategiaSaludMental_ingles.pdf
80. Ministry of Health (2022b). Mental Health Action Plan 2022-2024. Madrid. https://www.sanidad.gob.es/areas/calidadAsistencial/estrategias/saludMental/docs/PlanAccionSaludMental2022_ingles.pdf
81. Becoña E. Bases teóricas que sustentan los programas de prevención de drogas. Madrid: Government Delegation for the National Plan on Drugs, 1999. https://pnsd.sanidad.gob.es/profesionales/publicaciones/catalogo/catalogoPNSD/publicaciones/pdf/bases.pdf
82. Becoña E. La prevención ambiental del consumo de drogas ¿qué medidas podemos aplicar? Madrid: Government Delegation for the National Plan on Drugs, 2021. https://pnsd.sanidad.gob.es/profesionales/publicaciones/catalogo/catalogoPNSD/publicaciones/pdf/2021_PrevencionAmbientalDrogas.pdf
83. Galician Regional Government. Procesos preventivos y cartera de servicios en materia de prevención del Plan de Galicia sobre Drogas, 2008. https://extranet.sergas.es/catpb/Docs/cas/Publicaciones/Docs/Drogodependencias/PDF-1774-es.pdf
84. Regional Government of Galicia. Instrumentos para la evaluación de los programas incluidos en la cartera de servicios en materia de prevención de las drogodependencias, 2011. https://www.sergas.gal/gal/DocumentacionTecnica/docs/SaudePublica/adicciones/Doc_Tco_INSTRUMENTOS_EVALUACION_PREV.pdf
85. Ministry of Health. Estrategia Nacional sobre Drogas 2009-2016: Informe de la Evaluación final, 2017. https://pnsd.sanidad.gob.es/pnsd/estrategiaNacional/docs/2017_Informe_Evaluacion_Final_Estrategia_Nacional_sobre_Drogas_2009_2016.pdf
86. Ministry of Health. Estrategia Nacional sobre Adicciones 2017-2024. https://pnsd.sanidad.gob.es/pnsd/estrategiaNacional/docs/180209_ESTRATEGIA_N.ADICCIONES_2017-2024__aprobada_CM.pdf
87. Ministry of Health. Plan de Acción sobre Adicciones 2018-2020. https://pnsd.sanidad.gob.es/pnsd/planAccion/docs/PLAD_2018-2020_FINAL.pdf
88. Ministry of Health. Plan de Acción sobre Adicciones 2021-2024. https://pnsd.sanidad.gob.es/pnsd/planAccion/docs/PlanASA_2021-24_aprobado.pdf
89. BOE. Extracto de la Resolución de 6 de julio de 2022, de la Secretaría de Estado de Sanidad, por la que se convoke la concesión de ayudas económicas a corporaciones locales para el

desarrollo de programas de prevención de las adicciones, con cargo al Fondo de bienes decomisados por tráfico ilícito de drogas y otros delitos relacionados. Official State Gazette, 162, of July 7, 2022. https://www.boe.es/boe/dias/2022/07/07/pdfs/BOE-B-2022-22179.pdf
90. BOE. Extracto de la Resolución de 18 de mayo de 2022, de la Secretaría de Estado de Sanidad, por la que se convoca la concesión de ayudaseconómicas a entidades privadas sin fines de lucro y de ámbito estatal,para la realización de programas supracomunitarios sobre adicciones en el año 2022. Official State Gazette, 129, of May 18, 2022. https://www.boe.es/boe/dias/2022/05/31/pdfs/BOE-B-2022-17376.pdf
91. BOE. Extracto de la Resolución de 17 de Agosto de 2022 por la que se convoca la concesión de subvenciones en régimen de concurrencia competitiva a entidades privadas sin fines de lucro y de ámbito estatal, para el desarrollo de proyectos en materia de prevención y tratamiento de adicciones correspondientes al año 2022 en el marco del Plan de Recuperación, Transformación y Resiliencia, financiado por la Unión Europea -Next GenerationEU. Official State Gazette, 203, of August 24, 2022. https://www.boe.es/boe/dias/2022/08/24/pdfs/BOE-B-2022-25670.pdf
92. DOG. ORDE do 14 de xullo de 2022 pola que se aproban as bases reguladoras da concesión de subvencións, en réxime de concorrencia competitiva, que incorpora fondos procedentes do tramo autonómico da asignación tributaria do 0,7 % do IRPF destinado á realización de programas de interese xeral para fins de carácter sociosanitario, para o cofinanciamento de proxectos de prevención de condutas adictivas promovidos por entidades privadas sen ánimo de lucro que desenvolven o seu labor no eido da prevención na Comunidade Autónoma de Galicia, e se procede á súa convocatoria (código de procedemento SA463F). Official Gazette of Galicia, 146, of August 2, 2022. https://www.xunta.gal/dog/Publicados/2022/20220802/AnuncioC3K1-150722-0003_es.html
93. DOG. ORDE do 21 de xullo de 2022 pola que se aproban as bases reguladoras da concesión de subvencións, en réxime de concorrencia competitiva, para o cofinanciamento de proxectos de prevención de condutas adictivas promovidos por concellos, mancomunidades de concellos ou agrupacións de concellos da Comunidade Autónoma de Galicia, e se procede á súa convocatoria (código de procedemento SA463G). Official Gazette of Galicia, 153, August 11, 2022. https://www.xunta.gal/dog/Publicados/2022/20220811/AnuncioC3K1-220722-0001_gl.pdf
94. Volkow ND, Torrens M, Poznyak V, Sáenz E, Busse A, Kashino W, *et al.* Managing dual disorders: A statement by the Informal Scientific Network, UN Commission on Narcotic Drugs. World Psychiatry. 2020;19(3):396–97. https://doi.org/10.1002/wps.20796
95. Colizzi M, Lasalvia A, Ruggeri M. Prevention and early intervention in youth mental health: Is it time for a multidisciplinary and trans-diagnostic model for care? Int J Ment Health Syst. 2020;14:23. https://doi.org/10.1186/s13033-020-00356-9
96. Castillo EG, Ijadi-Maghsoodi R, Shadravan S, Moore E, Mensah MO 3rd, Docherty M, *et al.* Community Interventions to Promote Mental Health and Social Equity. Curr Psychiatry Rep. 2019;21(5):35. https://doi.org/10.1007/s11920-019-1017-0
97. Genuis SJ, Genuis RA. Preconception Care: A New Standard of Care within Maternal Health Services. BioMed Rese Int. 2016;2016:6150976. https://doi.org/10.1155/2016/6150976
98. Cook JL, Green CR, de la Ronde S, Dell CA, Graves L, Ordean A, *et al.* Epidemiology and Effects of Substance Use in Pregnancy. J Obstet Gynaecol Can. 2017;39(10):906-915. https://doi.org/10.1016/j.jogc.2017.07.005
99. Substance Abuse and Mental Health Services Administration. Results from the 2020 National Survey on Drug Use and Health: Detailed Tables. Rockville, MD: Center for Behavioral Health Statistics and Quality, Substance Abuse and Mental Health Services Administration, 2022.
100. Pichini S, Puig C, Zuccaro P, Marchei E, Pellegrini M, Murillo J, *et al.* Assessment of exposure to opiates and cocaine during pregnancy in a Mediterranean city: Preliminary results of the "Meconium Project." Forensic Sci Int. 2005;153(1):59–65. https://doi.org/10.1016/j.forsciint.2005.04.013

101. García-Algar O, Vall Combelles O, Puig Sola C, Mur Sierra A, Scaravelli G, Pacifici R, *et al.* Prenatal exposure to drugs of abuse using meconium analysis in a low socioeconomic population in Barcelona. Anales de Pediatría. 2009;70(2):151–8. https://doi.org/10.1016/j.anpedi.2008.08.008
102. Friguls B, Joya X, Garcia-Serra J, Gómez-Culebras M, Pichini S, Martinez S, *et al.* Assessment of exposure to drugs of abuse during pregnancy by hair analysis in a Mediterranean island. Addiction (Abingdon, England). 2012;107(8):1471–79. https://doi.org/10.1111/j.1360-0443.2012.03828.x
103. Lendoiro E, González-Colmenero E, Concheiro-Guisán A, de Castro A, Cruz A, López-Rivadulla M. Maternal hair analysis for the detection of illicit drugs, medicines, and alcohol exposure during pregnancy. Ther Drug Monit. 2013;35(3):296–304. https://doi.org/10.1097/FTD.0b013e318288453f
104. Roca A, Jarque P, Gomila I, Marchei E, Tittarelli R, Elorza MÁ, *et al.* Clinical features and risk factors associated with prenatal exposure to drugs of abuse. Anales de Pediatria. 2021;95(5):307–20. https://doi.org/10.1016/j.anpedi.2020.08.003
105. Blount AJ, Adams CR, Anderson-Berry AL, Hanson C, Schneider K, Pendyala G. Biopsychosocial factors during the perinatal period: risks, preventative factors, and implications for healthcare professionals. Int J Environ Res Public Health. 2021;18(15):8206. https://doi.org/10.3390/ijerph18158206
106. Austin M-P, Highet N and the Expert Working Group. Mental Health Care in the Perinatal Period: Australian Clinical Practice Guideline. Melbourne: Centre of Perinatal Excellence, 2017. https://cesphn.org.au/wp-content/uploads/2022/09/Final-COPE-Perinatal-Mental-Health-Guideline-5.pdf
107. Howard LM, Khalifeh H. Perinatal mental health: A review of progress and challenges. World Psychiatry. 2020;19(3):313–27. https://doi.org/10.1002/wps.20769
108. Barrero-Castillero A, Morton SU, Nelson CA 3rd, Smith VC. Psychosocial Stress and Adversity: Effects from the Perinatal Period to Adulthood. NeoReviews. 2019;20(12):e686–96. https://doi.org/10.1542/neo.20-12-e686
109. Reyes AM, Akanyirige PW, Wishart D, Dahdouh R, Young MR, Estrada A, *et al.* Interventions addressing social needs in perinatal care: A systematic review. Health Equity. 2021;5(1):100–18. https://doi. org/10.1089/heq.2020.0051
110. Monk C, Dimidjian S, Galinsky E, Gregory KD, Hoffman MC, Howell EA, *et al.* The transition to parenthood in obstetrics: Enhancing prenatal care for 2-generation impact. Am J Obstet Gynecol MFM. 2022;4(5):100678. https://doi.org/10.1016/j.ajogmf.2022.100678
111. Freedman R, Hunter SK, Hoffman MC. Prenatal Primary Prevention of Mental Illness by Micronutrient Supplements in Pregnancy. Am J Psychiatry. 2018 Jul 1;175(7):607–19. https://doi.org/10.1176/appi.ajp.2018.17070836
112. Bekdash RA. Early life nutrition and mental health: The role of DNA methylation. Nutrients. 2021;13(9):3111. https://doi.org/10.3390/nu13093111
113. DeCapo M, Thompson JR, Dunn G, Sullivan EL. Perinatal nutrition and programmed risk for neuropsychiatric disorders: A focus on animal models. Biol Psychiatry. 2019;85(2):122–34. https://doi.org/10.1016/j.biopsych.2018.08.006
114. Adan RAH, van der Beek EM, Buitelaar JK, Cryan JF, Hebebrand J, Higgs S, *et al.* Nutritional psychiatry: Towards improving mental health by what you eat. Eur Neuropsychopharmacol. 2019;29(12):1321–32. https://doi.org/10.1016/j.euroneuro.2019.10.011
115. Izett E, Rooney R, Prescott SL, De Palma M, McDe-vitt M. Prevention of Mental Health Difficulties for Children Aged 0–3 Years: A Review. Front Psychol. 2021;11:500361. https://doi.org/10.3389/fpsyg.2020.500361
116. Siegenthaler E, Munder T, Egger M. Effect of preventive interventions in mentally ill parents on the mental health of the offspring: Systematic review and meta-analysis. J Am Acad Child Adolesc Psychiatry. 2012;51(1):8–17.e8. https://doi.org/10.1016/j.jaac.2011.10.018

117. Lannes A, Bui E, Arnaud C, Raynaud JP, Revet A. Preventive interventions in offspring of parents with mental illness: A systematic review and meta-analysis of randomized controlled trials. Psychol Med. 2021;51(14):2321–36. https://doi.org/10.1017/S0033291721003366
118. Caponnetto P, Casu M, Amato M, Cocuzza D, Galofaro V, La Morella A, *et al.* The effects of physical exercise on mental health: From cognitive improvements to risk of addiction. Int J Environ Res Public Health. 2021;18(24):13384. https://doi.org/10.3390/ijerph182413384
119. Sabe M, Chen C, Sentissi O, Deenik J, Vancampfort D, Firth J, *et al.* Thirty years of research on physical activity, mental health, and wellbeing: A scientometric analysis of hotspots and trends. Front Public Health. 2022;10: 943435. https://doi.org/10.3389/fpubh.2022.943435
120. Rankin J, Matthews L, Cobley S, Han A, Sanders R, Wiltshire HD, Baker JS. Psychological consequences of childhood obesity: Psychiatric comorbidity and prevention. Adolesc Health Med Ther. 2016;7:125–46. https://doi.org/10.2147/AHMT.S101631
121. Oral R, Ramirez M, Coohey C, Nakada S, Walz A, Kuntz A, *et al.* Adverse childhood experiences and trauma-informed care: The future of health care. Pediatric Res. 2016;79(1–2):227–33. https://doi.org/10.1038/pr.2015.197
122. Kessler RC, McLaughlin KA, Green JG, Gruber MJ, Sampson NA, Zaslavsky AM, *et al.* Childhood adversities and adult psychopathology in the WHO World Mental Health Surveys. Br J Psychiatry. 2010;197(5):378–85. https://doi.org/10.1192/bjp.bp.110.080499
123. Barnes AJ, Anthony BJ, Karatekin C, Lingras KA, Mercado R, Thompson LA. Identifying adverse childhood experiences in pediatrics to prevent chronic health conditions. Pediatr Res. 2020;87(2):362–70. https://doi.org/10.1038/s41390-019-0613-3
124. Loveday S, Hall T, Constable L, Paton K, Sanci L, Goldfeld S, *et al.* Screening for adverse childhood experiences in children: A systematic review. Pediatrics. 2022;149(2):e2021051884. https://doi.org/10.1542/peds.2021-051884
125. Das JK, Salam RA, Lassi ZS, Khan MN, Mahmood W, Patel V, *et al.* Interventions for adolescent mental health: An overview of systematic reviews. J Adolesc Health. 2016;59(4S):S49–60. https://doi.org/10.1016/j.jadohealth.2016.06.020
126. Das JK, Salam RA, Arshad A, Finkelstein Y, Bhutta ZA. Interventions for adolescent substance abuse: An overview of systematic reviews. J Adolesc Health. 2016;59(4S):S61–75. https://doi.org/10.1016/j.jadohealth.2016.06.021
127. Baughman, N, Prescott, S. L, & Rooney, R. The prevention of anxiety and depression in early childhood. Front Psychol. 2020;11:517896. https://doi.org/10.3389/fpsyg.2020.517896
128. Harrison L, Sharma N, Irfan O, Zaman M, Vaivada T, Bhutta ZA. Mental health and positive development prevention interventions: Overview of systematic reviews. Pediatrics. 2022;149(Suppl. 5):e2021053852G. https://doi.org/10.1542/peds.2021-053852G
129. Werlen L, Gjukaj D, Mohler-Kuo M, Puhan MA. Interventions to improve children's access to mental health care: A systematic review and meta-analysis. Epidemiol Psychiatr Sci. 2019;29:e58. https://doi.org/10.1017/S2045796019000544
130. Martel MM, Markon K, Smith GT. Research review: Multi-informant integration in child and adolescent psychopathology diagnosis. J Child Psychol Psychiatry. 2017 Feb;58(2):116–28. https://doi.org/10.1111/jcpp.12611
131. Nees F, Deserno L, Holz NE, Romanos M, Banas-chewski T. Prediction along a developmental perspective in psychiatry: How far might we go?. Front Sys Neurosci. 2021;15:670404. https://doi.org/10.3389/fnsys.2021.670404
132. García-Couceiro N, Gómez Salgado P, Kim-Harris S, Burkhart G, Flórez-Menéndez G, Rial Boubeta A. The SBIRT model as a prevention strategy against addiction with and without substance in teenagers. Rev Esp Salud Publica. 2021;95:e202105065.
133. Mersky JP, Topitzes J, Langlieb J, Dodge K A. Increasing mental health treatment access and equity through trauma-responsive care. Am J Orthopsychiatry. 2021;91(6):703–13. https://doi.org/10.1037/ort0000572

134. Levy SJ, Williams JF. Committee on Substance Use and Prevention. Substance use screening, brief intervention, and referral to treatment. Pediatrics. 2016;138(1):e20161211. https://doi.org/10.1542/peds.2016-1211
135. Davies C, Cipriani A, Ioannidis JPA, Radua J, Stahl D, Provenzani U, *et al.* Lack of evidence to favor specific preventive interventions in psychosis: A network meta-analysis. World Psychiatry. 2018;17(2):196–209. https://doi.org/10.1002/wps.20526
136. Thomas S, Jenkins R, Burch T, Calamos Nasir L, Fisher B, Giotaki G, *et al.* Promoting Mental Health and Preventing Mental Illness in General Practice. London J Prim Care. 2016;8(1):3–9. https://doi.org/10.1080/17571472.2015.1135659
137. Buitrago Ramírez F, Ciurana Misol R, Chocrón Bentata L, Carmen Fernández Alonso MD, García Campayo J, Montón Franco C, Tizón García JL; PAPPS Mental Health Group. Prevención de los trastornos de la salud mental en atención primaria. Actualización PAPPS 2018. Primary Care. 2018;50 (Suppl. 1):83–108. https://doi.org/10.1016/S0212-6567(18)30364-0
138. Leggett A, Zarit SH. Prevention of Mental Disorder in Older Adults: Recent Innovations and Future Directions. Generations. 2014;8(3):45–52. https://pubmed.ncbi.nlm.nih.gov/26290620
139. El Hayek S, Geagea L, El Bourji H, Kadi T, Talih F. Prevention Strategies of Alcohol and Substance Use Disorders in Older Adults. Clin Geriatr Med. 2022;38(1):169–79.
140. Bellón JA, Conejo-Cerón S, Rodríguez-Bayón A, Ba-llesta-Rodríguez MI, Mendive JM, Moreno-Peral, P. Enfermedades mentales comunes en atención primaria: dificultades diagnósticas y terapéuticas, y nuevos retos en predicción y prevención. SESPAS Report 2020. Gaceta Sanitaria. 2020;34(Suppl. 1):20–26. https://doi.org/10.1016/j.gaceta.2020.05.013
141. Mulvaney-Day N, Marshall T, Downey Piscopo K, Korsen N, Lynch S, Karnell LH, *et al.* Screening for behavioral health conditions in primary care settings: A systematic review of the literature. J Gen Intern Med. 2018;33(3):335–46. https://doi.org/10.1007/s11606-017-4181-0
142. Bellón JÁ, Conejo-Cerón S, Moreno-Peral P, King M, Nazareth I, Martín-Pérez C, *et al.* Intervention to prevent major depression in primary care: A cluster randomized trial. Ann Intern Med. 2016;64(10):656–65. https://doi.org/10.7326/M14-2653
143. Conejo-Cerón S, Moreno-Peral P, Rodríguez-Morejón A, Motrico E, Navas-Campaña D, Rigabert A, *et al.* Effectiveness of Psychological and Educational Interventions to Prevent Depression in Primary Care: A Systematic Review and Meta-Analysis. Ann Fam Med. 2017; 15(3):262–71. https://doi.org/10.1370/afm.2031
144. Souza AP, Rezende K, Marin M, Tonhom S, Damaceno DG. Ações de promoção e proteção à saúde mental do idoso na atenção primária à saúde: uma revisão integrativa. Ações de promoção e pro-teção à saúde mental do idoso na atenção primária à saú-de: uma revisão integrativa. Ciencia & Saude Coletiva. 2022;27(5):1741–52. https://doi.org/10.1590/1413-81232022275.23112021
145. Lee C, Kuhn I, McGrath M, Remes O, Cowan A, Duncan F, Baskin C, Oliver EJ, Osborn DPJ, Dykxhoorn J, Kaner E, Walters K, Kirkbride J, Gnani S, Lafortune L; NIHR SPHR Public Mental Health Programme. A systematic scoping review of community-based interventions for the prevention of mental ill-health and the promotion of mental health in older adults in the UK. Health Soc Care Community. 2022;30(1):27–57. https://doi.org/10.1111/hsc.13413
146. Murniati N, Al Aufa B, Kusuma D, Kamso S. A Scoping Review on Biopsychosocial Predictors of Mental Health among Older Adults. Int J Environ Res Public Health. 2022;19(17):10909. https://doi.org/10.3390/ijerph191710909
147. James P, Kawachi I. Emerging directions in the study of the environmental determinants of mental health: Commentary on the MINDMAP Project. J Epidemiol Community Health. 2021;75(5):417–19. https://doi.org/10.1136/jech-2021-216713
148. Wey TW, Doiron D, Wissa R, Fabre G, Motoc I, Noor-dzij JM, *et al.* Overview of retrospective data harmonization in the MINDMAP project: Process and results. J Epidemiol Community Health. 2021;75(5):433–41. https://doi.org/10.1136/jech-2020-214259

149. World Health Organization. Ageing and Health. 2022. https://www.who.int/news-room/fact-sheets/detail/ageing-and-health
150. Fishbein DH, Ridenour TA, Stahl M, Sussman S. The full translational spectrum of prevention science: Facilitating the transfer of knowledge to practices and policies that prevent behavioral health problems. Transl Behav Med. 2016;6(1):5–16. https://doi.org/10.1007/s13142-015-0376-2
151. Rezapour T, Rafei P, Baldacchino A, Conrod PJ, Dom G, Fishbein DH, *et al.* Neuroscience-Informed Classification of Prevention Interventions in Substance Use Disorders: An RDoC-based Approach, 2022. medRxiv. https://doi.org/10.1101/2022.09.28.22280342
152. World Health Organization, 2003. Advocacy for mental health. World Health Organization. https://apps.who.int/iris/handle/10665/333227
153. World Health Organization. 2004. Promoting mental health: Concepts, emerging evidence, practice: Summary report/a report from the World Health Organization, Department of Mental Health and Substance Abuse in collaboration with the Victorian Health Promotion Foundation and the University of Melbourne. World Health Organization.
154. World Health Organization. 2004. Prevention of mental disorders: Effective interventions and policy options: Summary report/a report of the World Health Organization Dept. of Mental Health and Substance Abuse; in collaboration with the Prevention Research Centre of the Universities of Nijmegen and Maastricht. World Health Organization. https://apps.who.int/iris/handle/10665/43027
155. World Health Organization. 2014. Health for the world's adolescents: A second chance in the second decade: Summary. World Health Organization. https://apps.who.int/iris/handle/10665/112750
156. World Health Organization. 2021. Comprehensive mental health action plan 2013-2030. World Health Organization. https://apps.who.int/iris/handle/10665/345301
157. Fusar-Poli P, Bauer M, Borgwardt S, Bechdolf A, Correll CU, Do KQ, *et al.* European college of neuropsychopharmacology network on the prevention of mental disorders and mental health promotion (ECNP PMD-MHP). Eur Neuropsychopharmacol. 2019;29(12):1301–11. https://doi.org/10.1016/j.euroneuro.2019.09.006
158. National Institutes on Drug Abuse (US). Common Comorbidities with Substance Use Disorders Research Report, 2020. https://www.ncbi.nlm.nih.gov/books/NBK571451/

CHAPTER 10

Other Topics of Interest in Dual Pathology

10.1 NEUROBIOLOGICAL FOUNDATIONS OF DUAL PATHOLOGY

M. C. García-Mahía, F. J. Vicente Alba, G. A. Castaño Pérez, and M. Vidal Millares

The high prevalence of dual pathology and its worse prognosis in relation to suffering from an addictive or psychiatric disorder in isolation make it increasingly necessary to expand knowledge in this area. One of the most necessary lines of research is that which aims to understand the underlying neurobiological mechanisms involved in the onset of addictive disorders and dual pathology.

Addictive disorders are more prevalent in patients with psychiatric disorders than in the general population, especially in those suffering from schizophrenia, depression, post-traumatic stress disorder, antisocial personality disorder, and borderline personality disorder. The high prevalence of mental illness in patients with drug addiction is not specific to certain drugs, but is associated with all addictive substances.[1,2]

Animal models of psychiatric disorders studied in addiction paradigms suggest a unitary nature of mental illness and vulnerability to addiction at both the neurobiological and clinical-behavioral levels. These models would provide the basis for exploring the interactive role of biological, environmental, and developmental factors in the neurocircuits fundamentally involved in psychiatric and addictive disorders.[1]

Preclinical research indicates that comorbidity between addictive disorders and other psychiatric disorders may involve two different neurotransmitter systems, notably dopamine (DA), a key neurotransmitter in the **brain's reward system**.

While the differential profiles of intoxication and withdrawal from drugs of abuse are associated with different effects, mediated by various neurotransmitters in different brain regions, there are common reinforcement mechanisms, more anatomically localized, with specific neurobiological mechanisms. The subcortical dopaminergic system, which consists of neurons that project from the **ventral tegmental area to the nucleus accumbens**, plays a fundamental role in natural motivation and is involved in the process of addiction as a common substrate.

DOI: 10.4324/9781003786153-10

Volkow and Koob,[3] in relation to addictive phenomena, point out that:

- Substance use disorders are complex, multistage diseases characterized by alterations in three main neurocircuits:
  - i. Binge/intoxication stage related to the basal ganglia
  - ii. Extended withdrawal/negative affect stage related to the amygdala
  - iii. A stage of preoccupation/anticipation related to the prefrontal cortex
- There are neurotransmitter- and neuromodulator-specific changes in neuroplasticity in 18 subsystems, including the mesocorticolimbic DA ascending system, the corticotropin-releasing factor in the central nucleus of the amygdala, and corticostriatal glutamate projections.
- During the binge/intoxication stage, previously neutral stimuli become associated with drug availability, promoting the development of habits that encourage excessive drug-seeking through increases in DA and glutamate action.
- The binge/intoxication stage triggers a decrease in reward function (DA and opioid peptide deficits) and increases the activity of the brain stress system through corticotropin-releasing factor and dynorphin.
- Excessive drug intake also leads to deficits in executive function through the dysregulation of glutamatergic, GABAergic, and dopaminergic neural networks in the prefrontal cortex, which perpetuate the dysregulation of reward and stress function and induce compulsive drug use.
- During the preoccupation/anticipation stage, a combination of positive and negative reinforcement processes would occur, driving the pathological pursuit of drugs.

Molecular genetic mediation and epigenetic changes in these same circuits would provide preexisting vulnerabilities to addiction, greater susceptibility to environmental risk factors, and targets for the development of new treatments and resilience to relapse.

Another factor in favor of common neurobiological processes in dual pathology would be the effect of stress. Psychological stress worsens the symptoms of mental illness and increases consumption or relapse in patients with addictions. Neurobiological mediators of stress affect brain functions involved in addiction or mental illness.[4] Furthermore, the main brain structures involved in cognition, motivation, affect, and memory are so interrelated that it is likely that the processes of psychiatric and addictive diseases are closely related and are probably, in many ways, indivisible.[5]

NEUROBIOLOGY AND PSYCHIATRIC DISORDERS

Three key neurotransmitters have been identified as being involved in mental illness: serotonin, norepinephrine, and DA. In addition, the role of the endocannabinoid system has been highlighted in schizophrenia.[6]

In **depressive disorders**, serotonin, norepinephrine, DA, corticotropin-releasing factor (CRF), GABA, glutamate, neuropeptide Y, and somatostatin have been identified as involved neurotransmitters,[7] along with anatomical structures such as the hippocampus, prefrontal cortex, and amygdala; in addition, there are changes in neuronal size and glial density.

Markou[7] and Calarco CA[8] observed that some of these neurotransmitters are also involved in the depressive symptoms associated with substance withdrawal.

Another major group of psychiatric disorders are **anxiety disorders**, whose genesis involves the raphe nuclei, locus coeruleus, amygdala, and hippocampus, as well as various neurotransmitters such as serotonin, GABA, adrenaline, and DA.

As for psychotic disorders, the brain areas most involved are the prefrontal cortex, substantia nigra, nucleus accumbens, ventral tegmental area of the midbrain, raphe nuclei, and locus coeruleus (Grace, 1991). Likewise, the neurotransmitter most involved appears to be DA (Mathysse, 1974), although other neurobiological hypotheses include serotonin, acetylcholine, and glutamate.[9,10]

The prevalence of dual pathology in schizophrenia is particularly high and is noted in the current literature. The anatomical, pathological, neurobiological, and neuroimaging correlates of schizophrenia have been incorporated into theories about its pathophysiology.[11]

The effects of acute DA release in the nucleus accumbens, whether endogenous or drug-induced, are determined by the functional integrity of the prefrontal cortex and the temporolimbic zone (amygdala and hippocampus).[12–14]

Given that neuroplasticity in the nucleus accumbens, including its long-term potentiation and its variants, depends on specific combinations of DA and glutamate discharge in these regions, the functional integrity of the prefrontal cortex, amygdala, and hippocampus could also influence the long-term course of behavioral changes attributed to repeated episodes of DA release. Data from animal and clinical experiments support the theory that cortical and temporolimbic impairment can alter drug-induced motivation and behavior. Functional alterations in the prefrontal cortex in humans correlate with abnormalities in volition, motivational planning, and impulsivity, as traits associated with an increased risk of drug dependence. Structural or functional abnormalities of the hippocampus have been recognized in schizophrenia and in most psychiatric disorders involved in dual pathology, such as major depression, bipolar disorder, post-traumatic stress disorder, and borderline personality disorder.[15–17]

COMMON NEUROBIOLOGICAL FINDINGS IN DUAL PATHOLOGY

Several studies indicate that psychomotor responses to drugs are involuntarily increased in animal models of psychiatric disorders involving temporolimbic dysfunction, leading to greater changes in brain neuroplasticity associated with addictive disorders.[18]

Although different drugs have different effects on neurobiological systems, it has been postulated that any substance of abuse has similar nonspecific mechanisms.[3] There are also great similarities in the mechanisms involved in different types of addictions and even in substance and non-substance addictions or behavioral addictive disorders.[19]

Additionally, the fact that different drugs are used successively, which is common in patients with addictions, as well as the involvement of DA concentrations in the nucleus accumbens in most addictions and the involvement of corticotropin-releasing factor (CRF) and the hypothalamic-pituitary-adrenal axis in different phases of drug dependence, suggests that there are great similarities within the different types and phases of addictive disorders.

Previous studies in this field point to the probable involvement of several neurotransmitter systems, including DA, glutamate, γ-aminobutyric acid (GABA), and acetylcholine.

The review conducted by Rojas and Cas-taño,[6] based on previous studies,[20,21] indicates that there is evidence that neurobiological factors related to the risk of developing addictive disorders are associated with the pathogenesis of different mental disorders; i.e., they would represent a common biological vulnerability for both disorders.

Preclinical studies provide data that explain the neurobiological mechanisms involved in the onset of dual pathology. It is known that the brain's reinforcement system, mainly the connections between the neural regions that form the mesocorticolimbic-dopaminergic system and certain neurotransmitters, are involved in both the symptoms of addictive behavior and those of certain psychiatric disorders, specifically schizophrenia and depression. It is also known that stress can affect these systems, being a factor capable of generating imbalances that could induce comorbidity.

Also, in the review conducted by Rojas and Castaño[6] indicates the likelihood that the dopaminergic, glutamatergic, GABAergic, opioid, endocannabinoid, and cholinergic-nicotinic systems may be involved in both addictive disorders and mental illnesses, due to the correlations that exist between neurobiological mechanisms, a relationship previously noted by Ambrosio and Roncero[22] and Szerman.[23]

A summary of the neurotransmitter systems and neurobiological substrates where psychoactive substances interact and mental disorders occur can be seen in Table 10.1.

NEUROIMAGING, GENETIC, AND ENDOCRINOLOGICAL STUDIES IN DUAL PATHOLOGY

Balhara *et al.*,[24] in a comprehensive review of publications on the neurobiology of dual pathology, highlight that only a few specific topics have been studied. Although various authors have conducted studies on different neurobiological aspects, none of the specific drugs or psychiatric disorders have been studied in depth, making it difficult to draw definitive conclusions.

Functional neuroimaging studies have found that the frontal cortex is significantly less active in patients with schizophrenia and drug dependence compared to patients with schizophrenia alone or healthy controls. Emotional memory and prefrontal function are relatively better preserved in patients with schizophrenia and cannabis abuse than in schizophrenic patients who do not use cannabis. Genetic and neuroendocrine studies offer diverse and disparate results, without achieving consistent findings. These authors point out the main shortcomings of neurobiological studies of dual pathology, which are basically methodological in nature.

TABLE 10.1 Neurobiological Correlations in Dual Pathology

Neurobiological substrates	Neurotransmitters	Mental disorders	Substance use disorder
Meynert's basal nucleus with projections to the cortex and limbic system, and in the reticular system whose axons extend to the cortex, limbic system, hypothalamus, and thalamus	Acetylcholine	Psychosis, anxiety, depression	Nicotine
Ventral tegmental area of the midbrain, nucleus accumbens, centromedial and dorsolateral prefrontal cortex, substantia nigra, raphe nuclei, and locus ceruleus	Dopamine	Psychosis, anxiety, depression	Cocaine, amphetamine, nicotine
Hippocampus, amygdala, and prefrontal cortex	Monoamines (serotonin)	Depression	Amphetamine and derivatives
Hypothalamus, diencephalon, pons, hippocampus, and midbrain	Endorphins, enkephalins, and dynorphins	Borderline personality disorder	Opiates, alcohol
Hippocampus	N-methyl-D-aspartate (NMDA)	Psychosis	Ketamine, phencyclidine (PCP)
Cortex, limbic system, and brainstem region	γ-aminobutyric acid γ-aminobutyric acid ($GABA_A$)	Affective disorders and anxiety	Barbiturates, benzodiazepines, alcohol
Basal ganglia, cerebellum, hippocampus, cerebral cortex, periaqueductal gray matter	Anandamide, CB1 receptor agonists	Psychosis, autism, major depression, PTSD, bipolar I disorder (BID), anxiety disorder	Cannabis
Raphe nuclei of the brainstem	$5\text{-}HT_{2A}$ receptor agonist	Depression, anxiety, psychosis, obsessive-compulsive disorder	LSD, mescaline, and derivatives

Taken from Rojas Bernal LA, Castaño Pérez GA. Neurobiology of dual pathology. Health and Addictions. 2017;17(2):101–14 (with permission from the authors). https://ojs.haaj.org/?journal=haaj&page=article&op=view&path%5B%5D=310&path%5B%5D=pdf

As a general conclusion, it would be necessary to intensify research into the neurobiological bases of dual pathology in greater detail, with large samples that allow for a greater understanding of the neurobiological processes involved, which would enable a better focus on therapeutic interventions and, in particular, pharmacological treatments.

REFERENCES

1. Chambers R. A. Animal modeling and neurocircuitry of dual diagnosis. J Dual Diagn. 2007;3(2):19–29.
2. Singh S, Balhara YPS. A review of Indian research on co-occurring psychiatric disorders and alcohol use disorders. Indian J Psychol Med. 2016;38(1):10–9.

3. Volkow ND, Koob G. Brain disease model of addiction: Why is it so controversial? Lancet Psychiatry. 2015;2(8): 677–9. doi: 10.1016/S2215-0366(15)00236-9
4. Brady KT, Sinha R. Co-occurring mental and substance use disorders: The neurobiological effects of chronic stress. Am J Psychiatry. 2005;162:1483–93.
5. Chambers RA, Krystal JH, Self DW. A neurobiological basis for substance abuse comorbidity in schizophrenia. Biol Psychiatry. 2001; 50:71–83.
6. Rojas Bernal LA, Castaño Pérez GA. Neurobiología de la Patología Dual. Health and Addictions. 2017;17(2):101–14.
7. Markou A, Kosten TR, Koob GF. Neurobiological similarities in depression and drug dependence: A self-medication hypothesis. Neuropsychopharmacol. 1998;18(3):135–74.
8. Calarco CA, Lobo MK. Depression and substance use disorders: Clinical comorbidity and shared neurobiology. Int Rev Neurobiol. 2021;157:245–309. doi: 10.1016/bs.irn.2020.09.004
9. Lewis DA, Hashimoto T, Volk DW. Cortical inhibitory neurons and schizophrenia. Nat Rev Neurosci. 2005; 6(4): 312–24.
10. Peralta V, Cuesta MJ. Negative symptoms in schizophrenia: A confirmatory factor analysis of competing models. A J Psychiatry. 1995;152(10):1450.
11. Ross S, Peselow E. Co-occurring psychotic and addictive disorders. Neurobiology and Diagnosis. Clin Neuropharmacol. 2012 Sep-Oct;35(5):235–43. doi: 10.1097/WNF.0b013e318261e193
12. Pennarth CMA, Groenewegen HJ, Lopez da Silva FH. The nucleus accumbens as a complex of functionally distinct neuronal ensembles: An integration of behavioral, electrophysiological, and anatomical data. Prog Neurobiology. 1994;42:719–61.
13. O'Donnell P, Greene J, Pabello N, Lewis BL, Grace AA. Modulation of cell firing in the nucleus accumbens. Ann NY Acad Sci. 1999;877:157–75.
14. Finch DM. Neurophysiology of converging synaptic inputs from the rat prefrontal cortex, amygdala, midline thalamus, and hippocampal formation onto single neurons of the caudate/putamen and nucleus accumbens. Hippocampus. 1996;6:495–512.
15. Brenner JD, Narayan M, Anderson ER, Staib LH, Miller HL, Charney DS. Hippocampal volume reduction in major depression. Am J Psychiatry. 2000;157(1):115–8.
16. Driessen M, Herrmann M, Anderson ER, Staib LH, Miller HL, Hill A, *et al.* Magnetic resonance imaging of the hippocampus and the amygdala in women with borderline personality disorder and early traumatization. Arch Gen Psychiatry. 2000:57(12):115–22.
17. Blumberg H. P, Kaufman J, Martin A, Whiteman R, Zhang JH, Gore J, *et al.* Amygdala and hippocampal volumes in adolescents and adults with bipolar disorder. Arch Gen Psychiatry. 2003;60:1201–8.
18. Chambers RA, Taylor JR. Animal modeling dual diagnosis schizophrenia: Sensitization to cocaine in rats with neonatal ventral hippocampal lesions. Biol Psychiatry. 2004;56(5):308–16.
19. Vanyukov MM, Tarter RE, Kirillova GP, Kirisci L, Reynolds MD, Kreek MJ, *et al.* Common liability to addiction and "gateway hypothesis": Theoretical, empirical and evolutionary perspective. Drug Alcohol Depend. 2012 Jun;123(Suppl 1):S3–17.
20. Lembke A. Time to abandon the self-medication hypothesis in patients with psychiatric disorders. Am J Drug Alcohol Abuse. 2012;38(6):524–9.
21. Samaha AN, Potvin S. Drugs of abuse and psychiatric disorders: Neurobiological and clinical aspects. Prog Neuropsychopharmacol Biol Psychiatry. 2014 Jul 3;52:1–3.
22. Ambrosio E, Roncero C. Neurobiología de la Patología Dual. Patología Dual: Fundamentos clínicos y terapéuticos (1ª ed). Spain: Merge Books.
23. Szerman N, Martinez-Raga J, Peris L, Roncero C, Basurte I, Vega P, *et al.* Rethinking dual disorders/pathology. Addict Disord Their Treat. 2013;12(1):1–10.
24. Balhara YPS, Kuppili PP, Gupta R. Neurobiology of comorbid substance use disorders and psychiatric disorders: Current state of evidence. J Addict Nurs. 2017;28(1):11–26. doi: 10.1097/JAN.0000000000000155

10.2 GENETIC AND EPIGENETIC FACTORS IN DUAL PATHOLOGY

J.M. Tamayo Jaramillo, A. Aparicio Zambrano,
M. Martínez Fernández and G.A. Castaño Pérez

GENETICS AND EPIGENETICS OF SUBSTANCE USE DISORDERS

Exposure to drugs does not trigger the same psychopathological progression toward substance use disorder (SUD) in all individuals. Rather, a more complex model of vulnerability to addiction is determined by genetic and environmental factors that interact at multiple levels of molecular, neuronal, and circuit organization. At the genetic level, single nucleotide polymorphisms (SNPs) of genes related to multiple components of the brain's reward circuit play a key role, and their relationships with molecular alterations are often mediated by epigenetic mechanisms that regulate gene expression. The resulting alterations at the circuit level play an important role in the development of specific behavioral endophenotypes, such as impulsivity, novelty-seeking, or increased sensitivity to reward and decreased executive control, which may underlie an increased likelihood of experimenting with substances of abuse or developing a compulsive and habitual pattern of SUD.[1]

Based on twin and adoption studies, estimates of heritability (h^2) among SUDs in general vary considerably, but genetic predisposition is estimated to account for approximately 50% of the risk on average.[2] Until the advent of genome-wide association studies (GWAS) more than 15 years ago, associations of genetic variants were not substantially established. In complex genetic disorders, like mental illnesses, the GWAS approach is much more powerful in distinguishing genetic loci associated with the disease than traditional twin and genetic linkage studies. Unfortunately, SNPs only explain part of the variance in substance addiction.[3,4]

Specifically, linkage disequilibrium score regression approaches, based on summary statistics from GWAS, have shown SNP heritability rates (h^2_{SNP}) of ~0.07–0.10 for problematic alcohol use (PAU); ~0.09 for nicotine use disorder (NUD); ~0.12 for cannabis use disorder (CANUD); ~0.11–0.28 for opioid use disorder (OUD); and ~0.27–0.30 for cocaine use disorder (CUD).[5] Due to the small effect size of each SNP, clinical utility and predictive potential are insufficient. To improve statistical power, polygenic risk scoring (PRS) has been established and applied in GWAS as a robust analytical tool. Despite this, the use of PRS is still limited to the field of research, particularly in the case of psychiatric disorders.[2]

On the other hand, epigenetics studies heritable changes in phenotype that are not caused by alterations in DNA sequence. Repeated stressful life events can cause epigenetic changes. Given that drug-dependent patients often report experiencing stressful events in their early years of life, this may explain why these individuals are more vulnerable to drug-induced neuroplastic changes.[3]

The regulation of neuronal gene expression underlying the pathogenesis of SUDs is mediated by epigenetic mechanisms, such as DNA cytosine methylation and hydroxymethylation (mC and hmC), alteration of microRNAs, non-coding RNAs, and histone modification profiles underlying neural and behavioral adaptations associated with interindividual differences in susceptibility to SUDs, such as novelty-seeking, indicative of prefrontal cortex (PFC) dysfunction.[6,7] Drugs have been shown to promote the formation of neural ensembles in the rodent brain (e.g., nucleus accumbens, amygdala, and cortex) through hypermethylation in synaptic plasticity genes, and their synchronous activation facilitates stimulus-specific memory retrieval and behavioral plasticity.[7]

GENETIC BASES OF DUAL DIAGNOSIS IN GENERAL

The genetic architecture of complex traits is mainly characterized by two phenomena: polygenicity (the cumulative contribution of thousands of risk alleles with very small individual effects) and pleiotropy (risk alleles are shared between diseases and traits/phenotypes). A GWAS observed a broad genetic correlation between psychiatric disorders, including SUDs, with a large number of pleiotropic genes including 5,884 associations and 2,424 unique genes. Differentially expressed pleiotropic genes were involved in the regulation of neurodevelopment, neurogenesis, and neuronal differentiation. The high comorbidity observed between SUDs and other psychiatric disorders reflects shared genetic and non-genetic risk factors linking them. The vast majority (75.8%) of psychiatric disorder pairs evaluated showed a positive genetic correlation. The greatest genetic overlap of SUDs was observed with major depressive disorder (MDD), anxiety disorders (AnxDs), post-traumatic stress disorder (PTSD), neuroticism, and risk behaviors.[8] This was also observed by Hatoum *et al.*,[9] applying a genomic structural equation model to GWAS summary statistics for individuals of European ancestry (n = 1,019,521). They found that the shared genetic predisposition for UPA, problematic tobacco use, TUCan, and TUO was characterized by a unidimensional addiction risk factor (FRAU), independent of SUD. TUO and TUCan showed the highest loads, while UPT showed the lowest load. FRAU was positively associated with genetic predisposition for risk-taking (β = 0.45) and neuroticism (β = 0.25), and negatively associated with executive function (β = −0.17). The FRAU was also positively associated with psychopathology unrelated to substance use (psychotic disorders (β = 0.45) and neurodevelopmental disorders (β = 0.74)) and negatively associated with compulsive disorders (β = −0.32). The FRAU has a unique genetic architecture not shared with SUD or non-substance-related psychopathology, suggesting that dual pathology is not simply a linear combination of SUD and other psychiatric disorders. A substantial fraction of genetic influences on psychiatric disorders transcend the boundaries of clinical diagnosis.

Estimating the genetic correlation between multiple psychiatric disorders using GWAS data has become a standard analysis following the primary GWAS. Although SNP-based heritability is low, these analyses have confirmed that SUDs are genetically correlated with other psychiatric disorders and behavioral traits. However, while there is sufficient data to make correlations with substances such as alcohol and cannabis, there is insufficient data for other substances such as opioids and cocaine.[8] The genetic correlation (r_g) between phenotypes is a measure of the average effect of pleiotropy across all causal loci and could be used as an index of polygenic overlap between phenotypes.[10] Positive correlations have been reported between UPA and TUN (rg = 0.55), TUCan (r_g = 0.39), TDM (r_g = 0.39), risk-taking (r_g = 0.30), attention deficit/hyperactivity disorder (ADHD), bipolar disorder (BD), and schizophrenia; between TUN and TUA (r_g = 0.56), TDM (r_g = 0.38), and schizophrenia

($r_g = 0.16$); between TUCan and TUA ($r_g = 0.55$), schizophrenia ($r_g = 0.31$), and TUN ($r_g = 0.66$); between TUO and ADHD ($r_g = 0.36$), TUA ($r_g = 0.73$), TUN ($r_g = 0.51$), and TDM ($r_g = 0.35$); and between TUCoc and ADHD ($r_g = 0.50$), TUN ($r_g = 0.34$), TDM ($r_g = 0.40$), risk-taking ($r_g = 0.35$), and schizophrenia ($r_g = 0.20$).[5]

Another way to determine the causal bidirectional relationships between SUD and psychiatric disorders is to use instrumental variables based on genetic information to distinguish simple association from causality through Mendelian randomization (MR). However, MA analyses have several limitations, such as the fact that they are based on specific assumptions and the difficulty in determining whether other unaccounted confounding factors are affecting the results. In addition, the low heritability based on SNPs, high polygenicity, and complex pleiotropy of SUD-related traits strongly affect the statistical power and reliability of MA methods.[8]

Using the results of meta-analyses GWAS, Jang *et al.*[11] determined that the genetic etiology of SUDs (smoking, alcohol, and cannabis use) and other psychiatric disorders (ADHD, anorexia nervosa [AN], MDD, BD, and schizophrenia) is highly pleiotropic and involves a shared pathway of neurodevelopment, neurotransmission, and intracellular trafficking. Of all 30 possible substance use–psychiatric phenotype pairs, SUD and ADHD had the highest number of shared loci (n = 40), followed by age of onset of smoking and ADHD (n = 22). Previously, Abdellaoui *et al.*[12] used GWAS summary statistics to estimate genetic correlations between all traits and found that SUD and TUN showed significant genetic correlations with several other psychiatric disorders, including ADHD (ADHD–SUD: $r_g = 0.46$; ADHD–TUN: $r_g = 0.54$), TDM (TDM–TUA: $r_g = 0.52$; TDM–TUN: $r_g = 0.45$), and schizoaffective disorder (schizophrenia–TUA: $rg = 0.35$). TUCan was only significantly associated with ADHD ($rg = 0.35$).

Finally, using data from 192 individuals of Mexican ancestry, a PRS calculation was performed to test for common genetic variation shared by SUD and other psychiatric disorders (autism spectrum disorder [ASD], ADHD, TB, TDM, and schizophrenia). The authors found that only patients with schizophrenia and MDD shared genetic etiology as part of a dual pathology ($p = 0.0423$ and $p = 0.0118$, respectively).[13]

GENETICS AND EPIGENETICS OF PSYCHIATRIC DISORDERS COEXISTING WITH SPECIFIC SUBSTANCE USE DISORDERS

Attention Deficit/Hyperactivity Disorder (ADHD) and Concurrent SUD

The clinical picture of ADHD is heterogeneous and is often affected by psychiatric comorbidity, including SUDs. During childhood, conduct disorder (CD) and oppositional defiant disorder (ODD) are the most common comorbidities of ADHD. Both ODD and CD are associated with an increased risk of SUD in individuals with and without ADHD.[14] A Danish registry-based study showed that ADHD increased the risk of SUD more in females than in males after adjusting for observation time, age, and calendar year at the time of first ADHD diagnosis (OR = 1.30; 95% CI: 1.11–1.51). Associations were observed with alcohol (OR = 1.26; 1.04–1.53) and cannabis (OR = 1.34; 1.10–1.64). The factors most strongly associated with SUD, across all types and levels of severity, were older age at first diagnosis ADHD diagnosis (OR = 3.28; 2.75–3.92) and comorbid ODD/CD (OR = 2.87; 2.53–3.26).[15]

Based on preexisting GWAS datasets, Vilar-Ribó *et al.*[16] found significant results when considering smoking initiation as exposure and ADHD as outcome (OR = 2.46). They also found evidence of causal effects of ADHD propensity on the risk of cannabis use (OR = 1.15) and vice versa (OR = 1.46), with no evidence of horizontal pleiotropy or heterogeneity in either direction. These authors found no evidence of causal effects of ADHD propensity on the risk of AUD, CUD, and vice versa. Similarly, Treur JL *et al.*[17] found strong evidence of causal effects of propensity for smoking initiation on the risk of ADHD (OR = 3.72; 3.10–4.44), with no horizontal pleiotropy or heterogeneity. They also found a causal effect of ADHD propensity on the risk of cannabis use initiation (OR = 1.13; 1.02–1.25). There was no clear evidence of a causal effect of ADHD propensity on the risk of alcohol use, but there was some weak evidence that ADHD propensity causally influences AUD (OR = 1.07; 1.01–1.14).

With regard to comorbidities between ADHD and SUD, in particular, studies such as that by Sánchez-Roige *et al.*[18] have confirmed the existence of a positive genetic correlation between ADHD and SUD (*rg* = 0.23), as well as that of Walters *et al.*[19] in individuals of European descent (*rg* = 0.444). Genetic risk factors that contribute to the presence of some of the phenotypic traits of ADHD (or even the most severe symptoms of ADHD) also increase the risk of SUD, according to an analysis by AM.[17] Several genes involved in neuronal development are related to the comorbidity of ADHD and SUD. One of these genes, ADGRL3 (Latrophilin 3), is involved in the development of glutamatergic synapses. SNPs in this gene have been repeatedly associated with alcohol consumption[20] and ADHD.[21]

Regarding the comorbidity between ADHD and CanUD, two significant loci related to ADHD have been identified: a locus on chromosome 7 (FOXP2, rs7783012; OR = 1.11; 1.07–1.15) and a locus on chromosome 8 (near CHRNA2 and EPHX2, rs4732724; OR = 0.89; 0.86–0.93). A GWAS meta-analysis confirmed that the chromosome 8 locus was associated with CanUD. However, there is no evidence of causal genetic correlations between susceptibility to CanUD and ADHD, according to an AM-related approach that can account for sample overlap between GWAS.[22] Even so, ADHD and CanUD are partially determined by genetic factors. Using a two-sample AM approach, ADHD was found to be causal for lifetime cannabis use compared to individuals without ADHD (OR = 7.9; 3.72–15.51).[23] In line with previous evidence supporting the co-occurrence of these two traits and the increased risk of cannabis use in individuals with ADHD, a highly significant genetic correlation was found between them. These two conditions share a background of common genetic variants (*rg* = 0.29), which may explain the phenotypic overlap observed in the clinical setting.[23]

Finally, people with ADHD or other psychiatric disorders show high rates of NUD. A high genetic correlation was found between SUD and ADHD (*rg* = 0.53) and, to a lesser extent, also between SUD and ODD (*rg* = 0.42) and SUD and schizophrenia (*rg* = 0.18).[24]

Bipolar Disorders and Concurrent SUD

In a study using PRS, the diagnosis of multiple SUDs was strongly associated with schizophrenia and BD. The authors noted that the risk of SUDs appears to be slightly lower for BD-PRS than for schizophrenia-PRS.[25] A systematic review of polymorphisms potentially related to TB comorbid with SUDs found 17 case studies and controls that identified different types of genes grouped into 4 categories:[26]

- **Serotonergic genes**: SUD and depression appear to be associated with the h5-HTR1B G861C locus.
- **Dopaminergic genes**: No association was found for any SNP in dopamine genes when comparing patients with TB + SUD with healthy controls (HC).
- **Circadian rhythm regulatory genes**: An association has been found between two SNPs, one in the ARNTL gene and the other in the PER3 gene, and an increased risk of TB + TUA in a group of male patients.
- **Other, unspecified genes**:
  - A strong association was observed between an SNP in the bradykinin B2 receptor (BDKRB2) and panic disorder (PD), SAD, and BD.
  - An SNP of a member of the steroid receptor superfamily—thyroid hormone—retinoids, NR4A3, is significantly associated with the risk of TUN and TB.
  - An SNP of TSPO, the gene present in the mitochondrial compartment of peripheral tissues, may contribute to the comorbidity of TB with TUA.
  - An SNP in the TACR1 gene, from a family of tachykinin receptors, was associated with TB + AUD.
  - In a Han population in Taiwan, the concurrent presence of TB and TUA may be related to an SNP of ALDH2 and ADH1B.

Regarding comorbidities between TB and SUD in particular, a GWAS identified shared genetic factors in TB and TUCan ($rg = 0.17$) and for TB and cannabis use ($rg = 0.27$).[22] A two-sample bidirectional AM study examined causal pathways between lifetime cannabis use and TB and found that genetic predisposition to TB was significantly associated with an increased risk of lifetime cannabis use, but not vice versa.[27] Comorbidity between TUCan or cannabis use and TB may depend on the presence of specific SNPs in the genes encoding the CB2 receptor and 5-HTTLPR (serotonin transporter).[28] In a community-based cross-sectional study, TB-II in probands was associated with an increased risk of TUCan in relatives (aOR = 2.57; 1.06–6.23). Surprisingly, TB-I and TDM in probands were not significantly associated with TUCan in relatives. In relatives, TUCan was associated with TB-II (aOR = 4.50; 1.72–11.77) and TDMaOR = 3.64; 1.78–7.45). These results suggest that TUCan may share a common underlying diathesis with TB-II.[29] Traumatic childhood experiences may also play a role in the association between cannabis use or TUCan and TB. In a UK birth cohort, cannabis was found to mediate the association between childhood sexual abuse and hypomania.[30]

Regarding comorbidity between BD and SUD, in a GWAS study, the most significant SNP associations with BD + SUD were found in or near genes involved in cell adhesion, neurotransmission pathways, enzyme activity, cell messengers, connective tissue, and cell regulation. However, none of them reached statistical significance.[31] Based on GWAS studies, PRS were calculated for US Army soldiers exposed to trauma or not. Polimanti *et al.*[32] found a significant interaction between PTSD and alcohol abuse. Furthermore, they reported a positive correlation between TB and alcohol abuse in soldiers exposed to trauma ($r = 0.029$) and a negative correlation in soldiers not exposed to trauma ($r = -0.071$). The genetic variants included in the TB × trauma interaction showed significant enrichments for genes related to high-voltage calcium channel activity and for the signaling pathways of adrenergic receptors β_1/β_2.

Depressive/Anxiety Disorders and Concurrent SUD

As with TB, part of the association between TDM and TAns and substance use can be explained by shared genetic vulnerability and neurocognitive mechanisms. Approximately 76% of the covariance between substance use and generalized anxiety disorder (GAD)/depression was explained by genetic factors with an $r_g = 0.60$. The covariance between substance use and PD and agoraphobia/social phobia was best explained by genetic factors (77%; $rg = 0.47$), and the association between substance use and phobias/obsessive-compulsive disorder (OCD) was best explained by genetic influences (53%; $rg = 0.24$).[33]

In a study comparing male individuals with polydrug dependence (PDD) comorbid with MDD, SUD alone, and CS, Chmielowiec *et al.*[34] reported that in the DRD4 exon 3 gene, the s (short) allele was more frequent in PDD + MDD than in the l (long) allele (82% vs. 18%) and compared to CS (75% vs. 25%; $p = 0.046$).

Most family studies and GWAS identified consistent positive genetic correlations between SUDs and depression or anxiety ($rg = 0.30$–0.66 and $rg = 0.56$–0.66, respectively). Data from the population-based multigenerational cohort study Lifelines (n = 162,439) revealed that depression, anxiety, and smoking showed positive familial co-aggregation, conferring greater risk to other family members. With the exception of the genetic correlation of depression and anxiety ($rg = 0.94$), most continuous traits of depression, anxiety, and smoking showed moderate genetic correlations ($rg = 0.16$–0.36).[35] Regarding comorbidities between MDD and anxiety disorders, the most common comorbidities were anxiety disorders with depressive symptoms (e.g., generalized anxiety disorder, panic disorder, and depression) and anxiety disorders with depressive symptoms and suicidal tendencies (e.g., depression with suicidal tendencies). moderate genetic correlations ($rg = 0.16$–0.36).[35] Regarding comorbidities between MDD or ANSs and SUDs, in particular, conditional genetic associations were significant between SUD and depression ($bg = 0.30$), and evidence of a causal effect of smoking onset on predisposition to MDD was found in AM analyses, but not was able to rule out bias.[36] A significant genetic correlation between TUCan and TDM was also demonstrated, indicating a shared genetic etiology. A large-scale GWAS meta-analysis found evidence of overlap in genetic vulnerability between TUCan and TDM ($rg = 0.32$).[22] Furthermore, using the TUA, TUN, TUCoc, and TUO gene database (ANCO-GeneDB) and the human gene database (GeneCards), Freda *et al.*[37] demonstrated that the phenotypes that overlap most with opioid-related traits are those related to nicotine/tobacco use, followed by schizophrenia and depression. The authors mention that, among the SNPs, rs4606, an exonic SNP in the RGS2 (Regulator of G protein signaling type 2) gene, was associated with both TUO and TAG. In the same vein, and focusing on epigenomic assays on histone H3K27ac, the canonical mark of active regulatory elements, Corradin *et al.*[38] observed modest but widespread hypoacetylation of H3K27 at convergent loci enriched for TUO and TAG risk genes in *postmortem* samples of dorsolateral PFC from individuals who had overdosed on opioids. A study measuring circulating exosomal miRNAs (non-coding RNAs that play an essential role in gene silencing and translation repression) found that these are differentially expressed between CS and patients with methamphetamine use disorder (MUD) and in patients with OUD (heroin). Several miR-RNAs were negatively correlated with anxiety severity in MUD, but not in patients with OUD (heroin).[39] Furthermore, higher TDM PRS was associated with a significantly higher risk of AUD according to the meta-analysis of four independent GWAS datasets. Candidate gene studies reported a number of genes that may underlie both disorders, such as CHRM2 (muscarinic cholinergic receptor 2), SLC6A4 (serotonin transporter), COMT (catechol-O-methyltransferase), and DRD2 (dopamine receptor 2).[40] The Most of the significant SNPs detected in samples from patients with MDD and ANS coexisting with AUE are located in regions of the genome that are mainly involved in the processes of growth, development, and neuronal differentiation, as well as in the coding of neurotransmitter receptors and the ion channels controlled by them.[4] In a trans-ancestral GWAS of TUA, a significant genetic correlation was observed in individuals of European ancestry for depression ($rg = 0.561$) among other psychiatric disorders and SUD.[19]

Eating Disorders (EDs) and Concurrent SUD

Genetic linkage studies on TCA and SUD suggest that SNPs in genes of the dopamine (rs1800497 in the *DRD2/ANKKI* gene, rs4680 in the *COMT* gene) and serotonin (rs6311 in the *SLC6A4* gene) systems may play a role in the comorbidity of TCA and SUD. However, candidate gene studies generally have low power and produce false positive associations.[41] Several GWAS have been published that support a potential relationship between an SNP in the *DRD4* gene and SUD and TCA associated with inappropriate reward-seeking behaviors. The 7R allele appears to increase susceptibility to multiple environmental factors, and therefore individuals carrying this polymorphic variant are more prone to overweight and dysfunctional eating patterns.[42]

Association analyses focused on 32 SNPs revealed small-magnitude significant associations between the scores on the scales for TCA and the SNP rs1800955 of the *DRD4* gene (Cohen's $d = 0.09$). Additionally, the authors found that the SNPs rs759364 of *FOXN3* and rs1549250 and rs2973033 of *GDNF* may constitute genetic risk factors for multiple addictive behaviors such as EDs, pathological gambling, bigorexia, and excessive Internet use, in association with SUDs.[43] In adolescent twins, a significant genetic correlation between substance use and the drive for thinness (I × D) was observed only in girls (using the Cholesky decomposition model) ($ra = 0.40$; 0.23–0.61), while for substance use × bulimia nervosa (BN), in both girls and boys, the genetic correlations were not significant.[44]

With regard to comorbidities between EDs and SUDs, in particular, in a sample of adolescent twins, phenotypic correlations between smoking and I × D were significant only for young women (*rs* = 0.18; 0.07–0.30). The significant negative *rg* between three TUN phenotypes (smoking initiation, current smoking, and cigarettes per day) and AN without binge eating suggest that increased genetic vulnerability to AN without binge eating is associated with decreased genetic vulnerability to multiple smoking behaviors.[45] On the other hand, although some previous studies revealed that most genetic vulnerability to AUD was independent of other disorders, Baker *et al.*[46] found that the genetic correlation between BN and TUA (*rg* = 0.53) was higher than that observed for SUD in general (*rg* = 0.37) and TUN (*rg* = 0.35). Other studies have also reported a significant correlation between BN and TUA (*rg* = 0.23).[47] Another study also found genetic and environmental overlap between BED and binge eating disorder (BED × BE) in young adult European and African American women (*rg* = 0.33), with no differences between the two ethnic groups.[48] Munn-Chernoff *et al.*[49] also found a significant genetic association between BED and AN. Previous twin studies had not reported significant genetic correlations between these traits, probably due to smaller sample sizes, but the study cited here uses a combination of two existing GWAS of BED. The point estimate for r_g between BED and binge eating AN was 0.18 and higher than that for BED and non–binge eating AN (0.01). Shared genetic factors also appear to influence comorbidity between BED, maladaptive compensatory eating behaviors, and PEA. Specifically, r_g estimates of 0.31 between the UPA and the T × A and 0.61 between the UPA and inappropriate compensatory behaviors.[50] These findings were replicated in another independent study, which also observed a significant genetic overlap between the alcohol dependence factor (AD-FS) score and T × A (*rg* = 0.29) and between AD-FS and compensatory behaviors (*rg* = 0.32).[51] Finally, a genetic correlation was observed between AN and cannabis use initiation, using data from two GWAS, for pure AN (*rg* = 0.23) and binge eating AN (*rg* = 0.27).[49]

Personality Disorders (PD) and Concurrent SUDs

Higher levels of borderline personality disorder (BPD) traits predicted a higher rate of increase in SUD and SUDs in general. Conversely, the presence of SUD or SUDs predicted a slower rate of decline in BPD traits between the ages of 14 and 24. Genetic correlations between BPD and SUD ranged from 0.33 to 0.56. Twin analyses revealed that shared environmental factors explained the association between BPD traits and substance use at age 14, but genetic factors explained the association at age 18.[52] Regarding other personality traits, the *DRD4* repeat allele 2 was associated with substance use in adulthood and delinquent behavior in adolescence (range of aORs/IRR = 1.08–3.78).[53] Conduct disorder and self-injurious impulsivity are the most important risk traits for SUD among the 80 DSM-IV TPer criteria, and they predict SUD better than other TPer diagnoses.[54]

On the other hand, after adjusting for age and gender, antisocial TPer (β = 0.26; 0.21–0.31) and TLP (β = 0.12; 0.06–0.18) were associated with TUCan.[55] Finally, antisocial TPer traits (OR = 4.24; 2.66–6.86) and BPD (OR = 2.19; 1.35–3.57) were the only significant predictors of **cocaine use disorder**. After eliminating criteria associated with substance use, antisocial TPer explained 65% of the total genetic variance in cocaine use, while BPD explained only 4%.[56]

Schizophrenia and Concurrent SUD

As mentioned above, in a study using ***rg***, the diagnosis of several SUDs was slightly more strongly associated with schizophrenia than with BD.[25] Schizophrenia shares more genetic predisposition with SUDs than BD, MDD, AD, ADHD, or ASD. Using ***rg*** based on GWAS samples from patients with schizophrenia, significant associations with SUDs were detected in two databases (OR = 1.53, 1.31–1.79 and 1.18, 1.03–1.37).[57] A longitudinal study in young participants with schizophrenia showed that a 1 SD increase in the genetic risk of schizophrenia was associated with a 16.3% relative increase in the probability of substance use ($\beta = 0.151$; OR = 1.163). In addition, they are 14% more likely to experience a greater increase in the probability of substance use as they age ($\beta = 0.138$; OR = 1.148).[58] Using three data sets (COGEND, COGA, FSCD), Hartz *et al.*[59] found that there is a strong relationship between the PRS for schizophrenia and that for SUDs, which is partially attributable to shared polygenic liability rather than specific risks for individual SUDs. However, statistically significant associations were also found between schizophrenia and specific SUDs: NUD, AUD, CanUD, and stimulant use disorder (StUD).

With regard to comorbidities between schizophrenia and SUDs in particular, the impact of cannabis use on the risk of schizophrenia has been proposed by Gage *et al.*[60] in an AM analysis (OR = 1.04; 1.01–1.07). Furthermore, in another AM analysis, Vaucher *et al.*[61] found in a GWAS that the ten main loci associated with cannabis use were related to an increased risk of schizophrenia (OR = 1.08; 1.02–1.14). Applying estimates based on the general population, this translates into a 37% increase in risk of schizophrenia for cannabis users versus non-users (OR = 1.37; 1.09–1.67). However, there is also evidence to support the hypothesis that genetic risk for schizophrenia predicts the onset of cannabis use (OR = 1.10; 1.05–1.14).[60] In a longitudinal cohort study of adolescents, high vulnerability to schizophrenia was associated with a greater increase in cannabis use after age 16. PRS explained between 4.5% and 32.0% of the variance in the increase in cannabis use during late adolescence. No clear evidence of a relationship between smoking and alcohol consumption and schizophrenia was found.[62] Several S-PrediXcan analyses demonstrated a positive genetic correlation between genetic risk factors for cannabis use and schizophrenia (*rg* = 0.24). The strongest finding across the different analyses was for the *CADM2* gene, which has been associated with substance use, risk-taking, body mass index, and reduced feelings of anxiety. The authors also found evidence of a positive causal influence of schizophrenia risk on lifetime cannabis use (OR = 1.16; 1.06–1.27).[63] Another GWAS analysis showed that genetic predisposition to TUCan was significantly associated with that of schizophrenia ($\beta = 0.29$; 0.11–0.46), even when cannabis use, tobacco use, and TUN were taken into account as simultaneous predictors. Multivariate analyses of AM also suggested a significant effect on the association ($\beta =$ 0.10; 0.02–0.18).[64] Finally, a cross-sectional study of 109,308 participants from the UK Biobank found a strong, dose-dependent relationship between cannabis use and psychotic experiences, particularly persecutory delusions. Participants with high scores on the schizophrenia PRS showed strong associations between frequency of cannabis use and auditory hallucinations, delusions of reference, psychotic experiences in general, and visual hallucinations. Ever-use of cannabis was associated with a 1.58 times higher adjusted probability of psychotic experiences in one-fifth of individuals with the highest schizophrenia PRS, compared to only a 1.39 times higher adjusted probability in one-fifth with the lowest schizophrenia PRS.[65]

Regarding SUDs and schizophrenia, a longitudinal study of young participants with schizophrenia showed that their PRS was not associated with an increased overall likelihood of concurrent alcohol and other substance use ($\beta = 0.04$). However, participants with higher genetic risk associated with schizophrenia experienced a greater increase in the likelihood of concurrent alcohol and other substance use as they aged ($\beta = 0.095$).[58] In a trans-ancestral GWAS of SUD, a significant genetic correlation was observed in individuals of European ancestry for schizophrenia ($rg = 0.357$), among other psychiatric disorders and SUD.[19] Many genetic variants of brain-derived neurotrophic factor (BDNF) protein are associated with comorbid schizophrenia and AUD, but not with AUD alone. The allelic association between rs7103411 and rs6265 of *BDNF* with comorbid AUD was identified and replicated in patients with schizophrenia.[66]

On the other hand, psychotic disorders were significantly more frequent in the group of males with PDD, including StUD, compared to the group of males with PDD without StUD. The homozygous s/s presentation of the *DRD4* Ex3 gene alleles was more common in the study group. In the *DRD2* promoter region, rs1799732, the allele was more frequent than the ins allele in the study group.[67]

Finally, a local genetic correlation analysis of 20 psychiatric and substance use phenotypes identified 80 significant bivariate correlations across 61 loci, 43 of which harbored genes whose gene expression was related to one or both phenotypes in question. Locus 15.46 harbored local genetic correlations for schizophrenia and smoking behavior, and had 13 genes with regulated gene expression levels in CPF.[68,69] Bivariate genetic correlations between smoking behaviors and psychiatric disorders showed that, after accounting for the genetic influences of covariates, conditional genetic associations (*bg*) were significant between daily cigarette consumption and schizophrenia (0.14). AM analyses yielded consistent results suggesting a causal effect of smoking initiation on vulnerability to schizophrenia. A significant but less susceptible causal effect of schizophrenia on smoking initiation was also found, indicating the presence of bidirectional pleiotropy.[36]

Other Psychiatric Disorders Concurrent with SUD

In patients with insomnia, a GWAS identified a new genomic risk locus on chromosome 8 (main SNP rs17052966), and a meta-analysis of two recent GWAS on insomnia identified 13 significant loci. A strong positive genetic correlation was observed between insomnia and alcohol consumption ($rg = 0.56$), nicotine consumption ($rg = 0.50$), and opioid consumption ($rg = 0.43$).[70] Gibson *et al.*[71] found negative genetic correlations between smoking initiation and sleep duration ($rg = -0.14$) and smoking cessation and chronotype ($rg = -0.18$), and positive genetic correlations between smoking initiation and insomnia ($rg = 0.27$) and daily cigarette consumption and insomnia ($rg = 0.15$). MA provided strong evidence that smoking more cigarettes causally decreases the likelihood of being a morning person by affecting the circadian rhythm. A significant genetic correlation was also observed between lifetime cannabis use and an evening chronotype (*rg* = 0.24), as well as between TUCan and shorter sleep duration (< 7 h; *rg* = 0.23) and insomnia (*rg* = 0.20). The PRS for insomnia predicted an earlier age of first cannabis use (*rg* = 0.92) and a greater number of TUCan symptoms throughout of life (*rg* = 1.09). One possible explanation for this genetic relationship could be that alterations in circadian rhythm genes could disrupt the reward processing system, which could influence substance use. Another explanation could be that the endocannabinoid system is involved in the circadian sleep-wake cycle.[72]

On the other hand, the use of twin data (CATSS cohort) reveals that additive genetic factors explained 68% of the covariance between OCD and SUD. The estimated genetic correlation between the phenotypes was 0.31.[73]

Finally, Delforterie *et al.* (2015) reported a genetic correlation of 0.45 between suicidal ideation and cannabis use. A small study of an urban homeless population in the United States showed that suicidal behaviors were significantly associated with the interaction between the 5–HTTLPR genotype, a repeat polymorphism of the serotonin transporter gene, and the drug use ($\beta = 0.41$). For those with lower or no drug use, the short allele (s) was the risk or vulnerability factor. However, for individuals with higher drug use, the long allele (l) was the risk factor for predicting suicidal behavior.[74] When comparing the transcriptome of 38 Mexican individuals who died by suicide and had dual pathology with that of suicides with SUD alone and suicides with mood disorders alone, a different gene expression profile was identified for genes involved in specific glial markers (with upregulation of *GFAP*, involved in the negative regulation of apoptosis), in glutamatergic neurotransmission (with upregulation of *SLC1A3*, glutamate transporter), and in GABAergic transmission.[75]

CONCLUSIONS

Vulnerability to drug addiction is determined by genetic and environmental/epigenetic factors that interact at multiple levels of molecular, neuronal, and circuit organization, which play an important role in the development of specific behavioral endophenotypes, such as impulsivity, novelty-seeking, or increased sensitivity to reward and decreased executive control. The co-occurrence of psychiatric disorders and SUDs is supported not only by clinical observations but also by genetic and molecular evidence. Although these results may be relevant for researchers or mental health professionals who treat patients with dual pathology, it is necessary to consider the limitations associated with the inclusion of different publication designs, study methodologies, and the relative lack of uniformity in diagnostic inclusion criteria and primary outcome measures reported. Furthermore, there is currently a significant lack of systematic evidence examining the co-occurrence of SUDs and other psychiatric disorders. Even so, the findings presented here allow us to conclude that there is genetic overlap between OCD and other psychiatric disorders, such as MDD, AN, PTSD, ADHD, BD, schizophrenia, and EDs, among others.

Table 10.2 shows that the highest correlation rates observed and replicated were, in descending order of magnitude, for MDD and AUD, for ADHD and SAD, for ADHD and AUD, and for MDD and SAD. Thus, nicotine and alcohol dependence appear to be

TABLE 10.2 Genetic Correlations (r_g) Between SUD and Other Psychiatric Disorders

	AUD	**CanUD**	**CUD**	**OUD**	**NUD**
mDD	0.52[2]; 0.564	0.327	0.401	0.351	0.381; 0.452; 0.426
BD		0.177			
Schizophrenia	0.352; 0.364	0.311; 0.2412	0.201		0.161; 0.186
ADHD	0.462; 0.233; 0.444	0.352; 0.295	0.501	0.361	0.542; 0.536
AN	0.1210				
BN	0.539; 0.239				0.359
T × A	0.3311				
Insomnia	0.5613	0.2014		0.4313	0.5013
Suicidal behavior		0.4515			

Abbreviations: AN, anorexia nervosa; BN, bulimia nervosa; anxiety disorders; BD, bipolar disorder; ADHD, attention deficit/hyperactivity disorder; MDD, major depressive disorder; AUD, alcohol use disorder; CanUD, cannabis use disorder; CUD, cocaine use disorder; OUD, opioid use disorder; NUD, nicotine use disorder (Abdellaoui *et al.*, 2021; Artigas *et al.*, 2020; Baker *et al.*, 2010; Deak *et al.*, 2021; Delforterie *et al.*, 2015; Johnson *et al.*, 2020; Munn-Chernoff *et al.*, 2015; Munn-Chernoff *et al.*, 2021; Pasman *et al.*, 2018; Sánchez-Roige *et al.*, 2019; Soler-Vink *et al.*, 2021; Trace *et al.*, 2013; Song *et al.*, 2020; Walters *et al.*, 2018; Winiger *et al.*, 2021).

genetically correlated with depression and ADHD. The table also shows that some psychiatric conditions have been studied more than others in terms of the risk of being part of a dual pathology. Such is the case with AUD, NCD, MDD, ADHD, schizophrenia, and insomnia. This highlights the need for many more studies in order to draw definitive conclusions about the role of genetics in dual pathology.

REFERENCES

1. Egervari G, Ciccocioppo R, Jentsch JD, Hurd YL. Shaping vulnerability to addiction - the contribution of behavior, neural circuits and molecular mechanisms. Neurosci Biobehav Rev. 2018;85:117–25. doi: 10.1016/j.neubiorev.2017.05.019
2. Ikeda M, Saito T, Kanazawa T, Iwata N. Polygenic risk score as clinical utility in psychiatry: A clinical viewpoint. J Hum Genet. 2021;66(1):53–60. doi: 10.1038/s10038-020-0814-y
3. Popescu A, Marian M, Drăgoi AM, Costea RV. Understanding the genetics and neurobiological pathways behind addiction (Review). Exp Ther Med. 2021;21(5):544. doi: 10.3892/etm.2021.9976
4. Stoychev K, Dilkov D, Naghavi E, Kamburova Z. Genetic basis of dual diagnosis: a review of genome-wide association studies (GWAS) focusing on patients with mood or anxiety disorders and co-occurring alcohol-use disorders. Diagnostics (Basel). 2021;11(6):1055. doi: 10.3390/diagnostics11061055
5. Deak JD, Johnson EC. Genetics of substance use disorders: A review. Psychol Med. 2021;51(13):2189–200. doi: 10.1017/S0033291721000969
6. De Sa Nogueira D, Merienne K, Befort K. Neuroepigenetics and addictive behaviors: Where do we stand? Neurosci Biobehav Rev. 2019;106:58–72. doi: 10.1016/j.neubiorev.2018.08.018
7. Kaplan G, Xu H, Abreu K, Feng J. DNA epigenetics in addiction susceptibility. Front Genet. 2022;13:806685. doi: 10.3389/fgene.2022.806685
8. Gelernter J, Polimanti R. Genetics of substance use disorders in the era of big data. Nat Rev Genet. 2021;22(11):712–29. doi: 10.1038/s41576-021-00377-1

9. Hatoum AS, Johnson EC, Colbert SMC, Polimanti R, Zhou H, Walters RK, *et al.* The addiction risk factor: A unitary genetic vulnerability characterizes substance use disorders and their associations with common correlates. Neuropsychopharmacol. 2022;47(10):1739–45. doi: 10.1038/s41386-021-01209-w
10. Lee PH, Feng YA, Smoller JW. Pleiotropy and cross-disorder genetics among psychiatric disorders. Biol Psychiatry. 2021;89(1):20–31. doi: 10.1016/j.biopsych.2020.09.026
11. Jang SK, Saunders G, Liu M; 23 and Me Research Team; Jiang Y, Liu DJ, Vrieze S. Genetic correlation, pleiotropy, and causal associations between substance use and psychiatric disorder. Psychol Med. 2022;52(5):968–78. doi: 10.1017/S003329172000272X
12. Abdellaoui A, Smit DJA, van den Brink W, Denys D, Verweij KJH. Genomic relationships across psychiatric disorders including substance use disorders. Drug Alcohol Depend. 2021;220:108535. doi: 10.1016/j.drugalcdep.2021.108535
13. Martínez-Magaña JJ, Gonzalez-Castro TB, Genís-Men-doza AD, Tovilla-Zárate CA, Juárez-Rojop IE, Sauce-do-Uribe E, *et al.* Exploratory analysis of polygenic risk scores for psychiatric disorders: Applied to dual diagnosis. Revista de Investigación Clínica. 2019;71(5):321–9. doi: 10.24875/RIC.19003013
14. González RA, Vélez-Pastrana MC, Blankers M, Bäcker A, Konstenius M, Holtmann M, *et al.* Onset and severity of early disruptive behavioral disorders in treatment-seeking substance use disorder patients with and without attention-deficit/hyperactivity disorder. Eur Addict Res. 2020;26(4-5):211–22. doi: 10.1159/000508653
15. Wimberley T, Agerbo E, Horsdal HT, Ottosen C, Brikell I, Als TD, *et al.* Genetic liability to ADHD and substance use disorders in individuals with ADHD. Addiction. 2020;115(7): 1368–77. doi: 10.1111/add.14910
16. Vilar-Ribó L, Sánchez-Mora C, Rovira P, Richarte V, Corrales M, Fadeuilhe C, Arribas L, *et al.* Genetic overlap and causality between substance use disorder and attention-deficit and hyperactivity disorder. Am J Med Genet B Neuropsychiatr Genet. 2021;186(3):140–50. doi: 10.1002/ajmg.b.32827
17. Treur JL, Demontis D, Smith GD, Sallis H, Richardson TG, Wiers RW, *et al.* Investigating causality between liability to ADHD and substance use, and liability to substance use and ADHD risk, using Mendelian randomization. Addict Biol. 2021;26(1):e12849. doi: 10.1111/adb.12849
18. Sanchez-Roige S, Palmer AA, Fontanillas P, Elson SL; 23 and Me Research Team, the Substance Use Disorder Working Group of the Psychiatric Genomics Consortium; Adams MJ, Howard DM, Edenberg HJ, Davies G, Crist RC, Deary IJ, McIntosh AM, Clarke TK. Genome-wide association study meta-analysis of the alcohol use disorders identification test (AUDIT) in two population-based cohorts. Am J Psychiatry. 2019;176(2):107–18. doi: 10.1176/appi.ajp.2018.18040369
19. Walters RK, Polimanti R, Johnson EC, McClintick JN, Adams MJ, Adkins AE, *et al.* Transancestral GWAS of alcohol dependence reveals common genetic underpinnings with psychiatric disorders. Nat Neurosci. 2018;21(12):1656–69. doi: 10.1038/s41593-018-0275-1
20. Martinez AF, Abe Y, Hong S, Molyneux K, Yarne-ll D, Löhr H, *et al.* An ultraconserved brain-specific enhancer within ADGRL3 (LPHN3) underpins attention-deficit/hyperactivity disorder susceptibility. Biol Psychiatry. 2016;80(12):943–54. doi: 10.1016/j.biopsych.2016.06.026
21. Bruxel EM, Moreira-Maia CR, Akutagawa-Martins GC, Quinn TP, Klein M, Franke B, *et al.* Meta-analysis and systematic review of ADGRL3 (LPHN3) polymorphisms in ADHD susceptibility. Mol Psychiatry. 2021;26(6):2277–85. doi: 10.1038/s41380-020-0673-0
22. Johnson EC, Demontis D, Thorgeirsson TE, Walters RK, Polimanti R, Hatoum AS, *et al.* A large-scale genome-wide association study meta-analysis of cannabis use disorder. Lancet Psychiatry. 2020;7(12):1032–45. doi: 10.1016/S2215-0366(20)30339-4

23. Soler Artigas M, Sánchez-Mora C, Rovira P, Richarte V, Garcia-Martínez I, Pagerols M, Demontis D, Stringer S; ADHD Group of the Psychiatric Genomics Consortium, International Cannabis Consortium; Vink JM, Børglum AD, Neale BM, Franke B, Faraone SV, Casas M, Ramos-Quiroga JA, Ribasés M. Attention-deficit/hyperactivity disorder and lifetime cannabis use: genetic overlap and causality. Mol Psychiatry. 2020;25(10):2493–2503. doi: 10.1038/s41380-018-0339-3
24. Vink JM, Treur JL, Pasman JA, Schellekens A. Investigating genetic correlation and causality between nicotine dependence and ADHD in a broader psychiatric context. Am J Med Genet B Neuropsychiatr Genet. 2021;186(7):423–29. doi: 10.1002/ajmg.b.32822
25. Reginsson GW, Ingason A, Euesden J, Bjornsdottir G, Olafsson S, Sigurdsson E, *et al.* Polygenic risk scores for schizophrenia and bipolar disorder associate with addiction. Addict Biol. 2018;23(1):485–92. doi: 10.1111/adb.12496
26. de Marco A, Scozia G, Manfredi L, Conversi D. A systematic review of genetic polymorphisms associated with bipolar disorder comorbid to substance abuse. Genes (Basel). 2022;13(8):1303. doi: 10.3390/genes13081303
27. Jefsen OH, Speed M, Speed D, Østergaard SD. Bipolar disorder and cannabis use: A bidirectional two-sample Mendelian randomization study. Addict Biol. 2021;26(6):e13030. doi: 10.1111/adb.13030
28. Kuhns L, Kroon E, Colyer-Patel K, Cousijn J. Associations between cannabis use, cannabis use disorder, and mood disorders: Longitudinal, genetic, and neurocognitive evidence. Psychopharmacology (Berl). 2022;239(5):1231–49. doi: 10.1007/s00213-021-06001-8
29. Quick CR, Conway KP, Swendsen J, Stapp EK, Cui L, Merikangas KR. Comorbidity and coaggregation of major depressive disorder and bipolar disorder and cannabis use disorder in a controlled family study. JAMA Psychiatry. 2022;79(7):727–35. doi: 10.1001/jamapsychiatry.2022.1338
30. Marwaha S, Winsper C, Bebbington P, Smith D. Cannabis use and hypomania in young people: A prospective analysis. Schizophr Bull. 2018;44(6):1267–74. doi: 10.1093/schbul/sbx158
31. Lydall GJ, Bass NJ, McQuillin A, Lawrence J, Anjorin A, Kandaswamy R, *et al.* Confirmation of prior evidence of genetic susceptibility to alcoholism in a genome-wide association study of comorbid alcoholism and bipolar disorder. Psychiatr Genet. 2011;21(6):294–306. doi: 10.1097/YPG.0b013e32834915c2
32. Polimanti R, Kaufman J, Zhao H, Kranzler HR, Ursano RJ, Kessler RC, *et al.* Trauma exposure interacts with the genetic risk of bipolar disorder in alcohol misuse of US soldiers. Acta Psychiatr Scand. 2018; 137(2):148–56. doi: 10.1111/acps.12843
33. Virtanen S, Kuja-Halkola R, Mataix-Cols D, Jaya-ram-Lindström N, D'Onofrio BM, Larsson H, *et al.* Comorbidity of substance misuse with anxiety-related and depressive disorders: A genetically informative population study of 3 million individuals in Sweden. Psychol Med. 2020;50(10):1706–1715. doi: 10.1017/S0033291719001788
34. Chmielowiec K, Chmielowiec J, Masiak J, Czekaj M, Krawczyk P, Soroka E, *et al.* *DRD4* exon 3 gene polymorphisms in patients diagnosed with polysubstance use disorder and co-occurrence of a depressive episode. Genes (Basel). 2021;12(11):1834. doi: doi.org/10.3390/genes12111834
35. Wang R, Snieder H, Hartman CA. Familial co-aggregation and shared heritability between depression, anxiety, obesity, and substance use. Transl Psychiatry. 2022;12(1):108. doi: 10.1038/s41398-022-01868-3
36. Barkhuizen W, Dudbridge F, Ronald A. Genetic overlap and causal associations between smoking behaviors and mental health. Sci Rep. 2021;11(1):14871. doi: 10.1038/s41598-021-93962-7
37. Freda PJ, Moore JH, Kranzler HR. The phenomics and genetics of addictive and affective comorbidity in opioid use disorder. Drug Alcohol Depend. 2021;221:108602. doi: 10.1016/j.drugalcdep.2021.108602

38. Corradin O, Sallari R, Hoang AT, Kassim BS, Ben Hutta G, Cuoto L, *et al.* Convergence of case-specific epigenetic alterations identify a confluence of genetic vulnerabilities tied to opioid overdose. Mol Psychiatry. 2022;27(4):2158–70. doi: 10.1038/s41380-022-01477-y
39. Chen F, Zou L, Dai Y, Sun J, Chen C, Zhang Y, *et al.* Prognostic plasma exosomal microRNA biomarkers in patients with substance use disorders presenting co-morbid with anxiety and depression. Sci Rep. 2018;8(1):9231. doi: 10.1038/s41598-021-84501-5
40. Andersen AM, Pietrzak RH, Kranzler HR, Ma L, Zhou H, Liu X, *et al.* Polygenic scores for major depressive disorder and risk of alcohol dependence. JAMA Psychiatry. 2017;74(11): 1153–60. doi: 10.1001/jamapsychiatry.2017.2269
41. Munn-Chernoff MA, Baker JH. A primer on the genetics of comorbid eating disorders and substance use disorders. Eur Eat Disord Rev. 2016;24(2):91–100. doi: 10.1002/erv.2424
42. Botticelli L, Micioni Di Bonaventura E, Del Bello F, Giorgioni G, Piergentili A, *et al.* Underlying susceptibility to eating disorders and drug abuse: genetic and pharmacological aspects of dopamine D4 receptors. Nutrients. 2020;12(8):2288. doi: 10.3390/nu12082288
43. Vereczkei A, Barta C, Magi A, Farkas J, Eisinger A, Király O, *et al.* FOXN3 and GDNF polymorphisms as common genetic factors of substance use and addictive behaviors. J Pers Med. 2022;12(5):690. doi: 10.3390/jpm12050690
44. Baker JH, Brosof LC, Munn-Chernoff MA, Lichtenstein P, Larsson H, Maes HH, *et al.* Associations between alcohol involvement and drive for thinness and body dissatisfaction in adolescent twins: A bivariate twin study. Alcohol Clin Exp Res. 2018;42(11):2214–23. doi: 10.1111/acer.13868
45. Baker JH, Johnson NK, Munn-Chernoff MA, Lichtens-tein P, Larsson H, Maes HH, *et al.* Illicit drug use, cigarette smoking, and eating disorder symptoms: Associations in an adolescent twin sample. J Stud Alcohol Drugs. 2018;79(5):720–4. doi: 10.15288/jsad.2018.79.720
46. Baker JH, Mitchell KS, Neale MC, Kendler KS. Eating disorder symptomatology and substance use disorders: Prevalence and shared risk in a population-based twin sample. Int J Eat Disord. 2010:43(7):648–58. doi: 10.1002/eat.20856
47. Trace SE, Thornton LM, Baker JH, Root TL, Janson LE, Lichtenstein P, *et al.* A behavioral-genetic investigation of bulimia nervosa and its relationship with alcohol use disorder. Psychiatry Res. 2013;208(3):232–7. doi: 10.1016/j.psychres.2013.04.030
48. Munn-Chernoff MA, Grant JD, Agrawal A, Koren R, Glowinski AL, Bucholz KK, *et al.* Are there common familial influences for major depressive disorder and an overeating-binge eating dimension in both European American and African American female twins? Int J Eat Disord. 2015;48(4):375–82. doi: 10.1002/eat.22280
49. Munn-Chernoff MA, Johnson EC, Chou YL, Coleman JRI, Thornton LM, Walters RK, *et al.* Shared genetic risk between eating disorder- and substance-use-related phenotypes: Evidence from genome-wide association studies. Addict Biol. 2021;26(1):e12880. doi: 10.1111/adb.12880
50. Slane JD, Burt SA, Klump KL. Bulimic behaviors and alcohol use: Shared genetic influences. Behav Genet. 2012;42(4):603–13. doi: 10.1007/s10519-012-9525-2
51. Munn-Chernoff MA, Duncan AE, Grant JD, Wade TD, Agrawal A, Bucholz KK, *et al.* A twin study of alcohol dependence, binge eating, and compensatory behaviors. J Stud Alcohol Drugs. 2013;74(5):664–73. doi: 10.15288/jsad.2013.74.664
52. Bornovalova MA, Verhulst B, Webber T, McGue M, Iacono WG, Hicks BM. Genetic and environmental influences on the codevelopment among borderline personality disorder traits, major depression symptoms, and substance use disorder symptoms from adolescence to young adulthood. Dev Psychopathol. 2018;30(1):49–65. doi: 10.1017/S0954579417000463
53. Yang JJ, Wang Z, Trucco EM, Buu A, Lin HC. Chronic pain and delinquency partially explain the effect of the DRD4 gene polymorphism on adult substance use. Am J Drug Alcohol Abuse. 2022;48(2):235–44. doi: 10.1080/00952990.2021.1977311

54. Rosenström T, Torvik FA, Ystrom E, Czajkowski NO, Gillespie NA, Aggen SH, *et al.* Prediction of alcohol use disorder using personality disorder traits: A twin study. Addiction. 2018:113(1):15–24. doi: 10.1111/add.13951
55. Gillespie NA, Aggen SH, Neale MC, Knudsen GP, Krueger RF, South SC, *et al.* Associations between personality disorders and cannabis use and cannabis use disorder: A population-based twin study. Addiction. 2018;113(8):1488–98. doi: 10.1111/add.14209
56. Gillespie NA, Aggen SH, Gentry AE, Neale MC, Knudsen GP, Krueger RF, *et al.* Testing genetic and environmental associations between personality disorders and cocaine use: A population-based twin study. Twin Res Hum Genet. 2018;21(1):24–32. doi: 10.1017/thg.2017.73
57. Gurriarán X, Rodríguez-López J, Flórez G, Pereiro C, Fernández JM, Fariñas E, Estévez V, Arrojo M, Costas J; GenPol Study Group. Relationships between substance abuse/dependence and psychiatric disorders based on polygenic scores. Genes Brain Behav. 2019;18(3):e12504. doi: 10.1111/gbb.12504
58. Mallard TT, Harden KP, Fromme, K. Genetic risk for schizophrenia is associated with substance use in emerging adulthood: An event-level polygenic prediction model. Psychol Med. 2019; 49(12):2027–35. doi: 10.1017/S0033291718002817
59. Hartz SM, Horton AC, Oehlert M, Carey CE, Agrawal A, Bogdan R, *et al.* Association between substance use disorder and polygenic liability to schizophrenia. Biol Psychiatry. 2017;82(10):709–15. doi: 10.1016/j.biopsych.2017.04.020
60. Gage SH, Jones HJ, Burgess S, Bowden J, Davey Smith G, Zammit S. Assessing causality in associations between cannabis use and schizophrenia risk: A two-sample Mendelian randomization study. Psychol Med. 2017;47(5):971–80. doi: 10.1017/S0033291716003172
61. Vaucher J, Keating BJ, Lasserre AM, Gan W, Lyall DM, Ward J, *et al.* Cannabis use and risk of schizophrenia: A Mendelian randomization study. Mol Psychiatry. 2018;23(5):1287–92. doi: 10.1038/mp.2016.252
62. Hiemstra M, Nelemans SA, Branje S, van Eijk KR, Hottenga JJ, Vinkers CH, *et al.* Genetic vulnerability to schizophrenia is associated with cannabis use patterns during adolescence. Drug Alcohol Depend. 2018;190:143–50. doi: 10.1016/j.drugalcdep.2018.05.024
63. Pasman JA, Verweij KJH, Gerring Z, Stringer S, San-chez-Roige S, Treur JL, *et al.* GWAS of lifetime cannabis use reveals new risk loci, genetic overlap with psychiatric traits, and a causal influence of schizophrenia. Nat Neurosci. 2018;21(9):1161–70. doi: 10.1038/s41593-018-0206-1
64. Johnson EC, Hatoum AS, Deak JD, Polimanti R, Murray RM, Edenberg HJ, *et al.* The relationship between cannabis and schizophrenia: A genetically informed perspective. Addiction. 2021;116(11):3227–34. doi: 10.1111/add.15534
65. Wainberg M, Jacobs GR, di Forti M, Tripathy SJ. Cannabis, schizophrenia genetic risk, and psychotic experiences: A cross-sectional study of 109,308 participants from the UK Biobank. Transl Psychiatry. 2021;11(1):211. doi: 10.1038/s41398-021-01330-w
66. Cheah SY, Lawford BR, Young RM, Connor JP, Phillip Morris C, Voisey J. BDNF SNPs are implicated in co-morbid alcohol dependence in schizophrenia but not in alcohol-dependent patients without schizophrenia. Alcohol Alcohol. 2014;49(5):491–7. doi: 10.1093/alcalc/agu040
67. Masiak J, Chmielowiec J, Chmielowiec K, Grzywacz A. DRD4, DRD2, DAT1, and ANKK1 gene polymorphisms in patients with dual diagnosis of polysubstance addictions. J Clin Med. 2020;9(11):3593. doi: 10.3390/jcm9113593
68. Ohi K, Kuwata A, Shimada T, Kataoka Y, Yasuyama T, Uehara T, *et al.* Genome-wide variants shared between smoking quantity and schizophrenia on 15q25 are associated with CHRNA5 expression in the brain. Schizophr Bull. 2019;45(4):813–23. doi: 10.1093/schbul/sby093
69. Gerring ZF, Thorp JG, Gamazon ER, Derks EM. A local genetic correlation analysis provides biological insights into the shared genetic architecture of psychiatric and substance use phenotypes. Biol Psychiatry. 2022;92(7):583–91. doi: 10.1016/j.biopsych.2022.03.001

70. Song W, Torous J, Kossowsky J, Chen CY, Huang H, Wright A. Genome-wide association analysis of insomnia using data from Partners Biobank. Sci Rep. 2020;10(1):6928. doi: 10.1038/s41598-020-63792-0
71. Gibson M, Munafò MR, Taylor AE, Treur JL. Evidence for genetic correlations and bidirectional, causal effects between smoking and sleep behaviors. Nicotine Tob Res. 2019;21(6):731–8. doi: 10.1093/ntr/nty230
72. Winiger EA, Ellingson JM, Morrison CL, Corley RP, Pasman JA, Wall TL, *et al.* Sleep deficits and cannabis use behaviors: An analysis of shared genetics using linkage disequilibrium score regression and polygenic risk prediction. Sleep. 2021;44(3):zsaa188. doi: 10.1093/sleep/zsaa188
73. Virtanen S, Kuja-Halkola R, Sidorchuk A, Fernández de la Cruz L, Rück C, Lundström S, *et al.* Association of obsessive-compulsive disorder and obsessive-compulsive symptoms with substance misuse in 2 longitudinal cohorts in Sweden. JAMA Netw Open. 2022;5(6):e2214779. doi: 10.1001/jamanetworkopen.2022.14779
74. Roane SJ, Kapoor S, Sun S, Cramer RJ, Lamis DA. The interactive effect of the serotonin transporter genotype and drug use on suicidal behaviors in patients diagnosed with bipolar disorder. J Affect Disord. 2020;262:49–54. doi: 10.1016/j.jad.2019.10.049
75. Cabrera-Mendoza B, Fresno C, Monroy-Jaramillo N, Fries GR, Walss-Bass C, Glahn DC, *et al.* Brain gene expression profiling of individuals with dual diagnosis who died by suicide. J Dual Diagn. 2020;16(2):177–90. doi: 10.1080/15504263.2019.1692160

APPENDIX. Abbreviations Used in Section 10.2

AD anxiety disorders
ADHD attention deficit hyperactivity disorder
AN anorexia nervosa
ASD autism spectrum disorder
BD bipolar disorder
BN bulimia nervosa
BPD borderline personality disorder
CanUD cannabis use disorder
CD conduct disorder
CUD cocaine use disorder
ED eating disorders
FRAU unidimensional addiction risk factor
GAD generalized anxiety disorder
GWAS genome-wide association studies
HC healthy controls
MDD major depressive disorder
MR Mendelian randomization
MUD methamphetamine use disorder
NUD nicotine use disorder
OCD obsessive-compulsive disorder
ODD oppositional defiant disorder
OR odds ratio
OUD opioid use disorder

PAU	problematic alcohol use
PD	panic disorder
PDs	personality disorders
PFC	prefrontal cortex
PPD	polydrug dependence
PRS	polygenic risk score
PTSD	post-traumatic stress disorder
rg	genetic correlation
SNP	single nucleotide polymorphism
StUD	stimulant use disorder
SUD	substance use disorder

10.3 APPLICATION OF PROTEOMICS IN DUAL PATHOLOGY

C. Spuch Calvar, T. Rivera Baltanás, P. Fernández Palleiro, A. Piñón Blanco, Y. Diz Chaves, D. S. Rodrigues Amorin, and J. M. Olivares Diez

INTRODUCTION

Proteomics is a term coined in 1994 by researcher Marc Wilkins of the University of New South Wales (UNSW) in Sydney, Australia, as a new science dedicated to the comprehensive analysis of proteins in biological systems.[1]

Since the Human Genome Project was declared complete in 2003, international scientific efforts have sought a revolutionary turning point in the field of genomics and the application of genomics and technological advances in DNA sequencing, which have enabled a major scientific and biomedical leap forward in understanding and explaining genetic alterations and how they alter cellular functioning.[2] Scientists are now able to identify and characterize various components of a cell, tissue, or organism and analyze them in their entirety—their "ome," whether it be the complete expression of genes (genome), proteins (proteome), transcripts (transcriptome), or metabolites (metabolome), at any given moment. Analyzing all this data helps us understand the molecular journey from genotype to phenotype and where it can go wrong, in the case of disease phenotypes.

The next big leap in understanding biological systems and diseases themselves will come from proteomics and the combination of the so-called omics fields, such as genomics, proteomics, metabolomics, and transcriptomics, within systems biology. As researchers gain access to an increasing amount of omics information, it has become clear that working with segregated data sets can limit their usefulness. The connectivity between the omic worlds is fundamental, but it has been a challenge until now.

The study of the proteome involves the systematic investigation of the proteins that exist in a system, their properties, structure, post-transcriptional modifications, function, and control of this biological system.[3] Proteomics is a field that began three decades ago, but for many years it faced the major handicap that the technology itself prevented the collection of real and reliable data from the biological systems under study. This has changed in recent years with the rapid development of technology, with the latest advances in mass spectrometry and computational tools for studying the protein content of complex samples. The goal of deciphering the molecular basis of biological functions in biomedicine is now within reach.

PROTEOMICS BASED ON MASS SPECTROMETRY

Mass spectrometry is an analytical technique that separates ionized particles, such as atoms, molecules, and molecular groups, by using the differences in the ratios between their charges and their respective masses (mass/charge), and can be used to determine the molecular weight of particles. Mass spectrometers are commonly used to identify unknown compounds (by determining their molecular weight), to quantify known compounds, and to determine the structure and chemical properties of molecules.[4]

At the beginning of proteomics development, it was performed using two-dimensional gel-based electrophoresis, including two-dimensional differential in-gel fluorescent electrophoresis, known as 2D-DIGE.[5]

These techniques had major problems, as the preparation of these gels is labor-intensive, they have the major limitation that protein separation is not good, and they only identify a small number of proteins. This meant that when certain biological samples were analyzed, they never gave the expected results due to the low number of proteins they identified. Currently, the most widespread workflow for discovery proteomics is called *shotgun* proteomics.[6]

An example of how it was possible to expand the knowledge of the human proteome is based on research conducted on human plasma, one of the most widely used clinical samples for biomedical and clinical research. In 2003, chromatographic separation techniques were used to identify 325 different proteins.[7] In 2016, data published in the Plasma PeptideAtlas described a total of 3,509 proteins in plasma.[8] Recently, by optimizing the shotgun technique and the new Orbitrap mass spectrometer, our group identified 4,657 proteins from 21,165 different peptides.[9]

The key to developing this technology in biomedical applications lies in sample preparation, the technology used for analysis, and, finally, the subsequent algorithms that perform the analyses using available databases. Thus, this process begins with a sample preparation step, in which a complex mixture of proteins is enzymatically digested into peptides. This step is followed by a combination of a liquid chromatography system that allows the separation of peptides over time and ionization using *electrospray* ionization technology, which allows the formation of charged molecules, followed by their analysis in the mass spectrometer (LC-MS). The peptides are fragmented and the results of these MS/MS spectra are run through sequence databases using search engines to identifypeptides using statistically defined criteria.[10]

One of the keys to considering the validity of this technology in biomedical applications, and specifically in the field of psychiatry, is that this technique allows working hypotheses to be obtained. In other words, the analysis of certain samples yields large protein profiles, where the application of certain algorithms allows us to obtain profiles of proteins, peptides, or post-translational modifications (PTMs) that significantly separate different groups. These differences provide us with working hypotheses that can be developed using other, cheaper and more affordable techniques to identify possible biomarkers that separate both groups, hypotheses of new metabolic or molecular pathways for a specific pathology, or possible molecular alterations in the PTMs of certain proteins (Figure 10.1).[11]

An example of the usefulness of this technique for discovering new signaling pathways or cellular functioning in a pathology is as follows. In recent years, we have made great strides in our understanding of DNA methylation and acetylation in different psychiatric pathologies, with significant advances in the discovery of mutations, polygenic risk factors, and genetic variants, such as insertions, deletions, and duplications of DNA segments (known as CNVs), and hundreds of articles have been published. A specific example is the PsyCoursese longitudinal study, which investigated the role of DNA methylation in

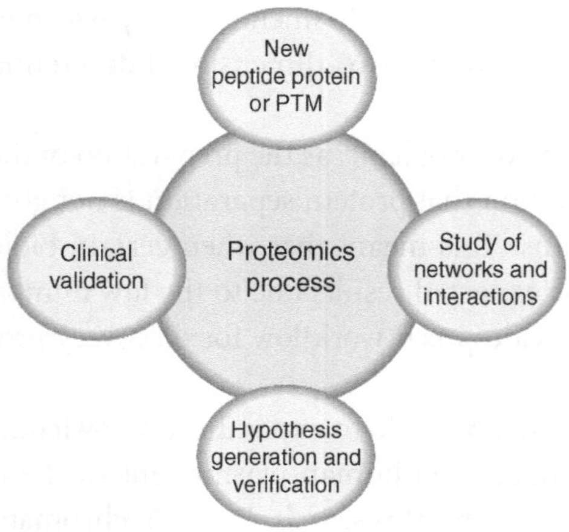

FIGURE 10.1 Diagram of the theoretical development process for the use of proteomics.Protein profiles are obtained from the analysis of several groups of samples and compared using different algorithms (*maxquant*, *labelfree*, *spider*, etc.). The list of selected proteins is then investigated in interaction analyses, such as STRING, where information can be obtained on the relationship of these proteins with many cellular, physiological, or pathological processes. With all this data, we obtain a working hypothesis that we need to verify by analyzing more samples or patients with more affordable methods (ELISA, *western blot*, SIMOA, etc.) to finally, if the hypothesis is confirmed, perform a clinical validation.

response to recent stressful life events in a cohort of bipolar patients.[12] If we transfer this to the study of proteins, where PTMs make them functional or not, or cause them to initiate a certain signaling or receptor recruitment. These mechanisms are yet to be discovered; very little is known about this part of systems biology, and ultimately, they are what give functions to cellular mechanisms. An example of this can be found in the work carried out on the formation of monoamine transporter clusters in the lymphocyte membrane in patients with psychiatric disorders. The way these proteins cluster in the membrane allows us to predict the therapeutic efficacy of antidepressants.[13,14]

USE OF PROTEOMICS IN DUAL PATHOLOGY

The use of proteomics in the field of dual pathology is very recent. Only a few years ago, accompanied by technological developments and advances in mass spectrometry analysis, the first studies began to be published in which proteomics was applied to the field of mental disorders. The first studies focused on investigating proteomic changes in the most common psychiatric pathologies, where we have many examples with schizophrenia,[11,15] psychotic disorders,[16] depression,[17,18] or bipolar disorder.[19] In recent years, proteomic studies have begun to investigate how certain psychiatric and neuropsychological treatments affect patients. Our group has carried out a couple of examples, where, on the one hand, we investigated the molecular changes induced by physical exercise in chronic patients with schizophrenia[9] and, on the other hand, we are currently investigating the changes induced by so-called "serious games," such as Trisquel[20] in patients with schizophrenia and substance abuse disorders.

The development of this field does not start from scratch, as it has a very strong foundation in all the genomic and epigenomic studies that have been carried out in the field of mental health. Proteomic research is a tool that must complement and expand on existing genomic studies in order to explore pathogenic changes in greater depth and contribute new hypotheses that seek to push the boundaries of knowledge in psychiatry and in the field of dual pathology, which attempt to reveal new diagnostic biomarkers, new molecules that can develop new treatments, or molecular information that can help clinicians apply certain therapies and also predict response to treatment.

> One indication of how novel proteomic research is in the field of substance abuse disorders is that if you search PubMed using the terms "proteomic" *AND* "substance abuse disorder," you will find no results. Only when the terms are entered without the *AND* separator do we obtain 313 articles, the vast majority of which are studies conducted on alcohol abuse disorder and animal models (Figure 10.2).

If we want to conduct in-depth research on patients with substance use disorder, we face a major obstacle that we must overcome: deciding what type of sample we are going to work with. According to the DSM-5 classification, substance use disorder is characterized by pathological behaviors and patterns that include one or more of the following problems with control over drug use, compulsive use, and continued use despite harm and withdrawal. Obviously, these pathological changes occur within the brain's circuitry, and if we want to investigate what happens inside the brain, the only way to do so is through neuroimaging techniques. If we seek to describe and demonstrate metabolic and molecular changes that allow us to discover what occurs in this pathology, we will encounter a problem with the working sample, since we will never be able to access a sample of brain tissue.

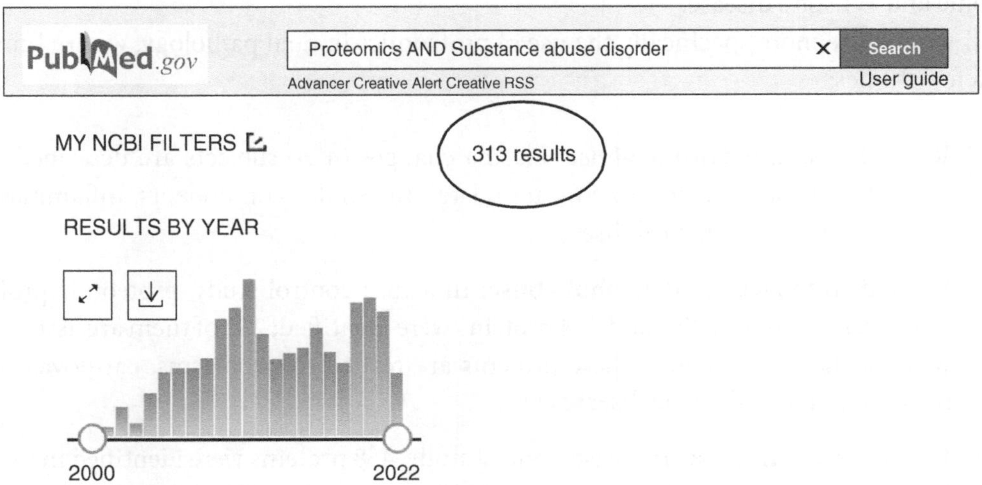

FIGURE 10.2 PubMed search for articles on proteomics in substance use disorders.

Therefore, in the field of dual pathology, we must make an effort to introduce complex systems biology analyses in order to access the secrets of the brain through peripheral samples, such as blood, lymphocytes, saliva, urine, sweat, or even, with more-invasive methods, cerebrospinal fluid (CSF) and skin biopsies.[21] However, when we set out to investigate the molecular mechanisms of addiction, we have to adapt to the types of samples that different centers can provide us with. As explained in other chapters of this book, patients with this type of pathology in Spain come from various drug addiction centers spread across day units, therapeutic communities, and, in severe cases, from the psychiatric unit of a hospital. This means that saliva is the most feasible sample to collect.

Saliva is a very attractive bodily fluid for the diagnosis of neurological and neuropsychiatric diseases for several reasons:

1. Saliva collection is usually inexpensive, safe, and easy, and can be done without the help of healthcare personnel (allowing samples to be taken at home).
2. It is considered an acceptable and non-invasive process by patients because it does not cause any pain (and can be easily collected in the case of pediatric patients).
3. Proteins of neuronal and glial origin can be found in saliva, and these are potential candidates as biomarkers for pathologies affecting the central nervous system.[22] In addition, saliva is a fluid where damage to the hypothalamus and neurovegetative system converges with neuroinflammation and neuroimmunological alterations.

Based on this type of test, biomarkers were sought in saliva that would predict Alzheimer's disease, such as lactoferrin or amyloid protein[23] or variations in the expression of aquaporin 5 in saliva and cerebral cortex.[24] The salivary proteome has been characterized in several diseases: oral squamous cell carcinoma and oral leukoplakia, chronic graft-versus-host disease in Sjögren's syndrome and other autoimmune disorders, such as SAPHO, schizophrenia and bipolar disorder, and genetic diseases, such as Down syndrome and Wilson's disease.

If we analyze more specifically the use of proteomics in dual pathology, we are limited to a few studies:

- **Related to amphetamine abuse**: Plasma changes in 20 subjects are described and suggest that the affected proteins are related to cellular components, inflammatory response, and neurological diseases.[25]
- **Related to tobacco and alcohol abuse**: In a case-control study, proteomic profiles were performed on saliva and 404 proteins were identified; 282 of them are associated with alcohol dependence. These proteins are related to neoplasms, cardiovascular, metabolic, and endocrine diseases.[26]
- **Related to cocaine use:** In a case-control study, 458 proteins were identified in saliva, including Statherin, TFGbeta-inducing protein, and NELF (*negative elongation factor*).[26]

In recent years, our group has been working on the application of different neurorehabilitation therapies in patients with substance abuse disorders as part of two projects funded by the Ministry of Health, Social Services, and Equality–Government Delegation for the National Plan on Drugs 2017I054 (entitled "Effectiveness of the Therapeutic Game 'El Trisquel' in the Treatment of Patients with Substance-Related Disorders: A Neuropsychological and Proteomic Study of Biomarkers Predictive of Treatment Response) and 2020I054 (entitled "Efficacy of the Social Cognition Rehabilitation Program 'Emotional Training 3.0' in the Treatment of Patients with Substance-Related Disorders and Development of Predictive Biomarkers of Response Using Proteomics"). In both projects, proteomic profiles are being carried out and analyzed in saliva samples from patients associated with these therapies. We are currently at different stages of development, but in the study conducted with El Trisquel, saliva samples from 53 participants with substance use disorder (El Trisquel vs. usual therapy) were analyzed using the shotgun LC-MS/MS technique and compared with a non-clinical control group ($n = 13$) (Figures 10.3 and 10.4).

We found that 39 of the 3,266 proteins identified and quantified showed significant differences when analyzing at least two individual peptides ($FDR > 2$) using the PEAKS program. This study describes for the first time the change in the expression pattern of proteins in the saliva of patients undergoing the "El Trisquel" neurorehabilitation program. The main changes found suggest that the "El Trisquel" intervention program mainly modifies the signaling pathways of the immune response, with changes found in the *Bactericidal/Permeability-Increasing Fold-Containing Family* (BPIF), the S-100 family, and the cystatin family, and in proteins linked to astrocyte and glial activity.

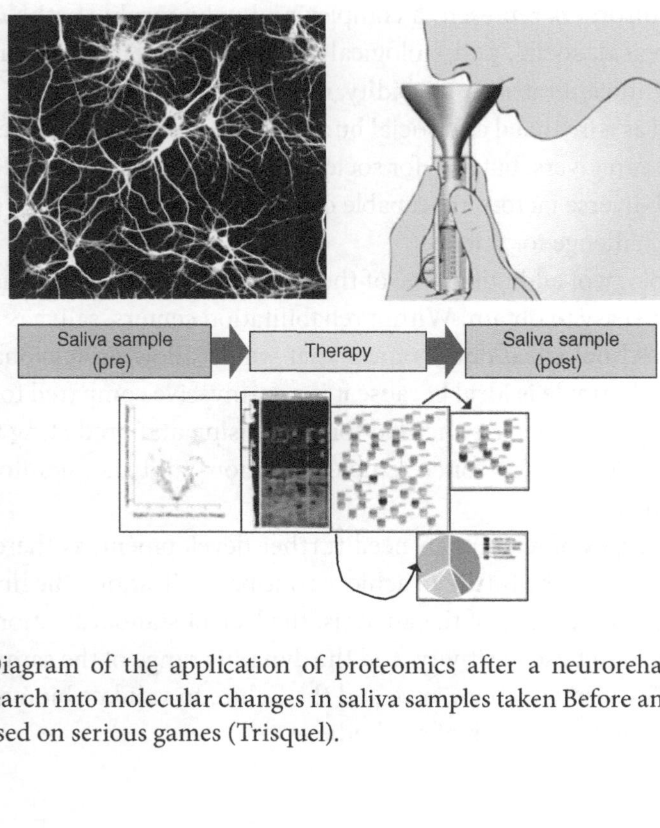

FIGURE 10.3 Diagram of the application of proteomics after a neurorehabilitation program. Summary of research into molecular changes in saliva samples taken Before and After a rehabilitation program based on serious games (Trisquel).

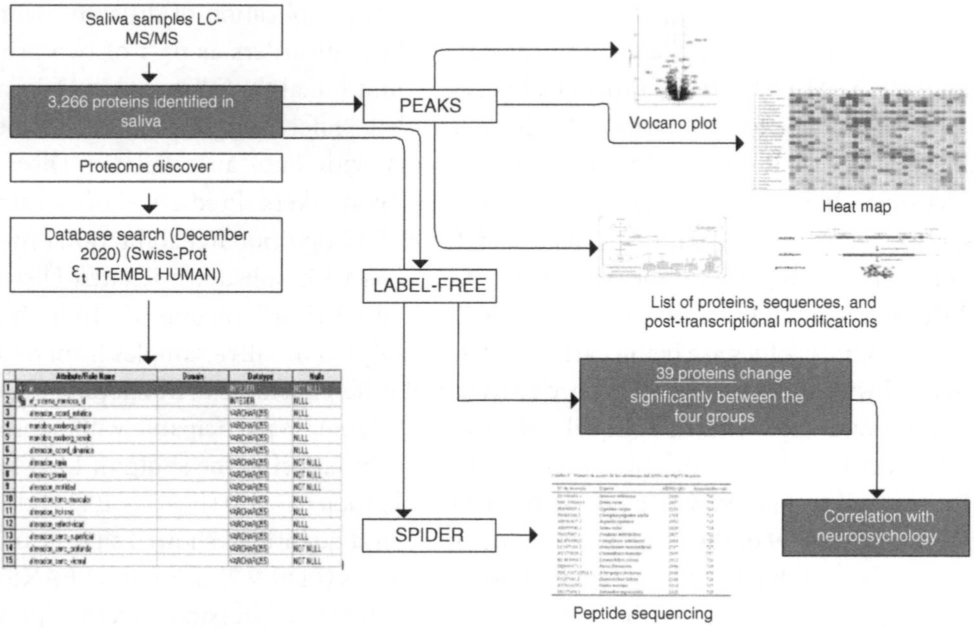

FIGURE 10.4 Schematic diagram of LC-MS/MS analysis in patients with substance use disorder after application of Trisquel neurorehabilitation therapy and control (usual therapy) and a non-clinical control group. After comparing all groups, we found that 39 of the 3,266 proteins identified and quantified exhibited significant differences when analyzing at least two individual peptides (FDR > 2) using the PEAKS program.

Substance use disorders represent a complex and polymorphic pathology with serious negative psychological, social, and biological consequences. Substance use disorders are responsible for significant rates of morbidity, mortality, and deterioration in quality of life worldwide, as well as a financial and social burden. They are a major challenge for patients, their doctors, and caregivers, but also for society and healthcare systems. Researching how such complex and diverse factors are capable of causing these pathologies and disability in individuals are a challenge for science.

In the neurobiology of addiction, one of the most promising areas is the search for new biomarkers that are easy to obtain. Within rehabilitation centers, saliva is the ideal sample for research and technological development that would allow professionals to use a biomarker. This type of sample is ideal because it is non-invasive compared to blood sampling or biopsies, making it an effective method for diagnosing and predicting the prognosis of multiple diseases, allowing for concrete determinations and the monitoring of patients undergoing treatment.

However, these types of techniques need further development, as there are limitations that must be overcome in the future to achieve routine application. The limitations of proteomics include the complexity of the analysis, the lack of standardization in sample processing, the risk of high false positivity, and the dynamic range of the sample, which limits the estimation of low protein abundance and the failure to validate biomarkers in a larger number of patients due to the lack of antibodies.

Although this mental health technique will be applied in the future, we hope that, at that time, the application of proteomic methods to psychiatric disorders, and especially to substance abuse disorders, will lead to clinical and healthcare improvements in the treatment of this population. Furthermore, the development of these biomarkers in saliva not only opens up a new clinical and healthcare aspect, but also paves the way, through the use of more sophisticated technologies such as nanotechnology and microfluidics, for the development of biosensors with Raman spectroscopy. These could be designed to be portable and implemented in drug addiction centers as advanced analysis systems that are easy to use and compact in design, so that they can be used by clinicians in all centers.

REFERENCES

1. Wilkins MR, Sanchez JC, Gooley AA, Appel RD, Humphery-Smith I, Hochstrasser DF, *et al.* Progress with proteome projects: why all proteins expressed by a genome should be identified and how to do it. Biotechnol Genet Eng Rev. 1996;13(1):19–50. https://doi.org/10.1080/02648725.1996.10647923
2. Craig Venter J, Adams MD, Myers EW, Li PW, Mural RJ, Sutton GG, *et al.* The sequence of the human genome. Science (New York, NY). 2001;291(5507):1304–51. https://doi.org/10.1126/SCIENCE.1058040
3. Patterson SD, Aebersold RH. Proteomics: the first decade and beyond Nat Genet. 2003;33:311–23. https://doi.org/10.1038/NG1106
4. Uzozie AC, Aebersold R. Advancing translational research and precision medicine with targeted proteomics. J Proteomics. 2018;189:1–10. https://doi.org/10.1016/J.JPROT.2018.02.021
5. Vidova V, Spacil Z. A review on mass spectrometry-based quantitative proteomics: Targeted and data independent acquisition. Analytica Chimica Acta. 2017;964:7–23. https://doi.org/10.1016/J.ACA.2017.01.059
6. Rodrigues-Amorim D, Rivera-Baltanas T, Del Carmen Vallejo-Curto M, Rodriguez-Jamardo C, de Las Heras E, Barreiro-Villar C, *et al.* Proteomics in schizophrenia: A gateway to discover potential biomarkers of psycho-neuroimmune pathways. Front Psychiatry. 2019;10:885. https://doi.org/10.3389/fpsyt.2019.00885
7. Pieper R, Gatlin CL, Makusky AJ, Russo PS, Schatz CR, Miller SS, *et al.* The human serum proteome: Display of nearly 3700 chromatographically separated protein spots on two-dimensional electrophoresis gels and identification of 325 distinct proteins. Proteomics. 2003;3(7):1345–64. https://doi.org/10.1002/PMIC.200300449
8. Geyer PE, Kulak NA, Pichler G, Holdt LM, Teupser D, Mann, M. Plasma proteome profiling to assess human health and disease. Cell Systems. 2016;2(3):185–95. https://doi.org/10.1016/J.CELS.2016.02.015
9. Vallejo-Curto MC, Rodrigues-Amorim D, Jardón-Gol-mar L, Blanco-Formoso M, Rivera-Baltanás T, Ro-driguez-Jamardo C, *et al.* Proteomic and metabolic profiling of chronic patients with schizophrenia induced by a physical activity program: Pilot study. J Psychiat Mental Health. 2021;14(3):125–38. https://doi.org/10.1016/J.RPSMEN.2021.07.002
10. Guerin CL, Guyonnet L, Goudot G, Revets D, Konstan-tinou M, Chipont A, *et al.* Multidimensional proteomic approach of endothelial progenitors demonstrate expression of KDR restricted to CD19 cells. Stem Cell Rev Rep. 2021;17(2):639–51. https://doi.org/10.1007/S12015-020-10062-1
11. Rodrigues-Amorim D, Rivera-Baltanás T, López M, Spuch C, Olivares JM, Agís-Balboa RC. Schizophrenia: A review of potential biomarkers. J Psychiatr Res. 2017;93:37–49. https://doi.org/10.1016/j.jpsychires.2017.05.009

12. Comes AL, Czamara D, Adorjan Anderson-Schmidt H, Andlauer TF M, Budde M, Heilbronner U. The role of environmental stress and DNA methylation in the longitudinal course of bipolar disorder. Intern J Bipo-lar Disord. 2020;12(8):1–9. https://doi.org/10.1186/S40345-019-0176-6
13. Rivera-Baltanas T, Olivares JM, Martinez-Villamarin JR, Fenton EY, Kalynchuk LE, Caruncho HJ. Serotonin 2A receptor clustering in peripheral lymphocytes is altered in major depression and may be a biomarker of therapeutic efficacy. J Affect Disord. 2014;163:47–55. https://doi.org/10.1016/j.jad.2014.03.011
14. Romay-Tallon R, Kulhawy E, Brymer KJ, Allen J, Rivera-Baltanas T, Olivares JM, *et al.* Changes in membrane protein clustering in peripheral lymphocytes in an animal model of depression parallel those observed in naïve depression patients: Implications for the development of novel biomarkers of depression. Front Pharmacol. 2018;9:1149. https://doi.org/10.3389/fphar.2018.01149
15. Guest PC. Proteomic studies of psychiatric disorders. Methods Mol Biol. 2018;1735:59–89. https://doi.org/10.1007/978-1-4939-7614-0_4
16. Mongan D, Föcking M, Healy C, Susai SR, Heurich M, Wynne McGuire P. Development of proteomic prediction models for transition to psychotic disorder in the clinical high-risk state and psychotic experiences in adolescence. JAMA Psychiatry. 2021;78(1):77–90. https://doi.org/10.1001/JAMAPSYCHIATRY.2020.2459
17. Qi YJ, Lu YR, Shi LG, Demmers JAA, Bezstarosti K, Rijkers E, *et al.* Distinct proteomic profiles in prefrontal subareas of elderly major depressive disorder and bipolar disorder patients. Transl Psychiatry. 2022;12(1):275. https://doi.org/10.1038/S41398-022-02040-7
18. Silva-Costa LC, Carlson PT, Guest PC, de Almeida V, Martins-de-Souza D. Proteomic Markers for Depression. In: Guest, P. (eds) Reviews on Biomarker Studies in Psychiatric and Neurodegenerative Disorders. Advances in Experimental Medicine and Biology, Vol. 1118. Springer, Cham, 2019. https://doi.org/10.1007/978-3-030-05542-4_10
19. Isgren A, Göteson A, Holmén-Larsson J, Pelanis A, Sellgren C, Joas E, *et al.* Cerebrospinal fluid proteomic study of two bipolar disorder cohorts. Mol Psychiatry. 2022;27(11):4568–74. https://doi.org/10.1038/S41380-022-01724-2
20. Pinón-Blanco A, Vergara-Moragues E, Fernández-Mar-tínez R, Gutiérrez-Martínez O, Alvarez-Counago M, Martínez-Reglero C, *et al.* Effectiveness of the "Trisquel" board game intervention program for patients with schizophrenia spectrum disorders. Actas Esp Psiquiatr. 2020 Sep;48(5):209–19. https://pubmed.ncbi.nlm.nih.gov/33210279/
21. Pennington K, Cotter D, Dunn MJ. The role of proteomics in investigating psychiatric disorders. Br J Psychiatry. 2005;187:4–6. https://doi.org/10.1192/BJP.187.1.4
22. Orive G, Lopera F, Carro E. Saliva is a good candidate to be the new gold-standard sample for neurodegenerative diseases. J Alzheimers Dis. 2022;87(4):1497–501. https://doi.org/10.3233/JAD-220144
23. Bermejo-Pareja, del Ser, T., Valentí, M., de la Fuente, M., Bartolome, and Carro, E. Salivary lactoferrin as a biomarker for Alzheimer's disease: Brain-immunity interactions. Alzheimers Dement. 2020;16(8):1196–204. https://doi.org/10.1002/ALZ.12107
24. Antequera D, Carrero L, Cunha Alves V, Ferrer I, Hernández-Gallego J, Municio C, *et al.* Differentially aquaporin 5 expression in submandibular glands and cerebral cortex in Alzheimer's disease. Biomedicines. 2022;10(7):1645. https://doi.org/10.3390/BIOMEDICINES10071645
25. Alasmari F, Alsanea S, Masood A, Alhazzani K, Alanazi IO, Musambil M, *et al.* Serum proteomic profiling of patients with amphetamine use disorder. Drug Alcohol Depend. 2020;214:108157. https://doi.org/10.1016/J.DRUGALCDEP.2020.108157
26. Chaiben CL, Batista TBD, Penteado CAS, Barbosa MCM, Ventura TMO, Dionizio A, *et al.* Salivary proteome analysis of crack cocaine dependents. Arch Oral Biol. 2021;121:104952. https://doi.org/10.1016/J.ARCHORALBIO.2020.104952

10.4 A QUESTION OF GENDER AND AGE IN DUAL PATHOLOGY

10.4.1 GENDER AND DUAL PATHOLOGY

J. M. Fernández

INTRODUCTION

The gender perspective is decisive in mental health: how it occurs, how it manifests itself, how it is responded to. It has been described that gender influences the prevalence of psychiatric disorders, pathoplasty, symptom expression, course, prognosis, demand, and response to treatment (Gearon, Nidecker, Bellack and Bennette, 2003b; Seedat, Scott, Angermeyer, Berglund, Bromet, Brugha *et al.*, 2009).

The literature indicates that women are particularly vulnerable to the consequences of alcohol and drug use, which is related to physiological, psychological, and sociocultural factors (Medina-Mora, 2011).

Most studies have evaluated gender differences in samples of patients with mental illness and substance use disorders (SUD) separately, with few studies on patients with dual diagnosis (DD). Although dual diagnosis is believed to be more common in men, women are considered to be at greater risk of developing both conditions. There is controversy about whether dual pathology is more common in men or women, with differences depending on where the studies are conducted; either in general psychiatric units, where there are more dual men than women, or in drug addiction units, where the opposite is detected. General epidemiological data, according to diagnosis, do not show significant variations between dual and non-dual patients. Men with dual pathology suffer a higher prevalence of schizophrenia and women with dual pathology suffer from affective and anxiety disorders, as is the case in the general population. Sociodemographically, there are no significant differences between dual pathology and women, except that dual pathology women have more children in their care, a higher risk of victimization, and fewer legal problems than dual-pathology men. All studies agree that male dual pathology patients exhibit a higher pattern of poly-substance use. On the other hand, no conclusions can be drawn about differences in substance use by gender in dual-pathology patients, given the variability of the samples.

International epidemiological studies (Kessler *et al.*, 1997) show that women who abuse or are dependent on alcohol have higher rates of other psychiatric disorders (OTP) than men with the same problem (65% vs. 44%) (Zilberman, Tavares, Blume, Guebaly, 2003). Among the psychiatric disorders identified as most prevalent in women with PD, affective disorders (except type I bipolar disorder) and anxiety disorders have been identified, as well as greater addiction to hypnotics, compared to men (Miquel, Roncero, López-Ortiz and Casas, 2011; Miquel *et al.*, 2013). On the other hand, women with psychotic disorders and concurrent substance use have greater difficulties in treatment prognosis, as they have a higher number of hospitalizations, more severe positive symptoms, greater exposure to some type of abuse, and decreased overall functioning compared to men (Miquel *et al.*, 2013).

GENDER DIFFERENCES IN THE PREVALENCE OF AXIS I PSYCHIATRIC DISORDERS IN DUAL-PATHOLOGY PATIENTS

The study published in the journal *Addictions* in 2011 by Miquel *et al.* describes significant gender differences in the prevalence of various axis I psychiatric disorders:

- ADHD (attention deficit hyperactivity disorder) is more common in girls and adolescent women than in boys of the same age.
- Affective disorders are more common in women, and depression is twice as common in women as in men.
- Substance use disorders, including smoking, are between 2 and 5 times more common in adult males than in adult females, but in adolescents, rates of consumption and addiction no longer tend to be as disparate based on gender. In patients with PD, gender differences tend to disappear, conferring greater clinical severity and a worse prognosis.
- The distribution of axis I mental disorders in dual patients, according to gender, remains similar to that of non-dual mental disorders in the general population.
- There is a higher prevalence of psychotic and bipolar disorders in men, and a higher prevalence of anxiety and affective disorders in women.
- Studies conducted on patients with dual pathology observed that schizophrenia is more common among men (57.7% vs. 38%).
- Women with dual psychosis have a prognosis similar to that of men with dual pathology and clearly worse than that of women with psychosis without SUD. In addition, they have a greater family burden, more history of aggression, and medical problems.
- Polydrug use is more common in men.
- In general psychiatric units, there are more dual pathology men than women (87.5% men and 12.5% women).
- Of every four patients in treatment, only one is a woman, and women suffer more from the stigma and social rejection associated with this illness; therefore, they also find it more difficult to overcome the barriers to seeking specialized help and requesting treatment.
- In relation to patients with an affective disorder who consume alcohol, women present consumption related to anxiety. They are at greater risk of attempting suicide or committing suicide and more frequently follow a pattern of self-medication and compulsive consumption. It might be hypothesized that there is a different etiopathogenic origin of SUD depending on gender, since most studies observe that affective disorders in women are primary, unlike in men, in whom they are predominantly secondary to consumption and more difficult to treat.

From a psychopathological perspective, the risk of developing a SUD varies according to gender. For example, bipolar women are at greater risk of developing a SUD than women in the general population, compared to men. When anxiety disorders are studied, it is found that dual pathology women have a similar prevalence of PTSD to those who only have a mental illness, but higher than those who have a SUD. Other disorders, such as GAD, which usually predominate in women, are more prevalent in men with dual disorders.

GENDER DIFFERENCES IN THE PREVALENCE OF AXIS II PSYCHIATRIC DISORDERS IN DUAL-PATHOLOGY PATIENTS

In the article by Szerman *et al.* on dual pathology in special populations, published in the *International Journal of Addiction Research* in 2015, reference is made to gender, highlighting the following data:

- With regard to personality disorders, Landhein *et al.* (2003) studied gender differences between polydrug users and pure alcoholics and found a higher overall prevalence of antisocial, passive-aggressive, and borderline personality disorders, while dependent disorder was more prevalent among alcoholics.
- Female poly-substance users had more borderline disorders, and men had more antisocial disorders.
- Women who were dependent only on alcohol were more likely to have Cluster C disorders, while men were more likely to have Cluster A disorders, especially schizoid disorder.

GENDER PERSPECTIVE: DIFFERENCES IN THERAPEUTIC NEEDS

In view of the results, the authors suggested that there are significant differences in therapeutic needs:

- Women face greater barriers to treatment for mental disorders than men; among those identified are late detection of the problem, diagnostic overshadowing, lack of treatment centers sensitive to women's needs, and social stigma. Furthermore, cumulative vulnerability contributes to the development of other, associated problems, such as the risk of losing custody of children, rejection by partners, and loss of family support (Galván and Marín Navarrete, 2011; Grella, 1996; Romero Mendoza *et al*, 2010) (Tables 10.3 and 10.4).
- Because violence, trauma, oppression, and stigma are common themes in the lives of women with this condition, several authors suggest that the development and implementation of gender-sensitive treatments could empower them to take a more active role in their treatment (Egeland and Erickson, 1990; Miquel *et al.*, 2013). Observations have shown that women respond better to interventions designed specifically for women with PD (Choi, Adams, Morse and MacMaster, 2015; Ruglass, Hien, Hu, Campbell, 2014). On the other hand, although women with PD tend to begin treatment when their symptoms and dysfunction in various areas are more severe, they remain in treatment longer than men with PD (Morse *et al.*, 2015).
- Pregnant women require special consideration (Grella, 1996), as the prevalence and vulnerability to PD is higher than in non-pregnant women; various systematic reviews on perinatal health and care have identified that this population

TABLE 10.3 Characteristic Elements of Drug Addiction Present in Women (Pantoja, 2007)

1. Later onset of use.
2. Addictive disorders progress more rapidly.
3. They consume smaller quantities, but the physical disorders resulting from consumption are more frequent and severe.
4. They suffer disproportionately from the impact of drugs on sexual and reproductive health.
5. The severity of addiction is greater.
6. They suffer from other psychiatric disorders associated with drug addiction at a higher rate than men.
7. They more frequently report the presence of psychiatric disorders prior to problematic drug use.
8. Reactions to depression, anxiety, and stress often appear as triggers for drug use.
9. They are more likely to have a history of physical or sexual abuse, suicide attempts, and physical or psychological abuse by their partner.
10. More often than not, the onset of drug use is related to specific stressors.
11. They have more family, work, and financial problems than men.
12. They have less family and social support to cope with problems.
13. They have fewer resources to access treatment.
14. They experience feelings of guilt and low self-esteem.

TABLE 10.4 Barriers to Treatment for Drug-Dependent Women (Sánchez, 2008)

1. The stigma or added shame that women endure.
2. Barriers derived from their responsibilities as mothers or wives, such as concern for the care of their children or fear of losing custody.
3. The presence of a drug-dependent partner.
4. Not realizing that substance-use disorders are a disease and/or believing that they can overcome this problem on their own.
5. Fear of withdrawal.
6. Waiting lists for access to certain services or inability to access them when they have minor children (mainly residential services).
7. Lack of information about treatment options.
8. The absence of services tailored to women's needs (for example, women who are drug addicts are denied access to shelters for abused women).

This group shows a particular vulnerability to anxiety disorders, depression, and somatic disorders. In addition, substance use and mental disorders significantly increase the risk of complications during childbirth or conditions that compromise the health of the product (e.g., fetal alcohol syndrome) (Bennet, Einarson, Taddio, Koren and Einarson, 2004; Fisher *et al.*, 2012; Ross, McLean, and Psych, 2006; Shaw, Levitt, Wong, and Kaczorowski, 2006).

GENDER PERSPECTIVE: ADOLESCENTS

At the VII Gender Conference "Women, Adolescence, and Dual Pathology," organized in Valencia by the Spanish Society of Dual Pathology (SEPD) in 2013, President Néstor Szerman and other experts called for greater attention to be paid to this at-risk population:

- Adolescence is a stage of life characterized by profound, significant, and continuous changes in the individual's neurobiological, physical, emotional, psychological, and social development. The use of psychoactive substances takes on special importance in adolescence due to its high prevalence and the frequent presence of dual pathology. During adolescence, "the experimental initiation of substance use occurs."

- Among the factors that influence vulnerability to progress from substance use to developing a substance use disorder (SUD) during adolescence, experts have identified a family history of mental illness or addiction—present in more than half of cases—the age of first use, the presence of certain temperamental traits (low self-esteem, negative emotionality, sensation-seeking, or low frustration tolerance), accompanied by cognitive factors (knowledge, attitudes, beliefs, and expectations), and the influence of peers or gender.
- In relation to gender, adolescent girls present a particular asymmetry compared to males due to the interaction of biological and psychosocial factors, and are at particular risk of developing dual pathology.
- According to specialists, the use of cannabis, cocaine, and designer drugs among adolescents has a decisive impact on school failure and explains that 25–30% of them do not finish their studies, as well as promoting the onset of psychiatric disorders at increasingly early ages. In this regard, they have pointed out that in more than half of cases, attention deficit disorder underlies the onset of eating disorders.
- Experts indicate that certain behaviors can provide clues as early as five or six years of age about future cases of dual pathology, such as poor academic performance, behavioral disorders, impulsivity and confrontation with parents and teachers, or inattention.
- The mental disorders that show the highest prevalence in adolescents with SUDs are, in descending order of frequency, disruptive behavior disorders, attention deficit hyperactivity disorder (ADHD), mood disorders, and post-traumatic stress disorder (PTSD).
- Some studies of adolescents with SUDs found that, compared to boys, girls tend to show more internalizing symptoms (depression, anxiety, low self-esteem), often related to traumatic experiences, while externalizing symptoms (aggression, antinormativity) are a common factor for both sexes (Poulin *et al.*, 2005).

The heterogeneity of adolescents with dual pathology requires treatments tailored to the needs of each individual (Martínez Raga):

> Adolescent girls with dual pathology clearly have different care needs than boys. In fact, certain disorders are more common in girls, such as eating disorders (anorexia or bulimia) or post-traumatic stress disorder, while ADHD—especially the hyperactive subtype—is more common among boys. Psychotic disorders are also more severe and occur earlier in boys who use substances than in girls who use substances.
>
> These mental disorders are associated with different patterns of substance use and, therefore, therapeutic needs vary depending on gender and the combination of dual pathology".

For all the reasons outlined above, further study of gender differences in dual pathology is needed, as variations have been observed that may influence diagnosis, treatment, and service planning.

REFERENCES

Arias F, Szerman N, Vega P, Mesias B, Basurte I, Morant C, *et al.* Estudio Madrid sobre prevalencia y características de los pacientes con patología dual en tratamiento en las redes de salud mental y de atención al drogodependiente. Addictions. 2013;25(1):118–27.

Bennet H, Einarson A, Taddio A, Koren G, Einarson TR. Depression during Pregnancy: Overview of Clinical Factors. Clin Crug Investig. 2004; 24(3):157–79.

Choi S, Adams S, Morse SA, MacMaster S. Gender differences in treatment retention among individuals with co-occurring substance abuse and mental health disorders. Substance Use & Misuse. 2015; 50(5):653–63.

Egeland B, Erickson M. Rising Above the Past: Strategies for Helping New Mothers Break the Cycle of Abuse and Neglect. Zero to Three. 1990; 11:29–35.

Fisher J, Cabral de Mello M, Patel V, Rahman A, Tran T, Holton S, Holmes W. Prevalence and determinants of common perinatal mental disorders in women in low- and lower-middle-income countries: a systematic review. Bull World Health Organ. 2011 Nov 24;90(2):139–149H. doi: 10.2471/BLT.11.091850

Galván J, Marín Navarrete R. Sobre la atención a mujeres usuarias de drogas: cifras, barreras y modelo de tratamiento. En: Romero Mendoza MP, Medina-Mora ME y Rodríguez Ajenjo CJ (Editores). Mujeres y Adicciones (2ª edición). México: Comisión Nacional contra las Adicciones (CENADIC), 2011, 160–78.

Gearon JS, Nidecker M, Alan B and Bennett M. Gender differences in drug use behavior in people with serious mental illnesses. Am J Addict. 2003; 12(3):229–41.

Goti J, Diaz R, Arango C. Adolescentes y patología dual. In: Szerman N, Roncero C, Casas M. (eds.), Protocolos de Intervención en Patología Dual. Barcelona: EdikaMed, 2016.

Grekin ER, Sher KJ, Wood PK. Personality and substance dependence symptoms: modeling substance-specific traits. Psychol Addict Behav. 2006;20:415–24.

Grella CE. Background and overview of mental health and substance abuse treatment systems: Meeting the needs of women who are pregnant or parenting. J Psychoact Drugs. 1996; 28:319–43.

Kessler RC, Crum RM, Warner LA, Nelson CB, Schulenberg J and Anthony JC. Lifetime co-occurrence of DSM-III-R alcohol abuse and dependence with other psychiatric disorders in the National Comorbidity Survey. Arch Gen Psychiatry. 1997; 54(4):313–21. doi: 10.1001/archpsyc.1997.01830160031005

Landheim AS, Bakken K, Vaglum P. Gender differences in the prevalence of symptom disorders and personality disorders among poly-substance abusers and pure alcoholics. Substance abusers treated in two counties in Norway. Eur Addict Res. 2003;9(1):8–17.

Medina-Mora ME. Introducción. En: Romero Mendoza MP, Medina-Mora ME, Rodríguez Ajenjo CJ (Editores). Mujeres y Adicciones (2ª edición). México: Comisión Nacional contra las Adicciones (CENADIC), 2011, 13–36.

Miquel L, Roncero C, López-Ortiz C, Casas M. Diferencias de género epidemiológicas y diagnósticas según eje I en pacientes con Patología Dual. Adicciones. 2011; 23(2):165–72. doi: 10.20882/adicciones.160.

Miquel L, Roncero C, García-García G, Barral C, Daigre C, Grau-López L *et al.* Gender Differences in Dually Diagnosed Outpatients. Subst Abus. 2013; 34(1):78–80.

Pantoja Vargas L (director). ¿Programas específicos de tratamiento para mujeres drogodependientes?: avances en drogodependencias. Deusto: Universidad de Deusto, Instituto Deusto de Drogodependencias, 2007.

Peris L. Patología Dual en Trastornos de Personalidad. In: Szerman N, Roncero C, Casas M (eds.), Patología Dual. Protocolos de intervención. Barcelona: EdikaMed, 2016.

Romero Mendoza M, Saldívar G, Loyola L, Rodríguez E, Galván J. Inequidades de género, abuso de sustancias y barreras al tratamiento en mujeres en prisión. Salud Mental. 2010; 33(6):499–506.

Ross LE and McLean LM. Anxiety disorders during pregnancy and the postpartum period: A systematic review. J Clin Psychiatry. 2006 Aug;67(8):1285–98. doi: 10.4088/jcp.v67n0818.

Ruglass L M, Hien DA, Hu MC, Campbell AN. Associations between post-traumatic stress symptoms, stimulant use, and treatment outcomes: A secondary analysis of NIDA's Women and Trauma Study. Am J Addict. 2014; 23(1):90–5.

Sánchez Pardo L. Drogas y perspectiva de género. Documento marco. Plan de atención integral a la salud de la mujer de Galicia. Género y Drogas. Protocols. 2008. Galician Health Service. Subdirectorate General for Mental Health and Drug Addiction.

Seedat S, Scott KM, Angermeyer, MC, Berglund P, Bromet EJ,Brugha TS, *et al.* Cross-national associations between gender and mental disorders in the World Health Organization World Mental Health Surveys. Arch Gen Psychiatry. 2009; 66(7):785–95. doi: 10.1001/archgenpsychiatry.2009.36

Shaw E, Levitt C, Wong S, Kaczorowski J. Systematic review of the literature on postpartum care: Effectiveness of postpartum support to improve maternal parenting, mental health, quality of life, and physical health. Birth. 2006; 33(3):210–20. doi: 10.1111/j.1523-536X.2006.00106.x.

Szerman N, Marín-Navarreta R, Fernández-Mondragón J, Roncero C. Patología dual en poblaciones especiales: una revisión narrativa. Revista Internacional de Investigación en Adicciones. 2015; 1(1):50–67. doi: 10.28931/riiad.2015.1.07

Szerman N, Marín-Navarrete R, Fernández-Mondragón J, Roncero C. Dual pathology in special populations: a narrative review. Int J Addiction Res. 2015;1(1):50–67.

Szerman N, Martínez-Raga J, Peris L, Roncero C, Basurte I, Vega P, *et al.* Rethinking dual disorders/pathology. Ad-dict Disord Treat. 2013;12(1):1–10.

Zilberman ML, Tavares H, Blume SB, el-Guebaly N. Substance Use Disorders: Sex Differences and Psychiatric Comorbidities. Can J Psychiatry. 2003;48(1):5–13. doi: 10.1177/070674370304800103

10.4.2 ADOLESCENCE AND DUAL PATHOLOGY

G. Rossi Gonnet, M. L. Villalba Ambrosoni, and N. Tailanian Hagopian

INTRODUCTION

Adolescence is a vulnerable stage of life, which can increase the likelihood of experimenting with substances and developing dependence and psychiatric disorders.

It is known that the consequences of repeated exposure to toxins in a developing brain are different from those in adults and have serious consequences.

Dual pathology, co-occurrence, or comorbid disorder (hereinafter used as synonyms) in adolescents and young adults encompasses drug use and mental health.

Although this is a very important issue, the consideration of drug use among children and adolescents as a public health concern is recent. The minimization of consumption by adolescents or their families, where consumption can often be normalized, can lead to underreporting, delayed consultations, and difficulties in detecting the problem.[1,2]

Dual pathologies, understood as problematic drug use associated with other psychiatric disorders, must be taken into consideration when designing public policies aimed at addressing these problems. In these cases, it is necessary to emphasize the importance of prevention programs aimed at children and adolescents, knowing that preventive intervention can have a positive impact on adolescents and their families, helping them to develop healthier relationships.

This section aims to review and update certain aspects of drug use among children and adolescents, reflect on its association with other mental health conditions, establish treatment guidelines, and help in raising awareness among health, education, and judicial system professionalsof a complex, difficult-to-manage problem that is often overlooked.[1–3]

ADOLESCENCE AND DRUG USE

Adolescence is a unique stage of life in which there are multiple and rapid changes, ranging from biological and cognitive to social and familial.

The search for their own identity, differentiating themselves from their adult role models, encourages adolescents to seek new role models outside the family and to question, confront, and oppose anything that implies authority. It is then that relationships with peers, integration into a group, and the gaze and acceptance of others become very important for the construction of a sense of self and identity.

Furthermore, from a biological point of view, bodily and hormonal changes increase psychological imbalance, promoting impulsivity and acting out, favoring action over mentalization or reflection on the consequences.

In the development of the adolescent nervous system, there is an overactivation of the brain systems geared toward experimentation and thrill-seeking, with a less developed corticofrontal system, which implies weaknesses in the systems of planning, self-regulation, and impulse inhibition.

All these characteristics are to be expected and necessary for growth, but it is not difficult to imagine how this translates into a quest that leads them to experiment and put themselves in risky situations. Among these, the use of psychoactive substances is particularly important, mainly in those who present a greater individual, environmental, or constitutional vulnerability.[3]

However, although adolescence is a stage of risk accumulation, it is also a stage of self-construction, where risks are not equivalent to the existence of a disorder.

One of the most important challenges in clinical practice in mental health in children and adolescents is to differentiate between behaviors that are expected and normal and those that fall within the realm of psychopathology. Drug use in adolescence can have multiple meanings, depending on the personal characteristics of the user and the particular circumstances in which it occurs, which allows us to speak appropriately of "consumption patterns."[4]

For this reason, if we set aside universalist claims that attempt to explain the reasons for all consumption, it is possible to identify a series of individual, family, historical, and social variables that are significant for thinking about a particular adolescent who consumes a certain substance in a particular context. "Adolescence takes place within a specific socio-cultural framework, where biological, psychological, and social changes are influenced by the social environment, microsocial phenomena, and the adolescent's own constitution. Each culture has an effect on the development of its adolescents. The expectations, demands, or permissiveness of adults influence and shape the tastes and everyday problems of a large part of adolescents."[4]

These factors are of fundamental importance when it comes to assessing, understanding, and preventing the dynamics and heterogeneous situations involved in substance use among adolescents.

Consequences of Drug Use in Adolescence

We can start from a confirmed premise: "Drug use always has harmful effects on the adolescent body," since they are still developing. Any use affects their growth in various ways.

There are two critical periods in relation to neurodevelopment and its link to the use of psychoactive substances: the period from conception to age 3 (in relation to substance use during pregnancy and attachment) and adolescence. In both cases, due to the rapid and significant changes that take place in the central nervous system, the impact is greater and has more serious consequences. Consumption in individuals under the age of 21 presents greater risks than for individuals who have already completed their neurodevelopment. In the adolescent brain, the functions performed by the frontal lobe, such as impulse control and emotions, are particularly affected.[4–9] Neuroimaging studies comparing adults and adolescents with chronic marijuana use have shown significant differences, suggesting greater sensitivity in adolescence to the effects of the substance on the brain, leading to greater impairment in functioning.[10] In particular, poorer performance has been demonstrated in executive functions, mainly in attention, cognitive processing, and memory. Structural alterations have also been observed, such as increased cortical thickness, suggesting a decrease in myelination.[9–11] In turn, initiating psychoactive substance use in early adolescence carries a number of additional risks compared to later ages. The earlier use begins, the more likely it is to have adverse consequences at all levels: cognitive, physical, emotional, academic, and social.

An important finding that has been documented is that starting to drink alcohol before the age of 16 is an indicator of a high risk of developing substance use disorders in the future and is associated with greater difficulties in treatment. In addition, early onset of alcohol consumption appears to be a precursor to the use of other drugs.[12]

Numerous studies have concluded that alcohol consumption during adolescence can have lasting effects and increase the risk of problematic alcohol consumption in adulthood.[13] These studies could explain the correlation between early use and a higher probability of developing dependence in adulthood.

Although it cannot be argued that all adolescents who get drunk today will be alcoholics tomorrow, the immediate impact of excessive consumption and its consequences on the developing adolescent brain must be recognized.[7] Furthermore, being under the influence of alcohol and other substances increases the likelihood of violent behavior, unprotected sex, and accidents.[4,5]

On the other hand, it should be noted that adolescents appear to be less vulnerable than adults to the sedative effects and impaired balance and motor coordination induced by alcohol consumption.[5] Findings suggest that, in comparative studies between adults and adolescents who have consumed the same amount of alcohol, the latter are able to stay awake longer and perform movements with greater coordination, and are more resistant to the intoxicating and aversive effects of alcohol, such as nausea, vomiting, anxiety, and speech disorders, which are often signals to stop drinking. These differences may lead to relatively higher tolerance and greater alcohol intake during adolescence.

Epidemiological Aspects

The prevalence and characteristics of substance use among adolescents are difficult to determine.[14] Existing studies are based on general surveys or analyze data that comes mainly from adolescents who seek care at specialized centers, so extrapolations to the universe of "all adolescents" should be made with caution.

However, it can be said that, in most national and international studies, alcohol, cannabis, and tobacco are the most commonly used substances at this stage, often showing a pattern of problematic poly-use of the three substances. In addition, in recent years, epidemiological studies of school populations have begun to show a high prevalence of energy-drink consumption.[3,15–17]

With regard to prevalence, surveys conducted in recent years on substance use among the student population have shown some stabilization in drug use among adolescents.[16] The 2019 ESPAD report states that although alcohol consumption among adolescents appears to have declined in many countries, the average remains very high: 80% of students report having consumed alcohol at least once and almost half in the last month.[15] With regard to other drugs, cannabis continues to be the most commonly reported in this study. Although the prevalence rates vary considerably among the different countries studied, with 16% of participants reporting having used cannabis at least once in their lifetime, while 7% reported having used it in the last month.

Some similar results can be observed in the *Monitoring the Future* project. The report published in 2019 (*Monitoring the Future, Key Findings on Adolescent Drug Use*) states that alcohol continues to be the substance most frequently consumed by adolescents. Compared to the results of the survey conducted in previous years, its use appears to have stabilized, with a gradual downward trend in recent years. Similarly, illicit drug use (marijuana is considered the most common) has not changed significantly since 2006. However, there has been a marked and continuous increase in consumption through "vaping" (inhaling vapor created by devices). In South American countries, studies also show comparable prevalences in substance use. According to various studies, it can be assumed that there is a qualitative and quantitative change in substance use among adolescents, which could be expressed according to the following formula: "Individuals who use drugs start doing so earlier in life and also use them more intensively" (Uruguayan Drug Observatory, 2020).[17] Alarming figures have been found for excessive consumption and intoxication. It can be observed that a pattern of alcohol consumption among young people has become established, characterized by exposure during the weekend and for the purpose of promoting leisure and social relationships among adolescents and young people. The problem with this pattern has to do with lifestyle, with the way of having fun, of being and of projecting oneself to the world.[18]

This pattern of consumption carries an added risk: it should be noted that the use of psychoactive substances can often be linked to psychiatric emergencies (such as suicide attempts) and is one of the most common reasons for visits to emergency departments by children and adolescents.[19,20] Finally, it should be noted that these data were analyzed in studies conducted before the advent of the COVID-19 pandemic, so it would be interesting to compare them in a few years when information is collected information from 2020 and 2021.

ETIOPATHOGENESIS OF SUBSTANCE ABUSE DISORDER AND DUAL DISORDER

Citing the intervention protocols for dual pathology, we can say that the onset and development of addiction and other comorbid mental disorders would result from the reciprocal interaction between individual vulnerability factors and environmental factors.

Clinical and epidemiological studies have shown that most individuals who use drugs will not develop dependence. This suggests that there is an individual vulnerability to the development of addiction, which has a solid basis in the interaction between environment and biology.

Therefore, it is interesting to highlight the available evidence that points to a clearly epigenetic origin, in which temperamental, genetic, individual, family, and sociocultural aspects are intertwined and constantly interact with each other.

It has been found that certain temperamental traits might be associated with a greater predisposition to substance use, such as extroversion, behavioral disinhibition, and novelty-seeking.[21]

Also, from a genetic point of view, evidence from family, twin, and adoption studies shows that heredity may play an important role in substance use disorder.

On the other hand, at the family level, conflict and family separation are associated with increases in problematic consumption and behavioral problems.[22] A certain association has also been found with the use of violence, punishment as a means of setting limits, very rigid or inconsistent parenting styles, insufficient parental control, and neglect.[22]

Substance abuse by parents is another important factor. It has been shown that parental drug use is strongly correlated with and predictive of substance abuse in adolescents and the development of substance use disorders.[23]

Parental personality factors and attitudes toward their child's drug use appear to play a significant role in drug use.[24] It has been objectively established that substance use and antisocial personality in parents are predictive factors for physical and verbal domestic abuse.[22] Another important indicator is adolescents' perception of their parents' tolerance of alcohol and marijuana use, with higher consumption observed among adolescents who perceive that their parents allow or tolerate it.[17]

Thus, intergenerational transmission may be influenced by genetic factors and/or reflect the parental model of drug use. Likewise, there are also indirect effects of adolescent drug use, such as choosing friends with families that allow drug use.[25]

On the other hand, peer groups exert a great deal of influence on adolescents and can act as a restraining force or, conversely, as a driving force for experimentation with drugs or involvement in behavioral problems that can be modulated in one direction or another by family dynamics.

Culture and legislation also have a significant impact. This relates to the accessibility and availability of substances, and is linked to the regulations in force in each country, social acceptance, and the impact of the media and advertising, which can encourage or discourage the use of different drugs.[24,25]

Another area that deserves special attention is the study of transdiagnostic vulnerability factors (independent of psychopathological symptoms themselves). These have been shown to contribute to the development of emotional syndromes characterized by mood disturbances and anxiety associated with substance abuse.[26] Three transdiagnostic factors may be relevant in the association between emotional disorders and substance use: stress tolerance, which is characterized by the ability to tolerate physical and psychological stress,[27] is associated with anxiety disorders and depression and predisposes individuals to substance use as a way of alleviating these symptoms. Anhedonia is the tendency to experience little pleasure in response to rewards and is positively linked to substance use, through the pursuit of pleasure in experimenting with substances as a way to counteract the inability to achieve pleasurable feelings.

Anxiety sensitivity involves experiencing anxiety symptoms and is a robust risk factor for the onset of anxiety disorders. It has been associated with substance use, possibly because the motivation to use drugs may mitigate anxiety symptoms.

Other factors that have been identified include negative and positive affectivity with substance use in adolescents.[26]

While these hypotheses seem interesting from a theoretical point of view, there are few studies documenting the association of these factors in adolescents, with some data supporting the association of stress tolerance, anhedonia, and anxiety sensitivity and others showing no association at all.

Further study of the role of these factors might be useful in developing strategies for the prevention of mental illness and substance use.

Clinical: Diagnostic Perspective

The use of psychoactive substances is strongly associated with psychiatric morbidity in children, adolescents, and adults. In the pediatric population, due to major changes in nervous system development, there is increased vulnerability. This results in a synergistic effect between drug use and mental health problems.

In childhood and adolescence, it is important to emphasize that in order to establish diagnoses, exhaustive assessments must be carried out with the child and their caregivers, and the enormous variables of normality must be well understood, since behaviors that may be normal at a certain age become pathological at other stages of development. At this age, experimental use, occasional use, and frequent intoxication are not the same thing.

Furthermore, it is essential in adolescence to consider the repercussions that consumption may have. Some reviews of the prognoses for these adolescents were associated with school absenteeism, rebellious behavior, academic problems, and educational dropout.[28,29] It is clear that these consequences can have an impact on the prognosis for these young people.

Despite all these considerations, there are some psychiatric disorders that are more frequently associated with substance use in adolescence. It has been given that there is a close relationship between behavioral disorders and drug use in adolescence. On the one hand, substance abuse is considered a risk factor for antisocial behavior, and on the other, adolescent users have a higher prevalence of oppositional defiant disorder and conduct disorder (CD). In addition, it has been found that childhood-onset conduct disorder is linked to a worse prognosis in relation to drug use.[30] This conceptualization is very important because, as Pérez de los Cobos points out, "externalized disorders, and especially early-onset CD, would be the rule in early dual disorders."

If we consider the symptoms, the main psychopathological predictor of early-onset addiction is the existence of alterations in the aggression/impulsivity spectrum, which can be considered causal factors for subsequent problematic drug use, determining a high vulnerability to this pathology.[44]

Another condition that requires special consideration is attention deficit hyperactivity disorder (ADHD). This is a neurodevelopmental disorder whose symptoms begin in childhood and have a heterochronic presentation, changing over time and with the development of the central nervous system (APA, 2013). Children with ADHD are more likely than other children to develop a personality disorder in adolescence and antisocial personality in adulthood, and consequently, the possibility of substance use and criminal behavior increases. [31] The risk of developing a substance use disorder is high in young people with ADHD, especially when a personality disorder or antisocial personality develops. Impulsivity has been found to be associated with early onset of alcohol use in adolescents, while hyperactivity has been linked to arrest in young adults on charges such as illegal drug possession, use, and sale. Although still under debate, there appears to be sufficient evidence that appropriate and timely treatment of ADHD could prevent the later development of problematic use of substances.[32] However, it can be concluded that children with ADHD should be systematically assessed, treated, and monitored as a way to prevent problematic drug use in the future.

On the other hand, internalized disorders may also mean vulnerability to drug use, although there are no conclusive specific data on adolescents. However, it is important to bear in mind certain considerations when dealing with these diagnoses in the early stages, as their timely detection and treatment could lead to more favorable outcomes.

Mood disorders, which are also associated with substance use, have different clinical presentations in the pediatric population than in adults, which is why they often go unrecognized and are diagnosed late, with obvious consequences. With regard to suicide, there is literature confirming an increase in the suicide rate among young people who use substances.[33]

Anxiety disorders are common in clinical populations of children and adolescents. However, due to their internalized nature, their symptoms are not easily detectable by others, including family members and educational references. Among anxious adolescents, the theory of self-medication can be considered a theoretical basis for understanding, according to which the choice to consume a substance "allows" the desired disinhibition. Within this conceptualization, adolescents seek to alleviate symptoms that involve deficits in affectivity, self-esteem, self-care, social relationships, or, in some cases, an already established anxiety or mood disorder.

It is also important to consider the high incidence of traumatic events and symptoms of post-traumatic stress disorder (PTSD) among adolescents with problematic drug use.[34] It has been found that the association between PTSD and problematic drug use is common and is associated with a more complex prognosis when compared to either condition separately.[34] According to various authors, the frequency of PTSD in adolescent users is significant, so it is important to inquire with due caution about exposure to traumatic events in the medical history, which may be even more prevalent among females.[34]

PREVENTION AND TARGETED INTERVENTIONS

The economic costs and damages associated with drug use are considerable. Although the evidence in favor of universal preventive measures is convincing, there is debate as to whether it is preferable to focus on universal interventions (legislative measures, laws, penalties, media campaigns) or to target specific high-risk groups (selective and indicated prevention).[25] In the latter case, programs targeting adolescents appear to be essential. The objectives of prevention are to reduce or delay initiation of use, delay progression from experimentation to problematic use, and avoid complications.[26] Educational institutions are optimal locations for implementing prevention programs, as they offer an effective way to reach young people and identify students who are using excessively, making it possible to implement a wide range of educational measures.[35,36] Prevention programs that focus on promoting social skills in adolescents rather than on the effects of drugs are more likely to report long-term benefits than other interventions.[37]

As a general rule, when dealing with adolescents, one must learn to wait for the "right moment" to intervene, recognizing that sometimes it is best to "do nothing." Interventions should not be rushed, and one should recognize that sometimes it is best to "do nothing." Interventions should not be rushed due to the need for quick answers; rather, the necessary time should be taken to carefully analyze each situation and define what should be done to respond appropriately to the problems of the adolescent drug user.

Problematic drug use among adolescents is often a complex issue. Any adolescent who shows signs of drug use should undergo a screening procedure.[38] One factor that often leads to inappropriate interventions is the prevailing prejudice that "Behind every adolescent who uses drugs there is a potential criminal, addict, or mentally ill person." It should always be borne in mind that the fact that an adolescent might be using drugs does not necessarily imply the existence of a disorder requiring intensive treatment.

Thus, it may be appropriate to establish an intervention proposal based on the risk detected in each individual or group. Three levels of intervention can be established on this continuum:[39]

- **Universal intervention**: As part of health promotion strategies
- **Selective intervention**: In people at risk, with the aim of preventing and reducing risks
- **Indicated intervention**: Related to treatment and rehabilitation

However, when an adolescent is identified as being at risk and a decision is made to implement specific treatment (an indicated intervention), the objectives must go beyond mere detoxification or cessation of use, facilitating understanding and attention to other related aspects. The therapeutic strategy, defined jointly with the patient and their family, should consider the treatment of psychiatric disorders, if any, and problematic drug use. These approaches should be carried out simultaneously, adapting the intensity of the intervention and resources to the severity of the problems.[3,40]

Specific programs for adolescents generally consist of adaptations of programs designed for adults with dual pathology. To date, the treatments that have proven most effective in studies involving this population are family-based ecological treatment and individual and group cognitive-behavioral therapy.[41,42]

However, there is consensus in all treatment plans that treatment should be integrated and coordinated, taking into account the link with the educational institution, paying attention to recreational, occupational, and leisure activities, peer relationships, and, fundamentally, the adolescent's bond with their family.

The family forms the core reference point and provides role models, but adolescents are still dependent on adult role models. Research on interventions with adolescents reports that approaches involving the family are essential, even in relation to those aimed at peer groups and individuals alone.[40]

On the other hand, evidence indicates that educational institutions are a protective factor.[17] In cases of dropout, it is necessary to assess the reasons that lead to this situation. Often, a situation arises in which the adolescent rejects the institution, but the institution also disregards the adolescent, frequently due to behavioral difficulties and difficulties adapting to educational norms.[43] These characteristics mean that prevention and intervention during adolescence must take into account the special characteristics of this stage, while maintaining close coordination within the framework of continuous evaluation.[44–46]

REFERENCES

1. Matalí Costa JL, Pardo Gallego M, Trenchs Sainz de la Maza V, Serrano Troncoso E, Gabaldon Fraile S, Luaces Cubells C. Drug use in adolescents. Ethical dilemma in the diagnostic-therapeutic approach. An Pediatr (Barc). 2009;70(4): 386–90.
2. Roberts RE, Roberts CR, Xing Y. Comorbidity of substance use disorders and other psychiatric disorders among adolescents: evidence from an epidemiological survey. Drug Alcohol Depend. 2007;88:S4–13.
3. Goti Elejalde, J, Diaz Hurtado R, Arango, C. Protocolos de intervención. Patología Dual. Barcelona (Spain): EdikaMed SL, 2016.
4. Rossi G, Carbajal M. Los adolescentes y sus comportamientos. In: G. Rossi, M. Carbajal, A. Bottrill (eds.), La Previa: El consumo de alcohol entre los adolescentes. Aguilar, 2011.
5. Spear L. Alcohol and the developing Brain (Chapter 5). In: J Saunders, JM Rey (eds.), Young People and alcohol: Impact, Policy, Prevention, Treatment. Wiley Blackwell, 2011.
6. White A. Alcohol: una amenaza para el desarrollo neuropsicológico de los adolescentes. Durham (United States): Duke University, 2004.
7. Tapert S. (2004). Consumo de alcohol en adolescentes: efectos sobre el cerebro. Pharmacists. 2007;330:13–14.
8. Rossi G. Programas de reducción de daños en el manejo del uso para niños y adolescentes en curso, Abordaje integral para la prevención y reducción de las consecuencias adversas del consumo de drogas en poblaciones en situación de alta vulnerabilidad: una estrategia de salud pública. COPOLAD, 2019.
9. Lopez-Larson MP, Bogorodzki P, Rogowska J, McGlade E, King JB, Terry J, *et al.* Altered prefrontal and insular cortical thickness in adolescent marijuana users. Behav Brain Res. 2011;220(1):164–72. doi: 10.1016/j.bbr.2011.02.001.
10. Blest-Hopley G, Giampietro V, Bhattacharyya S. Residual effects of cannabis use in adolescent and adult brains - A meta-analysis of fMRI studies. Neurosci Biobehav Rev. 2018;88:26–41. doi:10.1016/j.neubiorev.2018.03.008
11. Jager G, Block RI, Luijten M, Ramsey NF. Cannabis use and memory brain function in adolescent boys: a cross-sectional multicenter functional magnetic resonance imaging study. J Am Acad Child Adolesc Psychiatry. 2010;49(6):561–72.
12. Skidemore S, Juhasz R, Zucker R. Early onset drinking (Chapter 2). In: J Saunders, JM Rey(eds.), Young People and alcohol: Impact, Policy, Prevention, Treatment. Wiley Blackwell, 2011.
13. Center for Substance Abuse Treatment. Incorporating Alcohol Pharmacotherapies into Medical Practice. Treatment Improvement Protocol (TIP) Series 49. HHS Publication No. (SMA) 09–4380. Rockville, MD: Substance Abuse and Mental Health Services Administration, 2009.

14. Buckstein OG, Brent DA, Kaminer Y. Comorbidity of substance abuse and other psychiatric disorders in adolescents. Am J Psychiat. 1989;146:1131–41.
15. Mokinaro S, Vincente J, Benedetti E, Cerrai S, Colasante E, Arpa S, *et al.* ESPAD Report, 2019. Results from European School Survey Project on Alcohol and Other Drugs. Luxembourg: Publications Office of the European Union, 2020.
16. Johnston L, Miech R, O'Malley P, Bachman J, Schulenberg J, Patrick M. Monitoring the Future national survey results on drug use, 1975–2019: Overview, key findings on adolescent drug use. National Institute on Drug Abuse National Institutes of Health U.S. Department of Health & Human Services, 2020.
17. Uruguayan Drug Observatory (OUD). VIII Encuesta Nacional sobre Consumo de Drogas en Estudiantes de Enseñanza Media. Uruguay: National Drug Secretariat, 2020.
18. Maturana A. Adolescencia y Consumo de Drogas. Rev Med Clin Condes. 2011;22(1):98–109.
19. Gobbi G, Atkin T, Zytynski T, Wang S, Askari S, Boruff J, *et al.* Association of cannabis use in adolescence and risk of depression, anxiety, and suicidality in young adulthood: a systematic review and meta-analysis. JAMA Psychiatry. 2019;76(4):426–34.
20. Prinstein MJ, Nock MK, Simon V, Aikins JW, Cheah CS, Spirito A. Longitudinal trajectories and predictors of adolescent suicidal ideation and attempts following inpatient hospitalization. J Consult Clin Psychol. 2008;76(1): 92.
21. Albores-Gallo L, Márquez-Caraveo ME, Estañol B. ¿Qué es el temperamento? El retorno de un concepto ancestral. Mental Health. 2003;26(3):16–26.
22. Barea J, Benito A, Real M, Mateu C, Martín E, López N, *et al.* Estudio sobre aspectos etiológicos de la patología dual. Addictions. 2010;22(1):15–24.
23. Buckstein OG. Comorbidity and adolescent substance abuse. In: T. W. Estroff (ed.), Manual of Adolescent Substance Abuse Treatment. American Psychiatric Publishing, Inc, 2001:69–89.
24. Brook J, Brook D, Pahl K. The developmental context for adolescent substance abuse intervention (Chapter 2). In: Howard A Liddle, Cynthia L Rowe (eds.), Adolescent Substance Abuse: Research and Clinical Advances. Cambridge: Cambridge University Press, 2006.
25. Rey JM. Trastornos por consumo de sustancias. Abuso de Alcohol. IACAPAP Textbook, 2019.
26. Cheung W, Kit-sum Lam A, Hung S. Uso de otras sustancias. IACAPAP Textbook, 2017.
27. Leyro TM, Zvolensky MJ, Bernstein A. Distress tolerance and psychopathological symptoms and disorders: A review of the empirical literature among adults. Psychol Bull. 2010; 136(4):576.
28. Angold A, Costello EJ, Erkanli A. Comorbidity. J Child Psychol Psychiat. 1999;40:57–87.
29. Costello EJ, Mustillo S, Erkanli A, Keeler G, Angold A. Prevalence and development of psychiatric disorders in childhood and adolescence. Arch Gen Psychiatry. 2003;60(8):837–44.
30. Myers MG, Stewart DG, Brown SA. Progression from conduct disorder to antisocial personality disorder following treatment for adolescent substance abuse. Am J Psychiatry 1998;155: 479–85.
31. Rossi G. Evaluación del trastorno por déficit atencional con hiperactividad en población de usuarios problemáticos de drogas. Rev Psiquiatr Urug. 2009; 73 (1):109–18.
32. Wilens T, Biederman J, Spencer T. ADHD across the lifespan. Annu Rev Med. 2002;53:113–31.
33. Esposito-Smythers C, Spirito A. Adolescent substance use and suicidal behavior: a review with implications for treatment research. Alcohol Clin Exp Res. 2004;28(5 Suppl):77S–88S.
34. McCauley JL, Killeen T, Gros DF, Brady KT, Back SE. Posttraumatic stress disorder and co-occurring substance use disorders: Advances in assessment and treatment. Clin Psychol (New York). 2012;19(3):10. doi: 10.1111/cpsp.12006.
35. Porath-Waller AJ, Beasley E, Beirness DJ. A meta-analytic review of school-based prevention for cannabis use. Health Educ Behav. 2010;37(5):709–23.
36. Stormshak EA, Connell AM, Véronneau MH, Myers MW, Dishion TJ, Kavanagh K, *et al.* An ecological approach to promoting early adolescent mental health and social adaptation: Family-centered intervention in public middle schools. Child Dev. 2011;82(1):209–25.

37. Foxcroft DR, Tsertsvadze A. Universal school-based prevention programs for alcohol misuse in young people. Cochrane Database Syst Rev. 2011 May 11;(5):CD009113.
38. Winters K (editor). Screening and Assessing adolescents for substance use disorders. Treatment Improvement Protocol (TIP) Series. No.31. SAMHSA-CSAT, 1998.
39. Salvador Llivina T, de Silva Rivera A. Guía de buenas prácticas y calidad en la prevención de drogodependencias en la comunidad autónoma de la región de Murcia. Murcia: Regional Plan on Drugs, 2010.
40. Becoña E. Bases científicas de la prevención de las drogodependencias. Madrid: National Plan on Drugs, 2002.
41. Hogue A, Henderson C, Becker S, Knisht D. Evidence Base on Outpatient Behavioral Treatments for Adolescent Substance Use, 2014–2017: Outcomes, Treatment Delivery, and Promising Horizons. J Clin Child Adolesc Psychol. 2018;47(4):499–526.
42. García Delgado Marina. Adolescentes y jóvenes con patología dual. Intervención desde un Centro de atención a la drogodependencia. J Dual Pathol. 2015;2(3):17.
43. CONACE (Technical Area of Treatment and Rehabilitation. National Council for the Control of Narcotics). Tratamiento de Drogas. Guía de asesoría clínica para programas de tratamiento y rehabilitación en Drogas para población infantoadolescente y sus especificidades. Santiago (Chile): Editores e Impresores Aconcagua S.A., 2008.
44. Morrison J. DSM-5® Guía para el diagnóstico clínico. Mexico City (Mexico): Editorial El Manual Moderno, 2015.
45. Pérez de los Cobos Peris JL. Trastornos duales: adicciones relacionadas con trastornos mentales en la infancia o la adolescencia. Un reto de asistencia y prevención. Barcelona: Ars Médica, 2009.
46. World Health Organization. Neurociencia del consume y dependencia de sustancias psicoactivas: resumen. World Health Organization, 2004.

10.5 SUBSTANCES AND DUAL PATHOLOGY

10.5.1 PSYCHOACTIVE SUBSTANCES IN DUAL PATHOLOGY

C. Sena Vasconcelos

INTRODUCTION

Psychoactive substances are chemicals that act primarily on the central nervous system, altering brain function and creating temporary changes in perception, mood, behavior, and consciousness. In this chapter, we will analyze the main groups of psychoactive substances, their neurobiological characteristics, and their impact on physical and mental health. We will begin with a historical and geographical perspective.

HISTORICAL AND GEOGRAPHICAL PERSPECTIVE OF THE "PLANTS OF THE GODS"

The consumption of plants with psychoactive properties has accompanied humanity since its beginnings, and their type and characteristics were related to the native flora of the places that were successively occupied. Globalization promoted by trade routes (e.g., the Silk Road) and the conquest of territories did the rest.

The prehistory of the consumption of psychoactive substances from plants is very difficult to trace. However, the study of archeological remains, using modern methods of analysis, images, statues, and writings, sheds some light on a period of time spanning tens of thousands of years. In fact, with the exception of Antarctica, psychoactive substances exist in all regions of the world, in all cultures and peoples.

The oldest trace of a potentially psychoactive plant is *Ephedra altissima*, a species dating back to around 50,000 BC found in a Neanderthal deposit inside a cave in Kurdistan (northern Iraq). Another trace, of *Papaver somniferum* seeds, was found at the bottom of Lake Bracciano, at the site known as La Marmotta, near Rome. This remnant, from the early Neolithic period, is about 7,700 years old. There is also evidence in China regarding the use of cannabis in cord-marked pottery dating back to 10,000 BC (York and Garden, 2018).

Opium and wine appeared in Eurasia. Opium extracted from *P. somniferum* appears in civilizations in the Fertile Crescent regions (Nile and Ganges valleys); vineyards appear on the slopes of the Black Sea.

Cannabis sativa is planted in Asian steppes and some regions of China (York and Garden, 2018).

Some Swiss researchers also observed the indigenous use of the plant *Radula marginata* (which contains cannabinoids) in New Zealand, where it is endemic.[1]

The American territories were occupied by Siberian tribes, who crossed the Bering Strait (which, during the last ice age, connected Asia and America via an extensive ice sheet). These peoples were already familiar with the effects of the mushroom *Amanita muscaria*, which they used for shamanic purposes. Coca, hallucinogenic mushrooms, and tobacco were used by these peoples. The various civilizations that flourished in Mesoamerica demonstrated great knowledge and experience in the use of numerous hallucinogens[2] which they used in magical, therapeutic, and religious rituals.[3]

Hemp, iboga, khat, and kola nuts are found in Africa. In India, the Philippines, Taiwan, and Malaysia, betel (misnamed, because it is the areca nut that is consumed with leaves from the plant that produces the betel pepper) is chewed by a large percentage of the population. In Australia, Aboriginal tribes consume *pituri*, which is a mixture of dried *Nicotiana spp.* leaves (containing tobacco) with acacia or *eucalyptus* wood ash.

Historians speculate about the use of entheogens in ancient Judaism and early Gnostic Christianity—e.g., in Moses' visions of the "burning bush," which is the acacia tree, rich in dimethyltryptamine (DMT entheogens), a substance analogous to that found in ayahuasca.

The consumption of psychoactive substances has been linked since its inception to religious rituals and therapeutic procedures, which are closely associated. It was not until long after Hippocrates (5th century BC) that it began to be used for medical purposes unrelated to religion.[4]

The Bible refers to wine and its effects in an episode in Genesis 9:18–28. "Noah, who was a farmer, began to till the ground and planted the first vineyard. Having drunk wine, he became drunk and stripped naked inside his tent" (Figure 10.5).

Initial experiments with addictive substances produce euphoria and extremely pleasant sensations, which induce people to continue consuming these substances, despite the significant harm that this consumption causes. Continued consumption causes structural

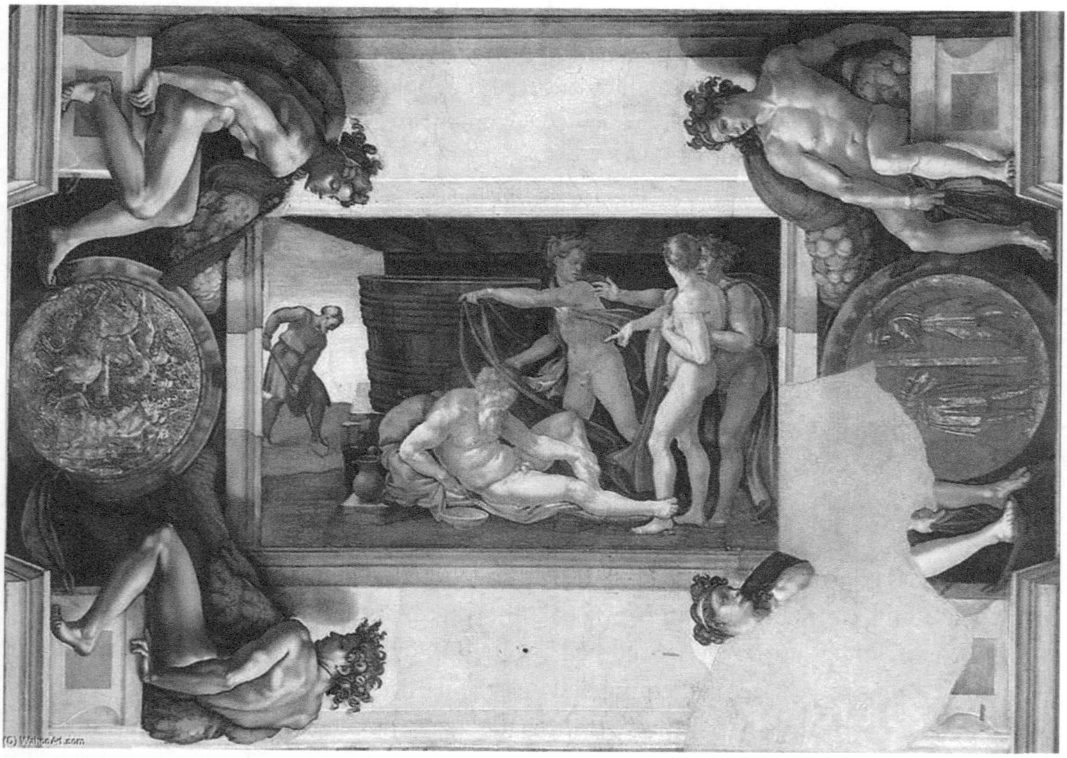

FIGURE 10.5 Michelangelo: Noah's drunkenness.

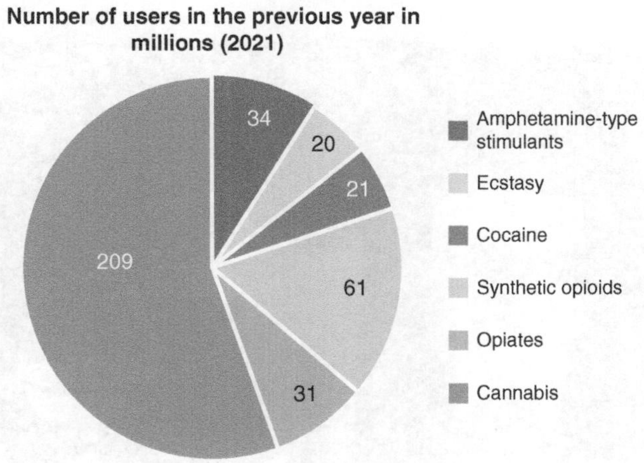

FIGURE 10.6 Psychoactive substance use worldwide in 2021, *World Drug Report*, 2022 (UNODOC).

and functional changes in the brain, called neuroadaptations. These neuroadaptations compromise brain function and cause a transition from occasional, controlled consumption to chronic consumption, which is difficult to control. Furthermore, these changes remain long after consumption has ceased, which explains the high percentage of relapse in the first year after treatment.[5]

Psychoactive Substance Use Worldwide

In 2021, 209 million people used cannabis, making it the most widely used illicit substance worldwide (see Figure 10.6). In comparison, 92 million people used opioids. Although smaller in number, this group accounted for 66% of drug-related deaths (overdoses) recorded in 2017 (estimated total number, 167,000 people) and represented 21 million years lost due to disability and premature death attributed to drug use. Stimulants, cocaine, and methamphetamine are experiencing sustained growth. Around 21 million people used cocaine in 2021 and 27 million used amphetamines.[6]

ALCOHOL

First you have a drink, then the drink has a drink, then the drink takes you.

F. Scott Fitzgerald, *The Great Gatsby*

Ethanol, also called ethyl alcohol, or simply alcohol, is an organic substance obtained from the fermentation of sugars. About 10 million years ago, human ancestors developed an enzyme capable of rapidly digesting alcohol: alcoholic dehydrogenase (from the ADH4 gene). This allowed early *Homo sapiens* to digest ethanol from naturally fermented fruit more than 100,000 years.[7] Alcoholic beverages were invented independently, and at various different times, on every continent except Antarctica. Alcoholic beverages made from fermented sugars from various types of fruit, cereals, or starchy roots have been present in different civilizations for the past 10,000 years.[8]

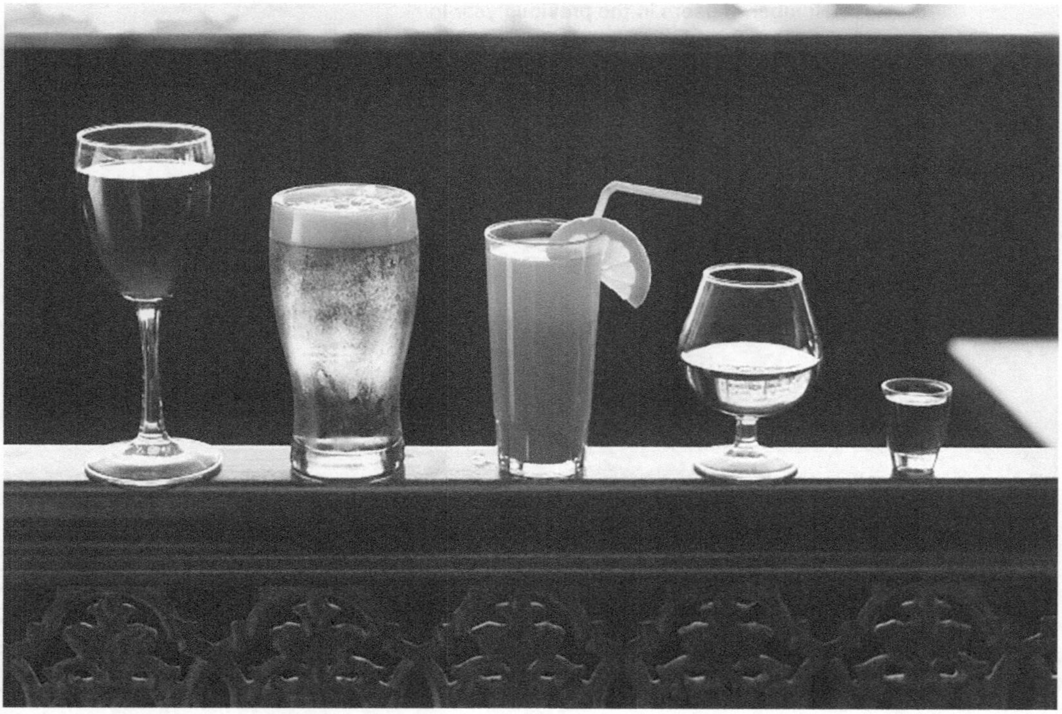

FIGURE 10.7 Standard "drinks" illustrated. Each container corresponds to one standard drink.

The fermentation of sugar into ethanol is, therefore, one of the earliest biotechnologies used by humankind.

It is customary to measure ethanol consumption using standard drink units, which are equivalent to 10–12 grams of pure ethanol. In Figure 10.7, each container is equivalent to one standard drink.

Ethanol is consumed worldwide by 2.4 billion people, making it the most widely consumed legal substance-drug in the world (Global Status Report, 2018 nd).

Action on Neurotransmission Systems

Ethanol consumption produces a wide variety of physiological and behavioral effects that depend on the amount consumed. From lowest to highest, and in a non-tolerant individual, these effects can include anxiolysis, muscle relaxation, analgesia, sedation, amnesia, hypothermia, and anesthesia, in succession. It causes changes in the cardiovascular, digestive, central and peripheral nervous systems, musculoskeletal system, and fetus. Ethanol causes profound depression of neuronal functions and decreases glucose metabolism in the human brain. It is now known that alcohol interacts with specific proteins in the neuronal membrane that are involved in signal transmission, causing changes in neuronal activity. Ethanol mainly interacts with membrane receptors, GABAA, NMDA, and GlyR. GABA is the main inhibitory neurotransmitter, and glutamate is the main excitatory neurotransmitter. With the combined effects of ethanol, the action of GABA and the antagonism of glutamate action are strengthened. Allosterically, ethanol potentiates the action of GABA or any activator of this system, such as BZD or barbiturates, stimulating chloride flux induced by GABAA receptors. These adaptations of the GABAA receptor may be important for understanding the marked increase in excitability that characterizes withdrawal. In addition, several GABAA gene polymorphisms have been found to be associated with dependence (especially its severity) and alcohol withdrawal.[9]

Chronic exposure to ethanol causes a decrease in the sensitivity of $GABA_A$ receptor-mediated responses, including sedative effects, motor incoordination, and acute cognitive impairment.[10] Chronic intermittent exposure to ethanol caused activation of tyrosine kinase phosphorylation regulation in laboratory animals in the su-β_2 and Y_2.[11]

The effect of alcohol on glutamatergic systems is based on the modulation of ionotropic glutamate receptors. The NMDA receptor forms a cation channel, whose activation increases the permeability of Na^+, K^+ and, especially, Ca^+, causing the depolarization of the neuronal membrane. The acute action of ethanol on this receptor reduces the flow through the channel and alters synaptic function, inhibiting the release of neurotransmitters. Chronic alcohol administration produces adaptive upregulation of the NMDA receptor. During withdrawal, these receptors undergo rebound activation, which can result in *delirium tremens* and, especially, seizures (the most serious complications of alcohol withdrawal).[12]

But other systems are also affected: dopaminergic, opioid (particularly in reward systems), serotonergic, noradrenergic, cannabinoid, and corticotropin-releasing factor systems. Alcohol activates the mesocorticolimbic dopaminergic system, increasing endorphin concentrations. and releasing dopamine in the *nucleus accumbens*. Alcohol acts directly on μ receptors and releases endogenous opioids, such as enkephalin. These actions of alcohol allow us to understand the use of opioid antagonists, such as naltrexone or nalmefene, to promote the blocking of μ receptors, with the aim of preventing relapses. Given the presence of presynaptic cannabinoid receptors in glutamatergic and GABAergic synapses, alcohol increases the release of endocannabinoids, which together with endogenous opioids, increase its euphoric effects. There are deficits in serotonergic transmission, including low serotonin content in the brain, a decrease in serotonin cells and fibers, an upregulatory compensation of 5HT1A receptors, and reduced availability of serotonin transporters.[12]

Changes in serotonin transmission appear to be more relevant in type II alcoholism, with antisocial personality traits, high heritability, and early onset of the disease, compared to type I alcoholism, characterized by anxious traits, late onset, and social traits.[12]

Ethanol Modulation of Signaling Systems

Ethanol can also modulate the function of intracellular signaling cascades that include cyclic AMP (cAMP), protein kinase A (PKA), and protein kinase C (PKC), among others. Significant advances have been made in this area, and this study may lead to new drugs of interest in the treatment of alcohol use disorders.[13]

Alcohol Consumption and Physical and Mental Health

There are multiple risk factors that can contribute to both psychosis and addiction. There are strong associations between substance use disorder and polygenic risk scores for schizophrenia, indicating that genetic susceptibility shared susceptibility may contribute to the co-occurrence of the two disorders. This has been confirmed by genomic studies.[12]

Ethanol consumption is the third leading preventable cause of death after smoking and hypertension. Around 38% of adults worldwide report drinking alcohol in the last 12 months. According to the World Health Organization (WHO), alcohol consumption is linked to more than 200 diseases and health problems related to injuries. Alcohol consumption accounts for approximately 4.2% of the total burden of disease measured in disability-adjusted life years (DALYs).[14]

TOBACCO

Quitting smoking is easy; I've done it a thousand times.

Mark Twain

Tobacco has been smoked in the Americas for at least 3,000 years (Figure 10.8). Tobacco was discovered during the voyages of Christopher Columbus and other navigators to America and brought to Europe.

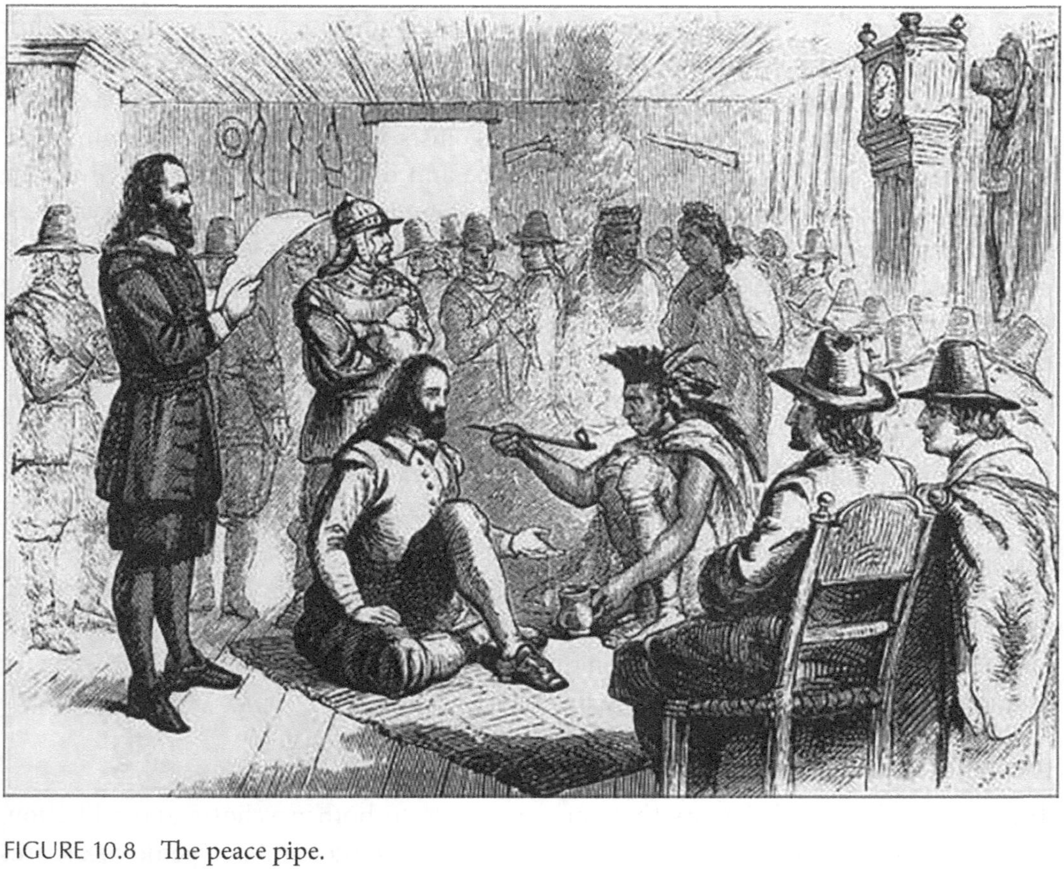

FIGURE 10.8 The peace pipe.

In 1560, Jean Nicot, French ambassador to Portugal, attributed special powers to the plant (and gave his name to the active substance, nicotine). Initially, smokers smoked cigars or pipes.[15] The cigarette was invented by Turkish soldiers who surrounded the city of San Juan de Acre in 1832. They put tobacco in the paper cylinders that wrapped the gunpowder and lit them to smoke them. Later, the machines of the Industrial Revolution did the rest: millions of cigarettes began to be produced. Nicotine is a tertiary amine consisting of pyridine and a pyrrolidine ring. (S)-nicotine, found in tobacco, binds stereoselectively to nicotinic cholinergic receptors. (R)-nicotine is a weak agonist at the nicotinic cholinergic receptor.

When a person inhales cigarette smoke, nicotine distilled from tobacco is carried in smoke particles to the lungs, where it is quickly absorbed into the pulmonary venous circulation. It then enters the arterial circulation and moves rapidly to the brain (in 10–19 seconds). Nicotine spreads rapidly in brain tissue, where it binds to nicotinic cholinergic receptors, which are ligand-gated ion channels. When the cholinergic agonist binds to the outside of the channel, it opens, allowing cations such as Na^+ and K^+[16] to enter (Figure 10.9). Nicotine produces stimulation and pleasure in humans and reduces stress and anxiety. Smokers consume nicotine to modulate their level of stimulation and control their mood in their daily lives. Smoking can increase concentration, reaction time, and performance in certain tasks. When a person stops smoking, nicotine withdrawal symptoms arise. These can include irritability, frustration or anger, depressed mood, restlessness, anxiety, problems in relationships with family and friends, difficulty concentrating, increased appetite and food intake, insomnia, and cravings to smoke. Nicotine withdrawal in untreated smokers produces mood changes comparable to those seen in psychiatric outpatients. Nicotine withdrawal and withdrawal from other drugs of abuse cause hedonic dysregulation, a feeling that there is little pleasure in life and that activities that were once rewarding are no longer so. It has been hypothesized that a relative deficiency in dopamine release,

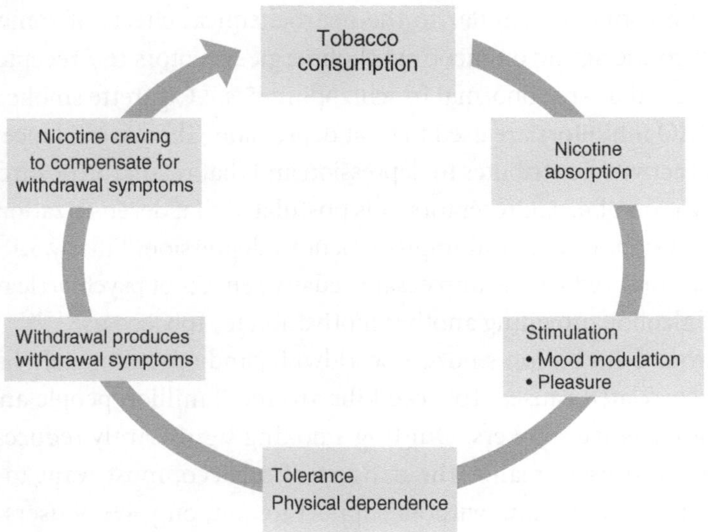

FIGURE 10.9 Nicotine addiction cycle (Prochaska and Benowitz).

after long-term exposure to nicotine, contributes to many mood disorders and anhedonia, as well as the urge to smoke, which can persist in smokers long after they quit. As a result, the pharmacological basis of nicotine addiction can be understood as a combination of positive reinforcements, such as improved mood and functioning, and avoidance of the negative consequences of previous substance use, which is the relief of withdrawal symptoms when nicotine is unavailable.

Smoking is a highly efficient way to administer a substance, as it enters the bloodstream quickly through the lungs and reaches the brain in seconds. Inhaled substances bypass first-pass intestinal metabolism and hepatic metabolism. The faster the rate of absorption and delivery of the drug to the brain, the greater the reinforcing effect of a drug. Inhalation produces high concentrations of a substance in the brain, comparable to those seen with intravenous administration. Because smokers regulate their nicotine intake to maintain their own nicotine levels in the body throughout the day, people who metabolize nicotine more quickly also absorb more cigarette smoke per day more quickly, compared to slower metabolizers. Genetically poor metabolizers (i.e., people with CYP2A6 gene variants associated with reduced enzyme activity) smoke fewer cigarettes per day on average and appear to be less dependent, based on the observation that the proportion of slow metabolizers decreases at higher ages in the smoking cohort, suggesting that this group may quit smoking more easily.[18]

Recent studies of the genome-wide association point to several genes that show promising signals as genetic determinants of nicotine dependence.

Tobacco addiction is much more common in people with mental illnesses and substance use disorders. Patients with more severe psychiatric symptoms are more likely to be smokers. Smokers with a history of major depression are at greater risk of relapse into depression after quitting smoking. Several mechanisms are thought to underlie the comorbidity between nicotine addiction and mental health disorders. There appears to be a shared genetic susceptibility with alcohol abuse and major depression. Nicotine may also be useful in treating certain psychiatric symptoms. For example, the serotonin and norepinephrine released in the brain by nicotine are similar to the neurochemical effects of some antidepressant medications. Nicotine acting on nicotinic cholinergic receptors α-7 receptors can improve the "sensory gates" that are abnormal in schizophrenics.[17] Cigarette smoke inhibits MAOA and MAOB. MAO inhibitors are used to treat depression. There is evidence that that excessive cholinergic activity contributes to depression and that regular exposure to nicotine can cause desensitization of nACh receptors. It is postulated that desensitization of these receptors causes mood stabilization and improvement in depression. Finally, nicotine, due to its stimulant effects, may reduce the unpleasant sedative effects of psychiatric medications and the sedation of alcohol, providing another motivation for tobacco use.[15,16]

There are around 1.3 billion smokers worldwide, and approximately half of them will die from tobacco-related causes. Tobacco kills around 8 million people annually, 1.2 million of whom are passive smokers. Quitting smoking significantly reduces the associated risks. When tobacco users realize the dangers of tobacco, most want to quit. However, nicotine is highly addictive, and without support to quit, only 4% of users who try to quit tobacco use will succeed. Professional support and proven smoking cessation medications can more than double a tobacco user's chances of successfully quitting the habit.[19]

CANNABIS

Two eminent scientists at the NIH said that the endocannabinoid system is involved in essentially all human disease. This is a very strong statement, but it seems to be correct. Today we know that the endocannabinoid system—the receptors, the endocannabinoids, the enzymes that form and break down the endocannabinoids—are involved in many physiological reactions and therefore in many disease states.

Mechoulam

Twelve-thousand years ago, as the last ice age was ending, primitive humans in the Upper Paleolithic period planted the first *cannabis sativa* crops on the border between what is now northern Mongolia and southern Siberia. The globalization of this culture followed the pace of trade with neighboring countries and the Silk Road, where caravans have been crossing Asia for millennia and reaching the Near East and from there, Eastern Europe. It was naturally integrated into Greek and Roman cultures. Bronze Age people were particularly important for the spread of this culture. It also reached India, where it was integrated into religious rituals and used as a component of drugs in Ayurvedic medicine. The expansion of this culture spread to sub-Saharan Africa. During the colonization of America, it accompanied black slaves, thus closing a global circuit.[20] Since then, hemp has been known for its age-old fiber, which has been used to make ropes, canvas, clothing, paper, shoes, and candles. The resin produced by the female plants is rich in cannabinoids.

Cannabis is one of the most popular recreational drugs in the world, with nearly 200 million people reporting its use. Over the past 30 years, there has been a major shift in attitudes toward its consumption. The vast majority of US states and a large number of nearly 50 countries around the world (including Portugal) have legalized cannabis in some form, both medical and recreational, and these numbers are growing.

Due to this high global consumption, intensive research efforts have focused on cannabis, with the aim of gaining more knowledge about its potential risks and/or health benefits. The discovery of a cannabinoid-stimulated system is relatively recent. Researchers such as Mechoulam, Howlett, Devine, and Hanus have made important contributions to our understanding of the endocannabinoid system, in terms of receptors, agonists, distribution in the body, and functions.[21]

The psychoactive component of cannabis that contributes most to its euphoric effects is delta-9-tetrahydrocannabinol (Δ9-THC), which is one of approximately 140 cannabinoids identified in the cannabis plant. There is significant knowledge about the pharmacological actions of some important cannabinoids in the cannabis plant, such as Δ9-THC, cannabidiol, cannabinol, cannabigerol, cannabichromene, and cannabidiolic acid. There are 440 other compounds, including terpenoids, that contribute to the complex effects of the plant. THC concentrations in common recreational plants have increased 7- to 20-fold in recent decades, with concentrations of 29% THC. As with all drugs of abuse, the higher the concentration of the psychoactive component, the greater the risk of developing a substance use disorder. It is estimated that about 10% of cannabis users meet the criteria for cannabis use disorder (CUD). Cannabis use does not cause fatal overdoses, but it has a significant psychiatric impact. CUD develops as a result of chronic neuroadaptations that occur over time with repeated cannabis use.[22] Cannabis use directly affects the natural endogenous system, the endocannabinoid system (ECB), which includes the receptors that mediate the direct actions of cannabinoids, as well as the ECB lipid bonds (arachidonoylethanolamide and N-acetylethanolamide), cannabinoid system (eCB), which comprises the receptors that mediate the direct actions of cannabinoids, as well as the eCB lipid compounds (arachidonoylethanolamide, also called anandamide, and 2-arachidonoylglycerol, also called 2-AG) and the associated enzymes responsible for their synthesis and degradation. Stimulation of cannabinoid receptors by THC initiates an extensive cascade of biological events, due to its abundant expression throughout the brain and body. The Gi/Go protein-coupled cannabinoid receptor subtype-1 is the predominant form in the brain, mediating the psychoactive effects of cannabis and expressed in multiple areas of the brain, such as the cerebral cortex, basal ganglia, hippocampus, cerebellum, amygdala, brainstem, and hypothalamus. CB2 receptors, although much less abundant in the brain, are involved in the neurobiological actions of THC relevant to addiction and are predominantly found in peripheral immune cells.[22,23]

The activation of cannabinoid receptors has a strong effect on multiple physiological functions and behaviors that extend beyond the effects of acute cannabis intoxication and may promote the development of CRS through changes in the neural systems that regulate cognition, memory, reward, mood, and sensitivity to stress.

The eCB system, being the prime site for THC action, has been the subject of PET neuroimaging studies, which consistently show that CB1Rs are dynamically altered depending on the phase of chronic opioid use. CB1Rs are generally downregulated in cannabis users, with the most intense and evident change observed shortly after cannabis use. These changes are predominantly found in the neocortex and limbic system, which regulate cognition and emotional processing, as well as in the ventral striatum, which is critically involved in the reward system and goal-directed behavior. Longer duration of use is associated with lower CB1 receptor densities. However, the reduction in CB1R in cannabis-dependent subjects is not permanent and normalizes 2–28 days after cessation of substance use. Return to apparently normal concentrations after delayed abstinence may not imply normalization of receptor function, as animal studies suggest that CB1R may remain functionally altered during abstinence. However, reduction of CB1R in the early stages of the disorder will have an impact on the cascade of neurobiological systems that may maintain persistent changes underlying the behaviors characteristic of SUD. In addition to CB1R, there is little in vivo evidence for other components of the eCB system, but preliminary data indicate reduced binding of fatty acid amide hydrolase (FAAH), the enzyme that metabolizes anandamide, suggesting that anandamide concentrations within corticolimbic brain regions may be altered in CUD. Acute THC consumption increases dopamine release in the striatal and prefrontal areas of healthy subjects. Early age of onset or longer duration of cannabis use is correlated with reduced levels of dopamine stimulation in the striatum. Low levels of dopamine release in the striatum of heavy cannabis users are related to inattention and increased negative symptomatology, and are inversely correlated with negative emotionality and severity of addiction. Decreased dopamine synthesis in cannabis-dependent individuals is associated with increased apathy. Measurements of dopamine transporters via PET, which are necessary for presynaptic dopamine reuptake, also reveal reduced availability in multiple areas of the brain, with the classic "amotivational syndrome" and negative affectivity characteristic of this disorder.[24]

The perpetuation of the addiction cycle is also characterized by changes in glutamate, which plays an important role in mediating inhibition control and drug-seeking behaviors. Glutamatergic transmission is highly regulated by endocannabinoid signaling (via CB1 receptors on presynaptic terminals that reduce glutamate release) and is sensitive to THC.

Some morphological changes resulting from cannabis use are reduced gray matter volume in the hippocampus and amygdala.[25]

The Current State of Medical Cannabis

We are at a point where medical cannabis has achieved great popularity. Furthermore, scientific evidence about its pharmacological potential is in line with the economic interests of this huge new market (valued at around US$13.5 billion in 2021, with projections pointing to US$70.6 billion in 2028), leaving aside some moral and social concerns.[26]

In addition to the classic methods of administration, such as smoking and inhaling, cannabis can be eaten, drunk, or mixed with other foods. From a pharmaceutical point of view, there are tablets and oromucosal sprays (nabiximols).

Some **therapeutic indications for cannabis** have been discovered:

1. Spasticity associated with multiple sclerosis or spinal cord injuries.
2. Nausea, vomiting (resulting from cancer chemotherapy and/or radiotherapy, combination therapy for HIV, and medication for hepatitis C).
3. Appetite stimulation in palliative care for patients with cancer or AIDS.
4. Chronic pain (associated with cancer or nervous system diseases, such as neuropathic pain caused by nerve injury, phantom limb pain, trigeminal neuralgia, or post-herpetic neuralgia).
5. Gilles de la Tourette syndrome.
6. Epilepsy and treatment of severe seizure disorders in childhood, such as Dravet and Lennox-Gastaut syndromes.
7. Glaucoma resistant to ophthalmological therapy.

Resolution No. 11/CD/2019, INFARMED, Portugal

OPIATES

Every person carries within them a dose of natural opium that is incessantly secreted and renewed.

Charles Baudelaire

The poppy (*Papaver somniferum*) is another old acquaintance of humankind. Five thousand years ago, the Sumerians used it to combat insomnia and diarrhea, and called it *hul gil*, the plant of joy. This plant, native to Asia Minor (the Fertile Crescent), was cultivated in adjacent regions.[27] The plant has a milky substance in its green bulb that produces opium.

In the 2nd century AD, Galen was an enthusiast of the virtues of opium, whose use became very popular in Rome, but he also realized the risks of excessive opium use through Emperor Antoninus, whose physician he was and who was a victim of drug addiction. It was with the Romans that the analgesic properties of opium became recognized.[28]

Islamic civilization flourished between the 9th and 16th centuries, and medicine was one of its hallmarks. Opium, which the Arabs called *af-yun*, was, for Avicenna, the most powerful of painkillers. This substance was administered both orally and rectally in the treatment of earaches and joint pain, especially in gout. In the 9th century, references appear to *spongia somnifera*, a mixture of opium, mandrake, hemlock, and hyoscyamus, used by Arab doctors to facilitate inhalation anesthesia for surgical procedures. Later, *spongia somnifera* was used in Palermo for the same purpose. During the golden age of Islamic civilization, the Arabs dominated trade in the Indian Ocean and introduced opium to India and later to China, where it was called *o-fu-yung*. For about 1,000 years, the Chinese used opium primarily to control diarrhea.

Paracelsus, a Swiss physician who lived between 1493 and 1541, was credited with reintroducing the medical use of opium in Western Europe. Sydenham's laudanum was the main liquid preparation containing opium. It was used in England in the 17th century and was widely accepted in Europe and the Americas until the early 20th century.

In the 16th century, the first book on opium abuse was written by the Persian scholar Imed al-Din Mahmed, entitled Afyunieh (this being the first book on addiction in history).[27]

It was not until 1700 that John Jones, a London physician, published a book called *Mysteries of Opium Revealed*. In the book, the author warns about the risks of excessive use of this drug.[28]

It is now known that a quarter of the weight of opium powder is composed of at least 25 alkaloids, which were classified into two distinct groups for chemical and pharmacological reasons.

The most important group is represented by phenanthrene derivatives, which act mainly on the central nervous system (CNS) (Figure 10.10). Morphine (isolated by Seturner in 1806) accounts for 10% of opium alkaloids. Codeine (methylmorphine) was isolated by Robiquet in 1832, and thebaine (dimethylmorphine) was isolated by Pelletier and Thiboumèry in 1835.

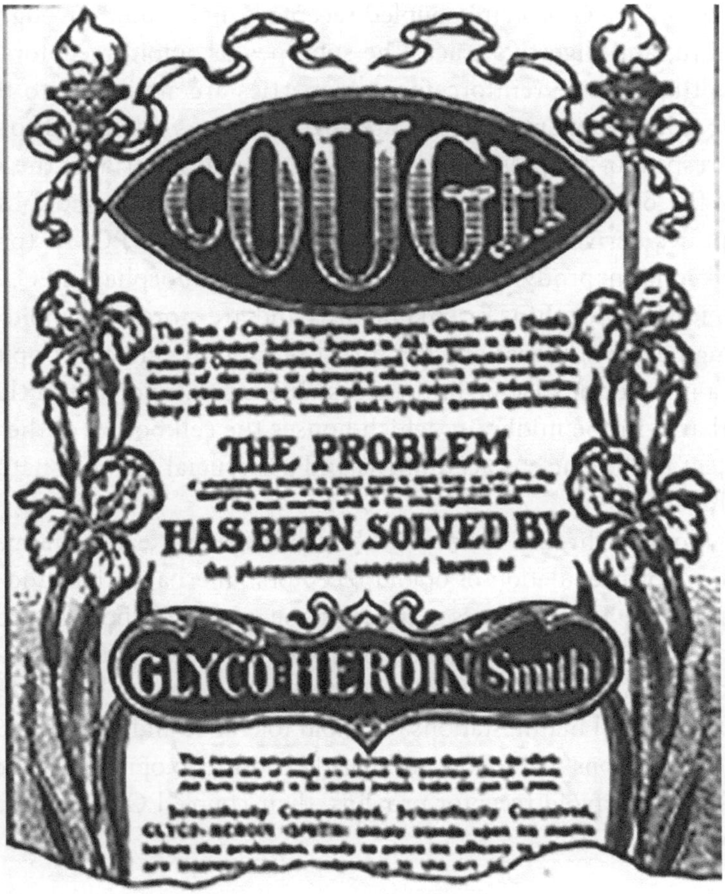

FIGURE 10.10 Glycoheroin.

Codeine and thebaine account for 0.5% and 0.2% of opium alkaloids, respectively.[29] Morphine was widely used as an anesthetic during the American Civil War (1861–1865). Many American soldiers subsequently developed physical dependence. In order to solve the problems of morphine dependence, Bayer Laboratories introduced heroin in 1898, which was intended to be a painkiller without the risk of addiction: "safe for children" and available over the counter. Throughout the 20th century, the Germans developed oxycodone in 1916, hydrocodone in 1920, and methadone in 1939. Paul Janssen, researcher Belgian scientist Peter Fentanyl synthesized fentanyl in 1959.

Exogenous opioids can have an analgesic effect (such as codeine and morphine) or are drugs of abuse (such as heroin) and act as agonists on μ, κ, and δ, especially μ. Euphoria is the main opioid reinforcement property. Opioids induce a very intense but brief euphoria, followed by a deep sense of calm, then drowsiness, mood swings, lethargy, apathy, and slowed movements. In the event of an overdose, these agents act as respiratory depressants and induce coma. These effects can be reversed by synthetic opioid antagonists such as naloxone and naltrexone.[30]

Opioid receptors are G protein–coupled receptors distributed throughout the brain, spinal cord, skin, and digestive tract. The subtypes of opioid receptors are μ, κ, and δ, and nociceptin. Positive reinforcement properties are attributed to the connection with μ and, to a lesser extent, δ. There are specific effects attributed to each receptor: euphoria and respiratory depression for the μ receptor, dysphoria for the κ receptor, and anxiolysis for the δ receptor. The brain produces endogenous opioid-like substances. These are peptides derived from precursor proteins, such as POMC (proopiomelanocortin), proenkephalin, prodynorphin, and pronociceptin/orphanin FQ. These proteins are cleaved to form endorphins or enkephalins and are stored in opioid neurons to be released during neurotransmission. The direct reinforcing effects of opioids appear to be limited to a number of specific brain areas. The most important of these is the ventral tegmental area in the midbrain, which houses the cell bodies of the dopaminergic cells that project to the nucleus accumbens and are crucial for both natural and drug-motivated behaviors.[31]

In cellular models, chronic exposure to opioid agonists causes numerous adaptive changes, such as downregulation of opioid receptors, internalization, and uncoupling of inhibitory G proteins. These processes appear to be related to the desensitization of opioid receptors. Another adaptive response to prolonged exposure to opioids is the hypersensitization of the cAMP-dependent signal transduction system. These adaptive changes contribute to the clinical manifestations of opioid tolerance and dependence. The cellular and molecular adaptations that follow prolonged exposure to opioids are the result of state of phosphorylation of opioid receptor proteins, their coupled G proteins, and numerous related effector proteins.[30]

What Are the Most Important Opioids with Clinical Applications? (Table 10.5)

TABLE 10.5 Equianalgesic Relationship Between Oral Morphine and Various Opioids Used to Treat Chronic Pain

Oral morphine	Transdermal buprenorphine	75:1 to 95:1
	Oral codeine	1:6 to 1:10
	Transdermal fentanyl	100:1 to 150:1
	Oral hydromorphone	5:1
	Intravenous morphine	3:1
	Subcutaneous morphine	2:1
	Oral oxycodone/naloxone	1.5:1 to 2:1
	Oral tapentadol	1:2.5
	Oral tramadol	1:5 to 1:10
	Tramadol IV/subcutaneous	1:5 to 1:10

The Prescription Opioid Epidemic

The situation in the United States, Canada, and Australia is paradigmatic of what could happen in other parts of the world, particularly in Europe.

The prescription of strong opioids for chronic non-cancer pain, particularly in fibromyalgia, has created favorable conditions for an epidemic of prescription opioids. Based on the assumption that patients with chronic pain will not develop opioid use disorder (OUD), large increases in opioid prescribing have effectively led to an increase in OUD. The case of the United States is paradigmatic, as several factors coincide to explain the "current epidemic of deaths from prescription opioids":

- High cost of prescription opioids
- Greater availability of purer, lower-priced heroin
- Difficulty in admitting OUD cases to treatment centers

The result was a huge increase in users of prescription and non-prescription opioids and opiates. The emergence of fentanyl (50 times more potent than heroin) and other highly potent synthetic analogues has only exacerbated the problem. In the United States, the number of deaths between 2010 and 2017 attributed to fentanyl overdose increased almost tenfold. It should be noted that these fentanyl or fentanyl-associated heroin overdoses are very difficult to treat with naloxone. The reasons are:

- The very high potency of fentanyl at the opioid μ receptor
- Its very rapid pharmacokinetics
- The longer duration of respiratory depressant effects and additive effects when combined with other drugs, such as heroin[32]

There are other opioids, such as buprenorphine and methadone, with a longer half-life, slower clearance rates, and cerebral absorption. Methadone is administered orally, slowing its entry into the brain. It is a full agonist of μ receptors and also has agonist effects on galanin receptors (which antagonize the effects on μ receptors, decreasing the rewarding effects).

The development of tolerance does not occur at the same time for the various pharmacological effects of opioids: it is faster for analgesic and hedonic effects and slower for respiratory depression. This explains why dose increases to maintain analgesia can increase the risks of respiratory depression and fatal overdose.

Antipsychotic Action of Opioids

Opioids are the only sedative drugs that have antipsychotic properties. This is quite evident in users who attend methadone maintenance programs with a history of psychotic episodes. The near-absence of relapses in these patients leads to the conclusion that these programs have a preventive effect. When a gradual reduction in the methadone dose is carried out, the onset of positive psychotic symptoms is observed in some cases. The action of methadone can be explained by its dopaminergic action (increase in prolactin after administration).[33]

COCAINE

If you want to hang out, you've got to take her out, cocaine

If you want to get down, get down on the ground, cocaine

She doesn't lie, she doesn't lie, she doesn't lie, cocaine

Eric Clapton

In the third millennium BC, cocaine was already being used by the ancient Incas who lived in the Andes mountains to counteract altitude sickness. Chewing a coca leaf is a remedy that is still used today in Andean countries to counteract altitude sickness.

Cocaine was isolated from coca leaves in the mid–19th century by German chemist Albert Niemann. In 1884, the father of psychoanalysis, Sigmund Freud, who was a cocaine user, wrote that cocaine "cured depression and sexual impotence."

In the same decade, the inventor of Coca-Cola, John Pemberton, used coca leaves as an ingredient in this drink. Coca-Cola became widely known as a drink that produced euphoria and increased energy.

At the beginning of the 20th century, cocaine use was a widespread problem, with thousands of deaths recorded as related to its consumption. It was banned in 1922. Since the 1970s, it has experienced renewed growth, which has continued unabated to this day.

Cocaine is a stimulant that has no therapeutic use in psychopharmacology. It has two main properties: it is a local anesthetic and an inhibitor of transporters, particularly dopamine, but also serotonin and norepinephrine. Compared to other stimulants used in clinical practice (e.g., methylphenidate), cocaine has a faster, more potent, and more complete action on the dopamine transporter.[31]

During the process of extracting cocaine from the leaves of the coca plant, two forms are produced: a base and a salt.

The base is created by heating the salt form in an organic solvent, which has a basic pH, in a process known as *free-basing*, which causes *crack* to form. This has a low melting point (98°C) and vaporizes quickly before the active compound is destroyed. As a result, it can be smoked but cannot be injected due to its insolubility in water.

In contrast, the salt form of cocaine is a white powder that cannot be smoked because it melts at a much higher temperature than the base form and is destroyed before it vaporizes. However, it is quickly inhaled through the nasal mucosa and dissolves, and it is also easily injected.

Cocaine is rapidly absorbed through the oral and nasal mucosa, and through the respiratory, gastrointestinal, and genitourinary tracts. After ingestion, it is rapidly distributed and absorbed by many organs, including the brain, heart, kidneys, adrenal glands, and liver. It can be measured in blood, urine, hair, sweat, and milk, and analysis of these fluids can be used for legal, employment, or treatment purposes.

The average purity of cocaine in salt form is approximately 50%, and various additives or adulterants may be mixed with cocaine powder. These additives may be inert, such as lactose, dextrose, or flour, or they may be active, such as benzocaine, procaine, hydroxyzine, diltiazem, phenacetin, or lidocaine. Psychoactive adulterants, such as amphetamines, caffeine, phencyclidine, or ephedrine, and may increase or complicate the effects.

When cocaine is administered by smoking (pulmonary) or injection, the maximum effect and its onset occur within minutes and last for 15–30 minutes.

When administered nasally (snorted), the onset of action is slower, occurring in 30–45 minutes, with a longer maximum effect and a more gradual decrease to baseline (around 60–90 minutes).

Once absorbed, cocaine is rapidly metabolized, forming two metabolites (benzoylecgonine and ecgonine methyl ester). These substances are water-soluble and are rapidly excreted in urine. The serum half-life of cocaine is 45–90 minutes, so it can be found in serum or urine only for a few hours after consumption. The metabolites can be found in the blood and urine for up to 24–36 hours after consumption, and toxicological tests that measure the metabolites benzoylecgonine and ecgonine show evidence of recent use.

Cocaine is known to affect brain cells in several ways: some effects are quickly reversed, while others can persist for weeks after use is discontinued. Finally, with repeated exposure to cocaine, the sum of these effects can lead to other effects that can last for months, years, or even become irreversible.[34]

The main effect of cocaine, when it enters the bloodstream and penetrates the brain, is the accumulation of dopamine. Dopaminergic pathways are very ancient in evolutionary terms (they are found in worms and flies, which takes us back two billion years).

The speed at which a stimulant enters the brain dictates the degree of intense euphoria it causes. This is why drugs that are inhaled, snorted, or injected, which enter the brain quickly and explosively, are generally much more reinforcing than the same drugs taken orally, because the rate of entry into the brain is significantly slowed down by the process of gastrointestinal absorption.

Cocaine is not even active when taken orally, so users have learned to consume it intranasally, bypassing the liver and thus achieving an even faster onset than intravenous administration. The fastest and most robust way to "get" drugs to the brain is to smoke those that are compatible with this route of administration because it avoids first-pass metabolism in the liver. The faster the entry into the brain, the more potent the reinforcing effects are, probably because this form of drug administration triggers phasic dopamine releases, which are associated with reward and salience.[31]

Cocaine interferes with the dopamine transporter, preventing reuptake and thus causing an accumulation of dopamine and hyperactivation of receptor cells. The limbic system is particularly sensitive to the action of cocaine because dopaminergic cells are mainly concentrated there. The nucleus accumbens (NAC), hippocampus, amygdala, and frontal cortex are important elements of this system, whose functioning is affected by cocaine. The frontal cortex acts as a brake on the other regions of the limbic system (when one decides to give up a pleasure to avoid its negative consequences), so when someone becomes addicted, the frontal cortex is compromised and cannot inhibit the impulses to consume. Cocaine also affects several transcription factors, such as ΔFosB, which are extremely high when cocaine is consumed.[34]

Methylphenidate, amphetamines, and cocaine share the inhibitory action of the dopamine transporter. High doses of stimulants can induce paranoia and hallucinations. Cocaine is a potent vasoconstrictor and poses a particular risk of injury to the cardiovascular and cerebrovascular systems (hypertension, tachycardia, ventricular arrhythmias, myocardial infarction, thrombosis, etc.).

SEDATIVES AND HYPNOTICS

She goes running for the shelter
Of her mother's little helper

And it helps her on her way
Gets her through her busy day

Rolling Stones, "Mother's Little Helper"

Sedatives and hypnotics include barbiturates, chloral hydrate, benzodiazepines, and Z-hypnotics. (Z drugs are a group of benzodiazepine analogues with similar effects to benzodiazepines, used in the treatment of insomnia and whose names mostly begin with the letter "Z"; they may have advantages over benzodiazepines, since, while the latter worsen sleep architecture, Z-hypnotics do not usually alter this architecture significantly.) Benzodiazepines are the most important group and are generally prescription drugs.

The first benzodiazepine available on the market, dating back to 1960 (more than 60 years ago), was chlordiazepoxide, marketed under the trade name Librium, launched by the pharmaceutical company Hoffman-La Roche.

It was more of a serendipitous scientific event, as the compound RO-5-0690, discovered by researcher Sternbech, had been forgotten in a laboratory stall for 20 years. This researcher had a reputation for being quite messy. It was a laboratory cleanup ordered by the administration that led to the rediscovery of this synthetic product. It was tested on laboratory animals and the results were sensational: it had anticonvulsant, muscle-relaxant, and sedative properties. This led to the discovery of chlordiazepoxide, which was given the trade name Librium[35] (Figure 10.11). The synthesis of diazepam (Valium) came later. Sternbech also synthesized flunitrazepam (Rohypnol). Prescriptions for these drugs increased exponentially. Between 1978 and 1979, Americans consumed around 2.3 billion Valium tablets per year. By the 1980s, there was already a concern about the potential for abuse and dependence on this group of drugs.[35]

It should be understood that in the early 1950s there were only three drugs available to treat anxiety, depression, and insomnia: chloral hydrate, reserpine, and barbiturates. The first two had marked toxic effects. Barbiturates had a very narrow therapeutic range, and their abuse could lead to respiratory depression and death. It was later discovered that they acted on GABA receptors, common to future benzodiazepine drugs.

The mechanism of action of benzodiazepines (BZD) was only discovered some 15 years later: they are positive allosteric modulators for $GABA_A$ receptors. In other words, they act through a GABA potentiation mechanism. BZDs require the presence of GABA to exert

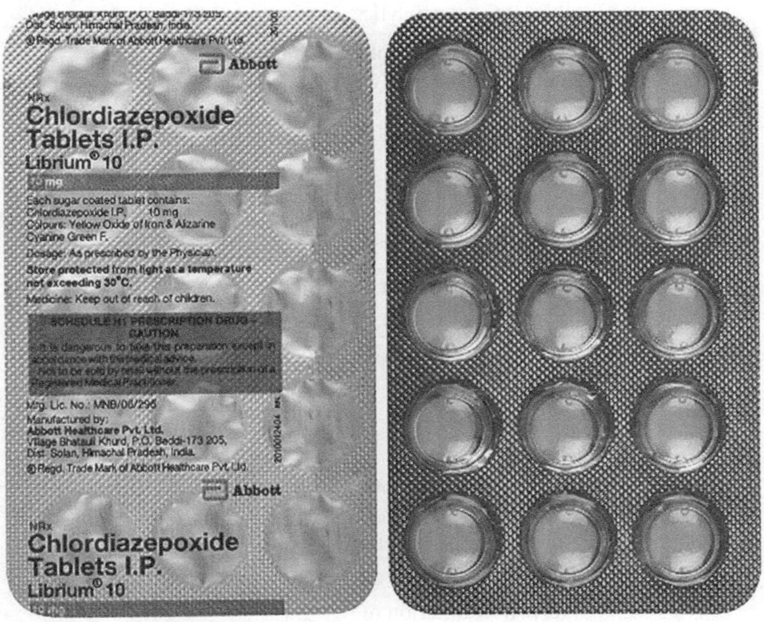

FIGURE 10.11 Chlordiazepoxide tablets.

their effects. The binding of BZD and GABA molecules in a chloride ion channel gives rise to the characteristic actions of BZDs: sedation, anxiety reduction, muscle relaxation, hypnosis, and anticonvulsant activity.[35]

αγBZD receptors were identified in 1977 by Möhler and Okada. Subsequent research concluded that benzodiazepines do not bind to the same active site as GABA, but to a separate site between the $GABA_A$ and $GABA_B$ subunits contained in the $GABA_A$ receptor.

Also in the same year, Braestrup and Squires found that diazepam binds to sites other than $GABA_A$.[35] These peripheral benzodiazepine receptors (PBRs) were located in mitochondrial membranes and tissue plasma throughout the body. These receptors had bonds such as porphyrin IX, heme, and endocannabinoids.[36] Endocannabinoids play an important role in steroid synthesis. But because these receptors were not specific to benzodiazepines, their name was changed to TSPO (18kDa translocator protein). These receptors are the subject of intense research. The discovery of specific benzodiazepine binding sites has led to the search for endogenous BZD ligands designated by the generic term endocannabinoids. The first endogenous ligand for BZD receptors was discovered in 1983 and designated DBI (diazepam-binding inhibitor). Endocannabinoids perform vital functions involving their involvement in anxiety and depressive disorders, homeostasis, neuroprotection, neurogenesis, tumorigenesis, and control of steroid and peptide hormone secretion. Their involvement in pathological situations is the subject of intense study, as new avenues for finding new drugs have been opened.

Given the addictive potential of BZDs, which became apparent shortly after their clinical use began, there are now recommendations that clinicians should follow. These recommendations relate to the non-routine use of benzodiazepines for the symptomatic

TABLE 10.6 Anxiolytics

Long duration of action (half-life of 24 hours or more)	Clobazam
	Clorazepate
	Chlordiazepoxide
	Clonazepam
	Cloxazolam
	Diazepam
	Ethyl loflazepate
Intermediate duration of action (12–24 hours)	Bromazepam
	Lorazepam
Short duration of action (6–12 hours)	Alprazolam
	Oxazepam

TABLE 10.7 Hypnotics

Short duration of action	Brotizolam
	Temazepam
Very short duration of action	Midazolam
	Triazolam
	Zolpidem
Intermediate duration of action	Estazolam
	Flunitrazepam
Long-acting	Flurazepam

treatment of anxiety, not using more than one anxiolytic or hypnotic BZD in the same patient, and establishing a time limit for their use, which is 8–12 weeks for anxiolytics and 4 weeks for hypnotics (Standard 055/201-Portuguese Directorate-General for Health).

The following tables present a summary of the benzodiazepinesavailable for clinical use and classified according to their half-life. The shorter the half-life, the greater the addictive potential. Some harmful practices involving the use of these substances include dilution and intravenous injection.

Some benzodiazepines, such as clonazepam and diazepam can be used as antiepileptics. Diazepam is used intravenously, diluted, to treat epileptic states. Diazepam and midazolam can be used as preanesthetics (Tables 10.6 and 10.7).

CLASSIC PSYCHEDELICS

The broad array of classic psychedelic compounds that have been universally ignored in pharmaceutical drug development may soon constitute a library of potential therapeutics. They may also help to inform the biological mechanisms of human consciousness.

Matthew W. Johnson, Peter S. Hendricks,
Frederick S. Barrett, and Roland R. Griffiths

Classic psychedelics are psychoactive compounds that exert their effects through agonist (and also partial agonist) activity at 5HT 2A receptors.[37] These compounds were initially called psychomimetics (because they are believed to induce psychosis), hallucinogens (because they can cause visions), psychedelics (because they can manifest or reveal the mind), and finally, entheogens (meaning that they can trigger the internal manifestation of the divine). The term *hallucinogen* is not ideal, because it has connotations of changes in perception, and the action of these compounds is much broader. Let us use *psychedelics*, studying the classic examples within this group. These have two general structures:

- One consists of variations in the structure of tryptamine, such as LSD, psilocybin, or DMT (dimethyltryptamine).
- The other has variations in the structure of phenylethylamine, such as mescaline. Synthetic compounds belonging to this second category will be discussed in the section on new psychoactive substances.

Psychedelics may be the oldest class of psychotropic drugs known to man. Mushrooms containing psilocybin have been used in faraway places, such as Mexico (by Aztec shamans) and Australia or Tanzania, for many thousands of years. Indigenous cultures in the Western Hemisphere have used compounds of both structural classes, such as ayahuasca, mushrooms containing psilocybin, and cacti containing mescaline.[38]

They produce a state of intoxication associated with changes in sensory experiences, such as dreamlike states, visual illusions, visual and auditory hallucinations, and synesthesia; changes in body image; altered self-perception; derealization; depersonalization; altered perception of time and space; altered thought content; changes in mood; anxiety; and nervousness. Emotions can range from ecstasy to pleasant and anxious sensations. There is greater awareness of external and internal stimuli and thoughts. "Psychedelic" is the term used for the subjective experience in which someone, due to increased sensory awareness and expansion of the mind, feels at one with humanity or the universe or has some kind of religious experience.[39]

What Are the Risks of Using Classic Psychedelics?

Any individual who takes a sufficiently high dose may have an anxious, dysphoric, or confused reaction and, rarely, an acute reaction called a "bad trip" (which can become dangerous in unsupervised environments). The second risk is the exacerbation of preexisting psychotic disorders or the onset of a prolonged psychotic reaction. Another risk is the possibility of a slight increase in blood pressure and heart rate.

Other changes include impaired judgment, fear of going crazy, anxiety, nausea, and increased body temperature. As intoxication increases, an acute confusional state called *delirium* may be experienced, in which the user is disoriented and agitated. This can progress to a state of overt psychosis and paranoia. Another unique dimension of psychedelic abuse is that it can cause the spontaneous recurrence of some symptoms of intoxication, which can last from a few seconds to a few hours, in the absence of recent hallucinogen use.

These recurrences (*flashbacks*) can occur days or months after discontinuing use and can be triggered by environmental stimuli. This might be explained by a neurochemical adaptation of the serotonergic system and its receptors, related to an extremely long-lasting inverse tolerance.

What Are the Prospects for Using These Substances in So-Called Psychedelic Psychotherapy?

Psychedelics attracted the interest of psychiatrists and psychologists as early as the 1950s. Studies published between 1949 and 1973 reported clinical improvement in almost 80% of subjects, but the absence of systems for classifying mental disorders, scales for measuring symptom severity, and randomization in these studies made them largely irrelevant. However, the clinical improvement and maintenance over time, as well as the safety of this type of intervention, were already well known.

There followed a period in which these studies became impossible due to the classification of these compounds as narcotics included in the United Nations's so-called Schedule I.[40] After a 20-year hiatus, clinical studies resumed, following a more careful experimental design.

There are clinical studies demonstrating the clinical efficacy of psychedelics in the treatment of anxiety and depression;[41] in treatment-resistant major depression;[42] and in cancer-related psychosocial disorders.[43]

Psychedelics induce mystical/religious experiences that can be profoundly transformative. Psychedelics may exert their therapeutic effects by destabilizing local network centers and global network connectivity at the brain level by amplifying neural avalanches, creating conditions for the *resetting* of the brain network.

REFERENCES

1. Veiga E. Conheça a radula , a planta que pode ser a maconha do futuro. From Milan to BBC News Brazil, 2018.
2. Carod-Artal FJ. Hallucinogenic drugs in pre-Columbian Mesoamerican cultures. Neurology (English Edition). 2015);30(1):42–9. https://doi.org/10.1016/j.nrleng.2011.07.010
3. Lathrap, D. The antiquity and importance of long-distance trade relationships in the moist tropics of pre-Columbian South America. World Archaeology. 1973;5(2):170–186.
4. Escohotado A. General History of Drugs. Espasa Calpe Publishing House, 2002.
5. Volkow ND, Koob GF, McLellan AT. Neurobiologic Advances from the Brain Disease Model of Addiction. N Engl J Med. 2016;374(4):363–71. https://doi.org/10.1056/nejmra1511480
6. United Nations Office on Drugs and Crime. (2019). The world drug report. In: United Nations publication (Issue January).
7. Carrigan MA, Uryasev O, Frye CB, Eckman BL, Myers CR, Hurley TD, *et al.* Hominids adapted to metabolize ethanol long before human-directed fermentation. Proc Natl Acad Sci U S A. 2015;112(2):458–63. https://doi.org/10.1073/pnas.1404167111
8. Keller M. A historical overview of alcohol and alcoholism. Cancer Research. 1979;39:2822–9.
9. Hall W. What has research over the past two decades revealed about the adverse health effects of recreational cannabis use? Addiction (Abingdon, England). 2015;110(1):19–35. https://doi.org/10.1111/add.12703
10. Perez de los Cobos J, Valderrama JCV, Cervera G Tratado SET de Toxicomanías (Sociedad). Madrid: Editorial Médica Panamericana, 2006.

11. Ravindran CRM, Ticku MK. Tyrosine kinase phosphorylation of $GABA_A$ receptor α_1, β_2 and γ_2 subunits following chronic intermittent ethanol (CIE) exposure of cultured cortical neurons of mice. Neurochemical Research. 2006;31(9):1111–8. https://doi.org/10.1007/s11064-006-9124-9
12. Erdozain AM, Callado LF. Neurobiological alterations in alcohol addiction: Addictions. 2014;26(4):360–70.
13. Newton PM, Messing RO. Intracellular signaling pathways that regulate behavioral responses to ethanol. Pharmacol Ther. 2006;109(1-2):227–37. https://doi.org/10.1016/j.pharmthera.2005.07.004
14. Hammer JH, Parent MC, Spiker DA. World Health Organization. Global status report on alcohol and health 2018. In: World Health Organization, 2018. https://doi.org/10.1037/cou0000248
15. Rosemberg J. Nicotine: Universal Drug. São Paulo: SES/CVE, 2003.
16. Prochaska JJ, Benowitz NL. Current advances in research in treatment and recovery: Nicotine addiction. Sci Adv. 2019;5(10). https://doi.org/10.1126/sciadv.aay9763
17. Benowitz NL. Pharmacology of nicotine: Addiction, smoking-induced disease, and therapeutics. Annu Rev Pharmacol Toxicol. 2009;49:57–71. https://doi.org/10.1146/annurev.pharmtox.48.113006.094742
18. Malaiyandi V, Sellers EM, Tyndale RF. Implications of CYP2A6 genetic variation for smoking behaviors and nicotine dependence. Clinical Pharmacology and Therapeutics. 2005;77(3):145–58. https://doi.org/10.1016/j.clpt.2004.10.011
19. WHO Report on the global tobacco epidemic, 2021. Addressing new and emerging products fresh and alive. (n.d.).
20. Warf B. High Points: An Historical Geography of Cannabis. Geographical Review. 2014;104(4):414–38. https://doi.org/10.1111/j.1931-0846.2014.12038.x
21. Crocq MA History of cannabis and the endocannabinoid system. Dialogues Clin Neurosci. 2020 Sep;22(3):223–28.
22. Ferland JN, Hurd YL. Deconstructing the neurobiology of cannabis use disorder. Nat Neurosci. 2020 May;23(5):600–10. https://doi.org/10.1038/s41593-020-0611-0
23. Lutz B. Neurobiology of cannabinoid receptor signaling. Dialogues in Clinical Neuroscience. 2020;22(3):207–22. https://doi.org/10.31887/DCNS.2020.22.3/BLUTZ
24. Chen DJ, Gao M, Gao FF, Su QX, Wu J. Brain cannabinoid receptor 2: Expression, function and modulation. Acta Pharmacol Sin. 2017;38(3):312–6. https://doi.org/10.1038/aps.2016.149
25. Lorenzetti V, Solowij N, Whittle S, Fornito A, Lubman DI, Pantelis C, *et al.* Gross morphological brain changes with chronic, heavy cannabis use. Br J Psychiatry. 2015;206(1):77–8. https://doi.org/10.1192/bjp.bp.114.151407
26. Pisanti S, Bifulco M. Modern History of Medical Cannabis: From Widespread Use to Prohibitionism and Back. Trends in Pharmacological Sciences. 2017;38(3):195–8. https://doi.org/10.1016/j.tips.2016.12.002
27. Moosavyzadeh A, Ghaffari F, Mosavat SH, Zargaran A, Mokri A, Faghihzadeh S, *et al.* (2018). The medieval Persian manuscript of Afyunieh: the first individual treatise on opium and addiction in history. J Integr Med. 2018;16(2):77–83. https://doi.org/10.1016/j.joim.2018.02.004
28. Freire Duarte D. Opium and opioids: A brief history. Revista Brasileira de Anestesiologia. 2005;55(1):135–46. https://doi.org/10.1590/S0034-70942005000100015
29. Schiff Jr PL. Opium and Its Alkaloids. American Journal of Pharmaceutical Education. 2002;66:186–94.
30. Nunes I, Santos C, Fortunato M. Bases moleculares da tolerância aos opioides. Portuguese Journal of Psychosomatics. 2005;7(1-2).
31. Stahl SM. Stahl's Essential Psychopharmacology (4th edition). Cambridge: Cambridge University Press, 2013.

32. Volkow ND, Blanco C. The changing opioid crisis: development, challenges, and opportunities. Molecular Psychiatry. 2021;26(1):218–33. https://doi.org/10.1038/s41380-020-0661-4
33. Maremmani AGI, Rovai L, Rugani F, Bacciardi S, De-ll'osso L, Maremmani I. Substance abuse and psychosis. The strange case of opioids. Eur Rev Med Pharmacol Sci. 2014;18(3):287–302.
34. Nestler EJ. The neurobiology of cocaine addiction. Sci Pract Perspect. 2005 Dec;3(1):4–10.
35. Wick JY. The history of benzodiazepines. Consultant Pharmacist. 2013;28(9):538–48. https://doi.org/10.4140/TCP.n.2013.538
36. Tonon M, Vaudry H, Chuquet J, Guillebaud F, Fan J, Masmoudi-kouki O, *et al.* Endozepines and their receptors: Structure, functions and pathophysiological significance. Pharmacol Ther. 2020;208:2081–56. https://doi.org/10.1016/j.pharmthera.2019.06.008
37. Nichols DE. Psychedelics. Pharmacol Rev. 2016 Apr;68(2):264–355.
38. Johnson MW, Hendricks PS, Barrett FS, Griffiths RR. Classic psychedelics: An integrative review of epidemiology, therapeutics, mystical experience, and brain network function. Pharmacol Ther. 2019;197:83–102. https://doi.org/10.1016/j.pharmthera.2018.11.010
39. Adams C. Psychedelics and holistic thinking: A tool for science. Drugs Alcohol Today. 2010;10(1):33–35. https://doi.org/10.5042/daat.2010.0126
40. United Nations, 1992. Conferencia de las Naciones Unidas para la aprobación de una convención contra el tráfico ilícito de estupefacientes y sustancias psicotrópicas: Viena, 25 de noviembre a 20 de diciembre de 1988: documentos oficiales.
41. Grob CS, Danforth AL, Chopra GS, Hagerty M, McKay CR, Halberstadt AL, Greer GR, *et al.* Pilot study of psilocybin treatment for anxiety in patients with advanced-stage cancer. Arch Gen Psychiatry. 2011;68(1):71–8. https://doi.org/10.1001/archgenpsychiatry.2010.116
42. Carhart-Harris RL, Bolstridge M, Day CMJ, Rucker J, Watts R, Erritzoe DE, *et al.* Psilocybin with psychological support for treatment-resistant depression: an open-label feasibility study. Lancet Psychiatry. 2016;3(7):619–27.
43. Griffiths RR, Johnson MW, Carducci MA, Umbricht A, Richards WA, *et al.* Psilocybin produces substantial and sustained decreases in depression and anxiety in patients with life-threatening cancer: A randomized double-blind trial. J Psychopharmacol. 2016;30(12):1181–97.
44. Nichols DE, Johnson MW, Nichols CD. Psychedelics as Medicines: An emerging new paradigm. Clin Pharmacol Ther. 2017;101(2):209–19.
45. Merlin MD. Archaeological Evidence for the Tradition of Psychoactive Plant Use in the Old World. Economic Botany. 2003;57(3):295–323. http://www.jstor.org/stable/4256701.

10.5.2 NEW PSYCHOACTIVE SUBSTANCES IN DUAL PATHOLOGY

J. P. Silva and F. Carvalho

New psychoactive substances (NPS) are, by convention, "new narcotic drugs or new psychotropic substances, in pure form or in a preparation, which are not controlled by the 1961 United Nations Single Convention on Narcotic Drugs or the 1971 United Nations Convention on Psychotropic Substances, but which may pose a threat to public health comparable to that posed by the substances covered by those Conventions. In this context, the term "new" refers mainly to the recent availability of such substances on the market. In general, the creation of NPS aims to mimic the effects of substances currently controlled under the aforementioned conventions, covering several groups, such as synthetic cathinones, synthetic cannabinoids, benzodiazepines, arylcyclohexylamines, and synthetic opioids.[1,2] According to the latest United Nations report, 1,047 NPS had been reported by December 2020, most of which were stimulants (specifically cathinones and phenethylamines), followed by synthetic cannabinoids and hallucinogens (e.g., tryptamines). In recent years, there has also been a substantial increase in new opioids (e.g., fentanyl) on the market.[2] However, since 2012, there has been a decline in both seizures and consumption of NPS, largely due to efforts by some countries to control these substances.[1,2]

The use of NPS presents several challenges for researchers and health professionals, since: (1) these substances are often consumed in a context of simultaneous abuse of multiple substances, making it difficult to correlate them with a specific adverse effect; (2) information on the acute effects of the use of NPS is limited and their long-term effects are largely unknown.[3] However, as with substances that mimic NPS (e.g., cannabis, cocaine, heroin, and methamphetamine), it has been associated with social and health problems, including psychiatric comorbidities (e.g., acute psychosis, depression, and anxiety).[2] It should be noted that not only can substance abuse in conjunction with these comorbidities lead to cognitive impairment, but preexisting cognitive dysfunction can promote greater vulnerability to addictive behavior.[4] The following sections describe the mechanisms of action of the main groups of NPS according to their chemical structure,[5] their main psychoactive effects, and their adverse psychological/psychiatric effects. These data are also summarized in Table 10.8.

SYNTHETIC CATINONES

Synthetic cathinones are chemical derivatives of cathinone, a natural amphetamine found in the *Catha edulis* plant (known as khat), commonly sold in crystalline or powdered mixtures in products labeled as "bath salts" or "fertilizers."[4] This group of NPS includes substances such as 4-methylmethcathinone (4-MMP, mephedrone), methylenedioxypyrovalerone (MDPV), and 3,4-methylenedioxy-N-methylcathinone (MDMC, methylone).[4] These substances account for 36% of NPS seizures in the European Union, with 130 molecules currently under the control of the European Monitoring Center for Drugs and Drug Addiction.[1] Like other psychostimulants, synthetic cathinones interact with monoamine membrane transporters and can act as blockers or substrates of dopamine, serotonin and

TABLE 10.8 Summary of the Main Mechanisms of Action of Some of the Most Prevalent Classes of New Psychoactive Substances (NPS) in Global Seizures

NPS class	Examples	Main mechanisms of action	Main psychoactive effects	Significant adverse effects	References
Arylcyclohexylamines	3-MeO-phencyclidine (3-MeO-PCP), 3-methoxyecyclizidine (3-MeO-PCE)	• Non-competitive NMDA receptor antagonists • Dopamine reuptake inhibitors • μ-opioid receptor agonists • σ receptor agonists • Nicotinic and muscarinic receptor antagonists	Dissociative anesthetics, hallucinogens, euphoriants	Respiratory failure, tachycardia, hypertension, urinary retention, myoclonic psychosis, audiovisual hallucinations, paranoia, increased agitation, catatonia, and death	(Bey & Patel, 2007; Morris & Wallach, 2014)[6,7]
Benzodiazepines	Etizolam, flualprazolam	• Positive allosteric modulators of GABA receptors	Sedatives/ hypnotics	Drowsiness, tiredness, and lethargy, aggressiveness, feelings of isolation and depression High doses: nausea, confusion, decreased psychomotor coordination, excessive sleepiness or sedation, memory loss, slow thinking, and emotional instability	(Griffin *et al.*, 2013; McKenzie *et al.*, 2014)[8,9]
Synthetic cathinones	3,4-DMMC, 4'-MePPP	• Blockers or substrates of monoamine transporters (e.g., dopamine, serotonin, and adrenaline) • Decreased expression of the GLT-1 glutamate transporter	Stimulants	Euphoria, high alertness, hyperthermia, tachycardia, paranoia, audiovisual hallucinations, extreme agitation, and violent behavior	(Baumann *et al.*, 2018; Gregg *et al.*, 2016; Murrie *et al.*, 2019)[10,11,12]
Synthetic cannabinoids	WIN55.212-2, CP55.940	• Agonists of CB1 and CB2 cannabinoid receptors CB2 receptor agonists, as well as other receptors such as TRPV, PPAR, GRP55, GPR18 • Some act as positive allosteric modulators of the serotonergic 5-HT1A receptor	Feeling of relaxation and increased well-being, social disinhibition, and increased appetite	Impaired cognitive function (e.g., memory, attention, and time perception disorders), motor incoordination, delirium and hallucinations, drowsiness, paranoia, confusion, psychosis, anxiety, stroke, seizures, heart attacks, muscle tissue failure muscle tissue failure, kidney damage, nausea and vomiting, and death	(Alexandre *et al.*, 2019; Di Forti *et al.*, 2019)[13,14]

Synthetic cocaine derivatives	pFBT, DMC	• Dopamine reuptake inhibitors • Voltage-dependent sodium channel blockers	Stimulants	Tachycardia, breathing difficulties, chest pain, vasoconstriction, insomnia, paranoia, anxiety, transient psychosis	(Meyer *et al.*, 2014; Zanda and Fattore, 2017)[15,16]
Herbal derivatives	Kratom, kava, *Salvia divinorum*	• Partial agonists of μ and δ opioid receptors • Monoamine oxidase inhibitors • Serotonin reuptake inhibitors	Hallucinogens Stimulants/depressants (depending on dose)	Kratom: anxiety, agitation, lethargy, profuse sweating, dizziness, diarrhea, nausea, dysphoria, tremors, anorexia, weight loss, seizures, psychosis Kava: lack of coordination, drowsiness, and muscle relaxation *Salvia divinorum*: perceptual disturbances	(González-Trujano *et al.*, 2016; Ujvary, 2014)[17,18]
Phenethylamines	Benzofurans, "2C" series	• 5-HT2 receptor agonists • Inhibition of monoamine reuptake (e.g., dopamine, serotonin, norepinephrine) • Some (e.g., 2C-B) act as agonists of adrenergic a1 receptors	Hallucinogens	Hallucinations, confusion, depression, nausea, vomiting, diarrhea, body aches, deep cerebral vasculopathy and serotonin syndrome	(Nelson *et al.*, 2014; Zanda and Fattore, 2017)[16,19]
Synthetic opioids	AP-237, isotonitazene	• μ-opioid receptor agonists	Antinociceptives	Increased relaxation, sedation, decreased heart rate, hypothermia, and respiratory failure	(Chen *et al.*, 2015; Vallersnes *et al.*, 2016)[20,21]
Piperazines	TFMPP	• Dopamine receptor agonists • Substrates of non-selective serotonergic receptor transporters/agonists	Stimulants, hallucinogens	Seizures, psychotic episodes, dissociative symptoms, anxiety, agitation, and drowsiness	(Arbo *et al.*, 2016; Austin and Monasterio, 2004; Baumann *et al.*, 2005) [22,23,24]
Tryptamines	AMT, 5-MeO-DMT	• 5-HT_{2A}receptor agonists	Hallucinogens, stimulants (α-methylated tryptamines α-methylated)	Auditory, visual, and sensory hallucinations, hypersensitivity, delirium, loss of sense of space and time, depersonalization/realization disorder, psychosis, paranoia, ataxia, confusion, increased agitation, and amnesia	(Araujo *et al.*, 2015; Fuse-Nagase and Nishikawa, 2013)[25,26]

3,4-DMMC, 3,4-dimethylmethcathinone; 4'-MePPP, 4-methyl-α-pyrrolidinopropiophenone; 3-MeO-PCP, 3-MeO-phencyclidine; 3-MeO-PCE, methoxyeticyclidine; 5-MeO-DMT, 5-methoxy-N,N-dimethyltryptamine; AMT, α-methyltryptamine; DMC, dimethocaine; GABA, γ-aminobutyric acid; GPR18, G protein–coupled receptor 18; GPR55, G protein–coupled receptor 55; NMDA, N-methyl-D-aspartate; pFBT, 3-(p-fluorobenzoxy)-tropane; PPAR, peroxisome proliferator–activated receptor; TFMPP, 1-(3-trifluoromethylphenyl)piperazine; DMT, N,N-dimethyltryptamine; TRPV1, transient receptor potential vanilloid type 1.

adrenaline.[10] For example, cathinones containing a pyrrolidine group in their structure (4-methyl-α -pyrrolidinopropiophenone, 4'-MePPP) block dopamine and adrenaline transporters with low affinity for the serotonin transporter, preventing their presynaptic reuptake, similar to cocaine. On the other hand, cathinones that have a methyl group in the aromatic ring (3,4-dimethylmethcathinone, 3,4-DMMC) act as non-selective substrates of monoamine receptors, enhancing the efflux (while blocking reuptake) of dopamine, serotonin, and/or adrenaline from presynaptic terminals, similarly to MDMA or methamphetamine.[10] Excess dopamine in the extracellular environment, for example, can significantly increase dopamine metabolism, with the simultaneous formation of dopamine-o-quinones and the induction of oxidative stress, and consequent cellular damage.[27] There is also evidence that some cathinones, such as MDPV, decrease the expression of the GLT-1 glutamate transporter. Since this transporter is responsible for removing any excess extracellular glutamate, decreased expression leads to increased extracellular glutamate concentrations, with consequent excitotoxicity.[11]

Regardless of whether they act as blockers or substrates, all synthetic cathinones increase the extracellular concentration of monoamines in signaling pathways associated with reward. For example, the locomotor and abuse susceptibility effects of synthetic cathinones observed *in vivo* appear to be related to elevated dopamine concentrations in the nucleus accumbens. However, these effects tend to vary depending on the selectivity of cathinones for dopamine and serotonin transporters (cathinones with greater selectivity for the dopamine transporter have a greater tendency to add, while cathinones with greater selectivity for the serotonin transporter have less additive potential).[10]

The consumption of small doses of synthetic cathinones is generally associated with euphoria and a heightened state of alertness, while regular consumption is responsible for more serious adverse effects such as hyperthermia, tachycardia, and, above all, psychotic episodes including paranoia, audiovisual hallucinations, extreme agitation, and violent behavior.[28,29]

SYNTHETIC CANNABINOIDS

Cannabinoids are a diverse group of NPS that mimic the psychoactive effects of tetrahydrocannabinol (THC, the main psychoactive component of cannabis), but with greater potency.[30] These substances accounted for a substantial proportion of NPS seizures between 2009 and 2019 and are marketed in powder form mixed with or sprinkled on plant material after being dissolved in organic solvents (e.g., acetone, methanol). The mixture is dried and packaged in attractive containers with appealing names (e.g., "Spice"). Although the number of new synthetic cannabinoids on the market declined between 2014 and 2018, their increasing association with serious intoxications and deaths compared to cannabis has made their use a major public health concern and a challenge for regulatory authorities.[1,2]

Like cannabinoids of natural origin, synthetic cannabinoids modulate the endocannabinoid system by binding to at least one of the main classical cannabinoid receptors: type 1 (CB1) or type 2 (CB2). Activation of these receptors, which belong to the G protein–coupled receptor family, leads to a reduction in adenylate cyclase activity and a consequent reduction in the formation of cyclic adenosine monophosphate (cAMP).[31] CB1 receptors are more common in the presynaptic terminals of neurons in areas such as the hippocampus or prefrontal cortex, although they may also be present in the basal ganglia and postsynaptic regions (e.g., neurons, astrocytes and other glial cells, and endothelial cells in the brain) at a lower density (Howlett and Abood, 2017). Activation of the CB1 receptor inhibits the opening of voltage-dependent calcium channels of the N and P/Q type, while activating the influx of potassium through the respective channels, which causes hyperpolarization of the presynaptic terminals, which in turn leads to inhibition of the release of neurotransmitters. Q-type voltage-dependent calcium channels, while activating potassium influx through the respective channels, causing hyperpolarization of presynaptic terminals, which in turn leads to inhibition of the release of various neurotransmitters (e.g., dopamine, glutamate, GABA). In turn, CB2 receptors are more common in peripheral tissues/organs (e.g., spleen, liver, lungs, tonsils, kidneys, and gastrointestinal tract), especially in immune system cells, playing a key role in immune modulation. These receptors are also present in the brain, mainly in microglia cells or postsynaptic neuronal terminals. It should be noted that overactivation of the CB2 receptor in the brain has been observed in some pathologies (e.g., inflammation, anxiety, addiction, epilepsy), suggesting that this receptor may play an important role in various psychiatric and neurological disorders (Howlett and Abood, 2017). In addition to cannabinoid receptors, synthetic cannabinoids are also capable of modulating the activity of other receptors, such as the vanilloid transient receptor potential type 1 (TRPV1) receptor, the peroxisome proliferator-activated receptor (PPAR) family, and G protein–coupled receptors 55 (GPR55) and 18 (GPR18).[31] Recently, Yano and colleagues (2020) observed that, unlike THC, synthetic cannabinoids containing an indole group in their structure (e.g., AM-2201, JWH-018) can act as positive allosteric modulators of the serotonergic receptor 5-HT1A receptor, thus demonstrating the ability of some synthetic cannabinoids to act directly on serotonergic receptors without activating cannabinoid receptors.

Although initially developed for scientific purposes, synthetic cannabinoids are increasingly being used for recreational purposes, and they are sought after for inducing various psychotropic effects that are more potent than cannabis, including feelings of relaxation and greater well-being, social disinhibition, and increased appetite. However, these substances can interfere with cognitive function (e.g., memory, attention, and time perception disorders) and motor coordination. Some neurological effects include delirium and hallucinations, drowsiness, paranoia, confusion, anxiety, sudden mood swings, and panic attacks, and have been associated with an increased risk of seizures and the development of psychosis-related illnesses.[32] Symptoms correlating synthetic cannabinoid use with dependence and withdrawal have also been described.[33]

BENZODIAZEPINES

In recent years, the market for benzodiazepines has expanded, making them the third most seized class of NPS in the European Union. In fact, the EMCDDA currently monitors 30 new substances in this group of NPS, 21 of which have been detected since 2015. The recreational use of these adulterated molecules (e.g., etizolam, flualprazolam), marketed in capsule or powder form, has been associated with severe intoxication and a high risk of death from overdose.[1]

Benzodiazepines act as positive allosteric modulators of γ-aminobutyric acid (GABA) receptors, promoting the binding of this neurotransmitter to its receptors. The binding of benzodiazepines to GABA receptors induces a change in their conformation, which in turn leads to a change in the conformation of the chloride channels associated with these receptors. This dysregulation of chloride ion flow leads to hyperpolarization of the cell, which determines the inhibitory nature of GABA receptors and is responsible for the relaxation effect normally associated with these substances.[8] For this reason, benzodiazepines are sometimes used to treat agitation resulting from psychosis, although this practice is increasingly discouraged, as its effectiveness has not been fully proven and there are possible adverse effects.[34] However, consuming these substances in high quantities, or in combination with other substances, can cause an exacerbated reduction in neural response time, which in turn can lead to the distortion of normal thought processes.[35] When not done under medical supervision, cessation of benzodiazepine use is associated with withdrawal symptoms, including psychosis.[36]

ARYLCYCLOHEXYLAMINES

Arylcyclohexylamines are a class of NPS composed of an aryl group attached to a cyclohexylamine unit. In some cases, the aryl group is a phenyl ring and may have additional substitutions. The amines present in these substances are usually secondary (e.g., methylamine, ethylamine) or tertiary (e.g., piperidines, pyrrolidines).[37]

These substances gained popularity for recreational purposes between 1960 and 1990 due to their hallucinogenic and euphoric dissociative effects. However, the anesthetic properties of arylcyclohexylamines were described earlier in the literature.[7] Currently, arylcyclohexylamines, which include ketamine analogues such as 3-MeO-phencyclidine (3-MeO-PCP), 3-methoxyeticyclidine (3-MeO-PCE) or 1-(3-methoxyphenyl)-N-propylcyclohexa-no-1-amine (3-MeO-PCPr), account for around 7% of total NPS seizures in the European Union.[1]

Arylcyclohexylamines can act as non-competitive antagonists of N-methyl-D-aspartate (NMDA) receptors, dopamine reuptake inhibitors, and opioid receptor agonists, with sigma receptor agonist effects also being reported (σ and antagonists of nicotinic and muscarinic receptors).[37] In particular, NMDA receptor blockade is generally associated with anesthetic, anticonvulsant, and neuroprotective effects[38] recognized for these substances. However, the use of arylcyclohexylamines has also been associated with cases of clinical intolerance,[39] acute poisoning including symptoms such as respiratory failure, tachycardia, hypertension, urinary retention, or myoclonus,[40] as well as neurological disorders, including psychosis, audiovisual hallucinations, paranoia, exacerbated agitation, and catatonia.[6] There have also been reports of deaths associated with the consumption of arylcyclohexylamines, either due to a direct effect on the body[41] or as a result of violent behavior induced by the consumption of these substances.[42] Withdrawal from these substances can lead to the onset of psychosis, strange behavior, or depression, which can appear within a day of stopping use and can last from days to weeks.[6]

SYNTHETIC OPIOIDS

The market for synthetic opioids has grown at an alarming rate. Since 2009, 57 new substances of this type have been detected in the European Union, eight of them in 2019 alone. These opioids are generally sold in powder form and can also be found in tablet or liquid form (for use in nasal sprays, for example). Although they currently represent only a small fraction of the NPS market (3%), these substances pose a serious risk of intoxication and overdose, which in turn can cause respiratory failure and death in users.[1,43] In 2017, there were more than 51,000 fentanyl overdoses in the United States and Canada alone.[2] While fentanyl derivatives have been predominant in synthetic opioid seizures until recently, since 2019, these have been replaced by other synthetic opioids, such as 2-fluoro-viminol, AP-237, 2-methyl-AP-237, piperidylthiobutene, furanyl UF-17, and isotonitazene, which are structurally different but have similar toxicity to fentanyl.[1,2,43]

Like endogenous or plant-derived opioids, synthetic opioids act as analgesics and are used in the treatment of chronic pain, such as that seen in, e.g., different types of cancer or post-surgical recovery. In addition, some synthetic opioids (e.g., methadone) are also used in the treatment of opioid dependence. Their pharmacological action results from binding to the μ opioid receptors present in nociceptors, a group of neuronal cells present in the brain and throughout the peripheral nervous system, with the ability to recognize chemical or mechanical stimuli.[44] μ-opioid receptors belong to the family of G protein–coupled receptors, so their activation by opioids leads to the dissociation of the G_{α} and $G_{\beta\gamma}$ subunits of the G protein, thereby activating different signaling pathways, which generally reduce neuronal function. The modulation of ion channels represents one of the highly conserved signaling pathways activated by opioid receptors. This process, initiated by the inhibition of the $G_{\beta\gamma}$ subunit, causes a decrease in the fusion of synaptic vesicles with the membrane terminal (a calcium-dependent mechanism) and the subsequent release of neurotransmitters. Similarly, opioids can also cause activation of the channels responsible for potassium influx in postsynaptic terminals.[45]

In addition to analgesia, the action of synthetic opioids can trigger various adverse effects, such as relaxation, sedation, decreased heart rate, hypothermia, and respiratory failure.[43] Discontinuation of these substances, when done without medical supervision, can lead to withdrawal syndrome, since, in the absence of the opioid, there is a dysregulation in the production of the molecules (i.e., endorphins) responsible for pain relief.[46]

OTHER NPS

In addition to the substances mentioned above, there are other NPS detected in seizures, but whose toxic and pharmacologic mechanisms are still poorly understood. Some of these groups of NSPs are described below.

Phenethylamines

Phenethylamines represent a group of NPS with stimulant, empathic, and hallucinogenic effects, with structures similar to amphetamines, catecholamines, synthetic cathinones, or other substances, and are usually sold in tablet or powder form.[19] These substances are divided into three groups: (1) classic phenethylamines (e.g., methylenedioxymethamphetamine [MDMA], methyldiethanolamine [MDEA]); (2) psychoactive phenethylamines, including mescaline derivatives (e.g., trimethoxyamphetamine [TMA], 2,5-dimethoxy-4-methylamphetamine [DOM]) ; (3) some newer molecules, such as benzofurans, phenethylamines containing an N-benzyl substituent, or phenethylamines of the "2C series" (e.g., 2C-I, 2C-E, 2C-B).[16] As with analogues, most phenethylamines show high affinity for different subtypes of serotonergic 5-HT2 receptors, and some inhibit the reuptake of monoamines (e.g., dopamine, serotonin, norepinephrine). Some of these substances (e.g., 2C-B) also act as agonists of adrenergic a1 receptors.[19,47] The consumption of phenethylamines can induce hallucinations, confusion, depression, nausea, vomiting, diarrhea, body aches, among other adverse effects.[19] It should be noted that intoxication caused by these substances can lead to severe cerebral vasculopathy and serotonin syndrome. The latter is characterized, among other symptoms, by altered mental status.[48] To date, few cases of related deaths have been reported. with the consumption of these substances.[19]

Piperazines

Piperazines emerged in the early 2000s, divided into two distinct classes: benzylpiperazines (e.g., N-benzylpiperazine [BZP], 1-(3,4-methylenedioxybenzyl)piperazine [MDBP]) and phenylpiperazines (e.g., 1-(3-chlorophenyl)piperazine [mCPP], 1-(4-fluorophenyl)piperazine [pFPP], 1-(3-trifluoromethylphenyl)piperazine [TFMPP]).[22] The most commonly used are BZP, which acts on dopamine receptors and transporters, and TFMPP, which acts presynaptically as a substrate for serotonin transporters and as a non-selective agonist of serotonergic receptors. These two piperazines are sometimes mixed in a single tablet, taking advantage of the stimulant effect (through dopaminergic action) of BZP, with the hallucinogenic effects (through serotonergic stimulation) of TFMPP.[24]

Piperazines are commonly consumed in capsule or tablet form, often combined with adulterants such as caffeine, vitamins, or other illicit substances such as ecstasy or cocaine,[49] and can reach high concentrations in both the brain and plasma. These high concentrations are often associated with seizures observed in users of these substances.[50] In addition, several clinical cases of neurological symptoms have been reported, including psychotic episodes, dissociative symptoms, anxiety, agitation, and drowsiness.[23,51,52] However, the mechanisms of neurotoxicity behind these effects triggered by piperazines are poorly understood. In one of the few studies available, Arbo *et al.*[22] demonstrated the neurotoxic potential of some of these substances (i.e., BZP, TFMPP, MeOPP, MDBP) in a human neuroblastoma cell line, observing that all the substances tested induced cell death by apoptosis, accompanied by a significant reduction in intracellular calcium concentrations and hyperpolarization of the mitochondrial membrane.

It should be noted that to date there is only one recorded death following the consumption of piperazine-based drugs (specifically BZP), but it was not possible to establish a direct link between this consumption and the cause of death, as the patient had simultaneously consumed ecstasy.[53]

Tryptamines

Tryptamines are a fairly diverse class of hallucinogenic PSBs that are structurally similar to serotonin and act primarily as agonists of the serotonergic 5-HT2A receptor (and less selectively for serotonergic receptors of the 5-HT1 or 5-HT2 subtypes), causing profound changes in mood, thinking, and sensory perception.[25] These substances can have different origins, namely natural, such as psilocybin and its derivatives (present in hallucinogenic mushrooms of the *Psilocybe* spp. species) or N,N-dimethyltryptamine (DMT, present in the fermented drink known as "Ayahuasca");[54] or synthetic, with lysergic acid diethylamide (LSD) being the best-known synthetic tryptamine.[55] However, the inclusion of these latter molecules in the 1971 United Nations Convention on Psychotropic Substances led to the emergence of other synthetic tryptamines, specifically α -methyltryptamine (AMT), 5-methoxy-N,N-dimethyltryptamine (5-MeO-DMT), and 5-methoxy-N,N-diisopropyltryptamine (5-MeO-DIPT).[25] Note that serotonin represents the simplest form of a tryptamine, differing from the others by the absence of a hydroxyl group in the aromatic ring.[56]

These substances are generally sold in tablet or powder form and are preferably consumed orally or, in the case of synthetic tryptamines, by inhalation and nasal insufflation, intravenous or intramuscular injection, or rectally.[57]

It is believed that the activation of serotonergic 5-HT2A receptors by tryptamines is primarily responsible for the hallucinogenic effects of these substances.[58] However, some tryptamines have the ability to bind to serotonergic receptors and activate them. For example, DMT has moderate affinity as an agonist of sigma-1 receptors (α_1).[59]

In addition to hallucinogenic effects, some tryptamines, specifically α-methylated compounds (e.g., DMT), can also induce stimulant effects. This effect appears to be related to the presence of the methyl group on the α carbon), a structural feature similar to amphetamines.[25]

To date, several cases of poisoning have been reported following the consumption of tryptamines. In addition to auditory, visual, and sensory hallucinations, users of these substances may experience hypersensitivity, delirium, loss of sense of space and time, or depersonalization/derealization disorder. Other neurological and neuropsychiatric effects include psychosis, paranoia, ataxia, confusion, increased agitation, and amnesia, among others.[25] In general, tryptamines have a low probability of causing death due to their low (or no) affinity for biological receptors with relevant vital functions. However, the use of these substances has been associated with deaths.[57]

Synthetic Cocaine Derivatives

Cocaine analogues have emerged, like most NPS, for use in research or for therapeutic purposes. For example, 3-(p-fluorobenzoxy)-tropane (pFBT) and dimethocaine [DMC, larocaine, 3-diethylamino-2,2-dimethylpropyl)-4-amino-benzoate] were initially developed for use as local anesthetics.[15] However, these substances were withdrawn from the market due to their stimulant effects, similar to those of cocaine.[60] Thus, the recreational use of synthetic cocaine derivatives as substitutes for cocaine gained popularity, and they began to be detected in products containing other stimulants (e.g., caffeine, cathinone derivatives) from 2008 onwards.[61,62] Recreational use of these substances is currently underreported and does not appear in the most recent reports on drug use.[1,2]

The toxicological and pharmacological effects of synthetic cocaine derivatives are virtually unknown. However, it is known that they can act as voltage-dependent sodium channel blockers, especially those containing a benzoxy group (e.g., (-)-1-methylcocaine) and/or as dopamine reuptake inhibitors by blocking the dopamine transporter (e.g., dimethococaine, phenyltropanes such as WIN35065-2, and WIN34,428).[60]

Previous studies had already shown that intraperitoneal administration of dimethocaine to rats caused an accumulation of dopamine and its metabolites, which in turn led to stimulation of the reward system,[63] which may explain the additive potential of these substances. In addition, some phenyltropanes (e.g., RTI-336) have been explored for the treatment of cocaine addiction due to their action on the dopamine transporter, the main neurotransmitter responsible for the addictive properties of cocaine.[64]

Synthetic cocaine derivatives are generally consumed intravenously or nasally, and ingestion can cause rapid hydrolysis. In addition, users of these substances tend to increase the dose consumed to achieve the same euphoric effects previously obtained. In turn, this development of tolerance increases the risk of adverse effects, which may include tachycardia, breathing difficulties, chest pain, vasoconstriction, insomnia, paranoia, anxiety, and transient psychosis.[16]

New Plant-Based Psychoactive Substances

The quantities of plant-derived NPS seized in the last three years were very similar to the quantities of synthetic NPS, also showing a downward trend in seizures.[2] Plant-based NPS represent a fairly diverse group, among which the plant *Mitragyna speciosa*, also known as kratom, was the most commonly reported in seizures (around 63% of total seizures of plant-based NPS). The leaves of this plant, grown mainly in Southeast Asia, contain more than 25 alkaloids, with mitragynine and 7-hydroxy-mitragynine considered the most active.[65] Mitragynine acts as a partial agonist of the μ- and δ-opioid receptors, and 7-hydroxy-mi-traginine is a μ-opioid receptor agonist, more potent than morphine.[66] On the other hand, kratom can induce stimulant or depressive effects, depending on the dose used: low doses (between 1 and 5 grams) produce a stimulant effect, increasing alertness, social disinhibition, and sexual appetite, reducing fatigue, and can also lead to anxiety and agitation. Intermediate doses (5–15 grams) promote pain relief and withdrawal symptoms, and finally, high doses (above 15 grams) can cause lethargy, excessive sweating, dizziness, diarrhea, nausea, and dysphoria. Prolonged use is associated with tremors, anorexia, weight loss, seizures, and psychotic symptoms.

The *Piper methysticum* (kava) plant is a broadleaf shrub that is prevalent in the South Pacific islands and is traditionally marketed as a dietary supplement and used in self-medication to treat anxiety, depression, and insomnia. It is also used in traditional medicine to treat fever, convulsions, respiratory problems, and urogenital problems. Ingesting small amounts of kava can induce mild euphoria and increase sociability. However, high doses promote lack of coordination, drowsiness, and muscle relaxation. It should be noted that kava has high hepatotoxicity and nephrotoxicity and can cause gastrointestinal problems and changes in vision.[18]

Sceletium tortuosum (kanna) is a plant native to South Africa, used by indigenous peoples to calm hunger and thirst. Its psychoactive effects are mainly due to the presence of alkaloids, including mesembry, a serotonin reuptake inhibitor. Antidepressant, anxiolytic, narcotic, and anti-addictive effects have been reported after consumption of kanna.[18]

This group of plant-based substances includes some with hallucinogenic properties. For example, the leaves of *Salvia divinorum*, known as "herb of the gods" or "Mary's leaves," are often used in some countries in Central and South America in shamanic rituals. The leaves of this plant are usually consumed orally (in the form of tea, which can also be chewed) or by inhalation. The main active compounds in this plant act as agonists of opioid receptors κ and are associated with the potential for addiction. Consumption of this plant has an anxiolytic and sedative effect, but it can also cause cognitive alterations, such as changes in perception.[17]

Ayahuasca is a hallucinogenic drink produced from the stems, bark, and leaves of the *Banisteriopsis caapi* plant, which is prevalent in seizures.[2] The hallucinogenic effects of this drink are essentially due to the alkaloids it contains, most of which are structurally similar to serotonin and inhibit the activity of monoamine oxidase. It should be noted that ayahuasca does not appear to induce symptoms of physiological dependence, tolerance, or withdrawal. Nor are there any reports that this drink can cause any type of physical or mental pathology.[67]

Tabernanthe iboga is a shrub that is predominantly found in West Africa, whose roots are used for their hallucinogenic properties, as well as for their stimulant and sedative effects. These effects are mainly caused by ibogaine, the main active alkaloid present in this plant, which has stimulant properties at low doses but hallucinogenic properties at high doses. Its consumption can cause tremors, ataxia, cardiovascular toxicity, and even death.[18]

CONCLUSIONS

In recent years, the number of NPS entering the market for substances of abuse has declined. However, the diversity of these substances is enormous, and new substances with psychoactive properties continue to appear every year. Although structurally different, NPS share a high potential for addiction due to their ability to interfere with the reward system in the brain, both by promoting short-term effects and by developing tolerance.

Furthermore, their use is often associated with adverse effects, the severity of which may depend on several factors such as the dose consumed or the regularity of use. This dose dependence is particularly notable in some naturally occurring NPS (e.g., *Salvia divinorum*, "kanna"), where low or high doses produce opposite effects. Furthermore, although the mechanisms responsible for their psychoactive effects are known, the neurotoxic effects of NPS are often unknown, making it difficult to correctly diagnose patients who are admitted to hospital emergency departments.

Overall, it is hoped that this review of different groups of NPS and their mechanisms of action, may make it possible to: (1) alert potential consumers of these substances to the risks associated with their use; (2) encourage researchers in the field of Substances of Abuse/Toxicology to seek to clarify the mechanisms of action responsible for the toxicological and pharmacological effects resulting from NPS use.

REFERENCES

1. EMCDDA-European Monitoring Centre for Drugs and Drug Addiction. European Drug Report 2020: Trends and Developments. Luxembourg: Publications Office of the European Union, 2020.
2. UNODC-United Nations Office on Drugs and Crime. World Drug Report 2020. United Nations Publications, 2020.
3. Dines AM, Wood DM, Yates C, Heyerdahl F, Hovda KE, Giraudon I, *et al.* Acute recreational drug and new psychoactive substance toxicity in Europe: 12 months data collection from the European Drug Emergencies Network (Euro-DEN). Clin Toxicol. 2015;53:893–900.
4. Leyrer-Jackson JM, Nagy EK, Olive MF. Cognitive deficits and neurotoxicity induced by synthetic cathinones: Is there a role for neuroinflammation? Psychopharmacol. 2019;236:1079–95.
5. Lukić V, Micić R, Arsić B, Nedović B, Radosavljević Ž. Overview of the major classes of new psychoactive substances, psychoactive effects, analytical determination and conformational analysis of selected illegal drugs. Open Chem. 2021;19:60–106.
6. Bey T, Patel A. Phencyclidine intoxication and adverse effects: A clinical and pharmacological review of an illicit drug. Cal J Emerg Med. 2007;8:9–14.
7. Morris H, Wallach J. From PCP to MXE: A comprehensive review of the non-medical use of dissociative drugs. Drug Test Anal. 2014;6:614–32.
8. Griffin CE 3rd, Kaye AM, Bueno FR, Kaye AD. Benzodiazepine pharmacology and central nervous system-mediated effects. Ochsner J. 2013;13:214–23.
9. McKenzie RR Jr, Madadi P, Sharma TR. Alprazolam withdrawal delirium and brief reversible psychosis: A case report. Prim Care Companion CNS Disord. 2014;16(5).
10. Baumann MH, Walters HM, Niello M, Sitte HH. Neuropharmacology of synthetic cathinones. Handb Exp Pharmacol. 2018;252:113–42.
11. Gregg RA, Hicks C, Nayak SU, Tallarida CS, Nucero P, Smith GR, *et al.* Synthetic cathinone MDPV down-regulates glutamate transporter subtype I (GLT-1) and produces rewarding and locomotor-activating effects that are reduced by a GLT-1 activator. Neuropharmacol. 2016;108:111–9.
12. Murrie B, Lappin J, Large M, Sara, G. Transition of substance-induced, brief, and atypical psychoses to schizophrenia: A systematic review and meta-analysis. Schizophr Bull. 2019; 46:505–16.
13. Alexandre J, Carmo H, Carvalho F, Silva JP. Synthetic cannabinoids and their impact on neurodevelopmental processes. Addict Biol. 2020; 25(2):e12824.
14. Di Forti M, Quattrone D, Freeman, TP, Tripoli G, Ga-yer-Anderson C, Quigley H, *et al.* The contribution of cannabis use to variation in the incidence of psychotic disorder across Europe (EU-GEI): A multicenter case-control study. Lancet Psychiatry. 2019;6:427–36.
15. Meyer MR, Lindauer C, Welter J, Maurer HH. Dimetho-caine, a synthetic cocaine analogue: Studies on its in-vivo metabolism and its detectability in urine by means of a rat model and liquid chromatography–linear ion-trap (high-resolution) mass spectrometry. Anal Bioanal Chem. 2014;406:1845–54.
16. Zanda MT, Fattore L. Chapter 29. Novel Psychoactive Substances: A new behavioral and mental health threat. In: Watson RR, Zibadi S (eds.) Addictive Substances and Neurological Disease. Academic Press, 2017:341–53.
17. Gonzalez-Trujano ME, Brindis F, Lopez-Ruiz E, Rami-rez-Salado I, Martinez A, Pellicer, F. Depressant effects of Salvia divinorumin involve disruption of physiological sleep. Phytother Res. 2016;30:1137–45.
18. Ujvary, I. Psychoactive natural products: Overview of recent developments. Annali dell'Istituto Superiore di Sanitá. 2014;50:12–27.
19. Nelson ME, Bryant SM, Aks SE. Emerging drugs of abuse. Emerg Med Clin North Am. 2014;32:1–28.

20. Chen K-J, Lu M-L, Shen WW. Tramadol-related psychosis in a patient with bipolar I disorder. Acta Neuropsychiatrica. 2015; 27:126–28.
21. Vallersnes OM, Dines AM, Wood DM, Yates C, Heyer-dahl F, Hovda KE, *et al.* Psychosis associated with acute recreational drug toxicity: A European case series. BMC Psychiatry. 2016;16:293.
22. Arbo MD, Silva R, Barbosa DJ, da Silva DD, Silva SP, Teixeira JP, *et al.* In vitro neurotoxicity evaluation of pipe-razine designer drugs in differentiated human neuroblastoma SH-SY5Y cells. J Appl Toxicol. 2016;36:121–30.
23. Austin H, Monasterio E. Acute Psychosis Following Ingestion of 'Rapture'. Australas Psychiatry. 2004;12:406–8.
24. Baumann MH, Clark RD, Budzynski AG, Partilla JS, Blough BE, Rothman RB. N-Substituted piperazines abused by humans mimic the molecular mechanism of 3,4-methylenedioxy-methamphetamine (MDMA, or 'Ecstasy'). Neuropsychopharmacol. 2005;30:550–60.
25. Araujo AM, Valente MJ, Carvalho M, da Silva DD, Gaspar H, Carvalho F, *et al.* Raising awareness of new psychoactive substances: Chemical analysis and in vitro toxicity screening of 'legal high' packages containing synthetic cathinones. Arch Toxicol. 2015;89:757–71.
26. Fuse-Nagase Y, Nishikawa, T. Prolonged delusional state triggered by repeated ingestion of aromatic liquid in a past 5-methoxy-N,N-diisopropyltryptamine abuser. Addict Sci Clin Pract. 2013;8:9.
27. Salim, S. Oxidative stress and the central nervous system. J Pharmacol Exp Ther. 2017; 360:201–5.
28. Araújo AM, Carvalho M, Bastos MdL, Carvalho F, de Pinho, PG. Metabolic signature of methylone in primary mouse hepatocytes, at subtoxic concentrations. Arch Toxicol. 2019; 93:3277–90.
29. Weinstein AM, Rosca P, Fattore L, London ED. Synthetic cathinone and cannabinoid designer drugs pose a major risk for public health. Front Psychiatry. 2017;8:156.
30. Pertwee RG, Howlett AC, Abood ME, Alexander SPH, Di Marzo V, Elphick MR, *et al.* International Union of Basic and Clinical Pharmacology. LXXIX. Cannabinoid Receptors and Their Ligands: Beyond CB1 and CB2. Pharmacol Rev. 2010;62:588–631.
31. Cristino L, Bisogno T, Di Marzo, V. Cannabinoids and the expanded endocannabinoid system in neurological disorders. Nat Rev Neurol. 2020;16:9–29.
32. Cohen K, Weinstein AM. Synthetic and non-synthetic cannabinoid drugs and their adverse effects—A review from a public health perspective. Front Public Health. 2018;6:162.
33. Uchiyama N, Kikura-Hanajiri R, Goda, Y. Identification of a novel cannabimimetic phenyl-acetylindole, cannabi-piperidiethanone, as a designer drug in a herbal product and its affinity for cannabinoid CB1 and CB2 Receptors. Chem Pharm Bull. 2011;59:1203–5.
34. Zaman H, Sampson SJ, Beck ALS, Sharma T, Clay FJ, Spyridi S, *et al.* Benzodiazepines for psychosis-induced aggression or agitation. Cochrane Database Syst Rev. 2017;12(12): CD003079.
35. Pétursson H. The benzodiazepine withdrawal syndrome. Addiction. 1994;89:1455–59.
36. Heather C Chapter III: Benzodiazepine Withdrawal Symptoms, Acute & Protracted. In: Ashton D (ed.) Benzodiazepines: How They Work and How to Withdraw. Institute of Neuroscience, Newcastle University, UK, 2013.
37. Wallach J, Colestock T, Cicali B, Elliott SP, Kavanagh PV, Adejare A, *et al.* Syntheses and analytical characterizations of N-alkyl-arylcyclohexylamines. Drug Test Anal. 2016;8:801–15.
38. Kalia LV, Kalia SK, Salter MW. NMDA receptors in clinical neurology: Excitatory times ahead. Lancet Neurol. 2008;7:742–55.
39. Lipton SA. Paradigm shift in neuroprotection by NMDA receptor blockade: Memantine and beyond. Nat Rev. Drug Disc. 2006;5:160–70.
40. Elliott SP, Brandt SD, Wallach J, Morris H, Kavanagh PV. First reported fatalities associated with the 'research chemical' 2-methoxydiphenidine. J Anal Toxicol. 2015;39:287–93.

41. Barton CH, Sterling ML, Vaziri ND. Phencyclidine intoxication: Clinical experience in 27 cases confirmed by urine assay. Ann Emerg Med. 1981;10:243–6.
42. McCarron MM, Schulze BW, Thompson GA, Conder MC, Goetz WA. Acute phencyclidine intoxication: Clinical patterns, complications, and treatment. Ann Emerg Med. 1981; 10(6):290–7.
43. EMCDDA-European Monitoring Centre for Drugs and Drug Addiction. Fentanils and synthetic cannabinoids: driving greater complexity into the drug situation. An update from the EU Early Warning System. Luxembourg: Publications Office of the European Union, 2018.
44. Schaefer CP, Tome ME, Davis TP. The opioid epidemic: A central role for the blood brain barrier in opioid analgesia and abuse. Fluids Barriers CNS. 2017;14:32.
45. Corder G, Castro DC, Bruchas MR, Scherrer G. Endogenous and exogenous opioids in pain. Ann Rev Neurosci. 2018;41:453–73.
46. Emery MA, Akil H. Endogenous opioids at the intersection of opioid addiction, pain, and depression: The search for a precision medicine approach. Ann Rev Neurosci. 2020;43:355–74.
47. Schifano F, Papanti, GD, Orsolini L, Corkery JM. Novel psychoactive substances: The pharmacology of stimulants and hallucinogens. Expert Rev Clin Pharmacol. 2016;9:943–54.
48. Ambrose JB, Bennett HD, Lee HS, Josephson SA. Cerebral vasculopathy after 4-bromo-2,5-dimethoxyphenethylamine ingestion. Neurologist. 2010;16:199–202.
49. Staack RF, Paul LD, Schmid D, Roider G, Rolf B. Proof of a 1-(3-chlorophenyl)piperazine (mCPP) intake-Use as adulterant of cocaine resulting in drug-drug interactions? J Chromatogr B. 2007;855:127–33.
50. Gee P, Gilbert M, Richardson S, Moore G, Paterson S, Graham, P. Toxicity from the recreational use of 1-ben-zylpiperazine. Clin Toxicol. 2008;46:802–7.
51. Kovaleva J, Devuyst E, Paepe PD, Verstraete A. Acute chlorophenylpiperazine overdose: A case report and review of the literature. Ther Drug Monit. 2008;30(3):394–8.
52. Wood DM, Button J, Lidder S, Ramsey J, Holt DW, Dargan PI. Dissociative and sympathomimetic toxicity associated with recreational use of 1-(3-trifluoromethyl-phenyl) piperazine (TFMPP) and 1-benzylpiperzine (BZP). J Med Toxicol. 2008;4:254–7.
53. Balmelli C, Kupferschmidt H, Rentsch K, Schneemann, M. Fatal brain edema after ingestion of ecstasy and benzyl-piperazine. Dtsch Med Wochenschr. 2001;126:809–11.
54. Cunningham, N. Hallucinogenic plants of abuse. Emerg Med Australas. 2008;20:167–74.
55. Nichols DE. Psychedelics. Pharmacol Rev. 2016;68:264–355.
56. Gibbons, S. 'Legal Highs' – novel and emerging psychoactive drugs: A chemical overview for the toxicologist. Clin Toxicol. 2012;50:15–24.
57. Corkery JM, Durkin E, Elliott S, Schifano F, Ghodse AH. The recreational tryptamine 5-MeO-DALT (N,N-dia-llyl-5-methoxytryptamine): A brief review. Prog Neuropsychopharmacol Biol Psychiatry. 2012;39:259–62.
58. Fantegrossi WE, Murnane KS, Reissig CJ. The behavioral pharmacology of hallucinogens. Biochem Pharmacol. 2008;75:17–33.
59. Fontanilla D, Johannessen M, Hajipour AR, Cozzi NV, Jackson MB, Ruoho AE. The hallucinogen N,N-dimethyltryptamine (DMT) is an endogenous sigma-1 receptor regulator. Science. 2009;323:934–7.
60. Wilcox KM, Kimmel HL, Lindsey KP, Votaw JR, Goodman MM, Howell LL. In vivo comparison of the reinforcing and dopamine transporter effects of local anesthetics in rhesus monkeys. Synapse. 2005;58:220–8.
61. Kavanagh P, Angelov D, O'Brien J, Fox J, O'Donnell C, Christie R, *et al.* The synthesis and characterization of 3β -(4-fluorobenzoyloxy)tropane (fluorotropacocaine) and its 3α e isomer. Drug Test Anal. 2012;4:33–8.
62. Reitzel LA, Dalsgaard PW, Müller IB, Cornett C. Identification of ten new designer drugs by GC-MS, UPLC-QTOF-MS, and NMR as part of a police investigation of a Danish Internet company. Drug Test Anal. 2012;4: 342–54.

63. Graham JH 3rd, Maher JR, Robinson SE. The effect of cocaine and other local anesthetics on central dopaminergic neurotransmission. J Pharmacol Exp Ther. 1995;274:707–17.
64. Carroll FI, Howard JL, Howell LL, Fox BS, Kuhar MJ. Development of the dopamine transporter selective RTI-336 as a pharmacotherapy for cocaine abuse. AAPS J. 2006;8:E196–E203.
65. Warner ML, Kaufman NC, Grundmann O. The pharmacology and toxicology of kratom: From traditional herb to drug of abuse. Int J Legal Med. 2016;130:127–38.
66. Schifano F, Orsolini L, Duccio Papanti G, Corkery, JM. Novel psychoactive substances of interest for psychiatry. World Psychiatry. 2015;14:15–26.
67. Santos RG. Ayahuasca: neuroquímica e farmacologia. SMAD - Electronic journal of mental health, alcohol, and drugs. 2007;3 (1): 1–11.
68. Yano H, Adhikari P, Naing S, Hoffman AF, Baumann MH, Lupica CR, *et al.* Positive allosteric modulation of the 5-HT1A receptor by indole-based synthetic cannabinoids abused by humans. ACS Chem Neurosci. 2020;11:1400–5.

Index

O

P

Q

R

S